Chronic Lymphocytic Leukemia

Editor

JENNIFER R. BROWN

HEMATOLOGY/ONCOLOGY CLINICS OF NORTH AMERICA

www.hemonc.theclinics.com

Consulting Editors
GEORGE P. CANELLOS
H. FRANKLIN BUNN

April 2013 • Volume 27 • Number 2

ELSEVIER

1600 John F. Kennedy Boulevard • Suite 1800 • Philadelphia, Pennsylvania, 19103-2899

http://www.theclinics.com

HEMATOLOGY/ONCOLOGY CLINICS OF NORTH AMERICA Volume 27, Number 2
April 2013 ISSN 0889-8588, ISBN 13: 978-1-4557-7101-1

Editor: Patrick Manley
Developmental Editor: Donald Mumford

Hematology/Oncology Clinics (ISSN 0889-8588) is published bimonthly by Elsevier Inc., 360 Park Avenue South, New York, NY 10010-1710. Months of issue are February, April, June, August, October, and December. Business and Editorial Offices: 1600 John F. Kennedy Blvd., Ste. 1800, Philadelphia, PA 19103–2899. Customer Service Office: 3251 Riverport Lane, Maryland Heights, MO 63043. Periodicals postage paid at New York, NY and at additional mailing offices. Subscription prices are $367.00 per year (domestic individuals), $599.00 per year (domestic institutions), $179.00 per year (domestic students/residents), $417.00 per year (Canadian individuals), $732.00 per year (Canadian institutions) $496.00 per year (international individuals), $732.00 per year (international institutions), and $241.00 per year (international and Canadian students/residents). International air speed delivery is included in all *Clinics* subscription prices. All prices are subject to change without notice. **POSTMASTER:** Send address changes to *Hematology/Oncology Clinics of North America*, Elsevier Health Sciences Division, Subscription Customer Service, 3251 Riverport Lane, Maryland Heights, MO 63043. Customer Service (orders, claims, online, change of address): Elsevier Health Sciences Division, Subscription Customer Service, 3251 Riverport Lane, Maryland Heights, MO 63043. Tel: 1-800-654-2452 (U.S. and Canada); 314-447-8871 (outside U.S. and Canada). Fax: 314-447-8029. E-mail: journalscustomerservice-usa@elsevier.com (for print support); journalsonlinesupport-usa@elsevier.com (for online support).

Reprints. For copies of 100 or more, of articles in this publication, please contact the Commercial Reprints Department, Elsevier Inc., 360 Park Avenue South, New York, New York 10010-1710; Tel.: 212-633-3813, Fax: 212-462-1935, E-mail: reprints@elsevier.com.

Hematology/Oncology Clinics of North America is covered in *MEDLINE/PubMed (Index Medicus), EMBASE/ Excerpta Medica, and BIOSIS.*

Printed and bound by CPI Group (UK) Ltd, Croydon, CR0 4YY

Transferred to digital print 2012

Contributors

CONSULTING EDITORS

GEORGE P. CANELLOS, MD
William Rosenberg Professor of Medicine, Department of Medical Oncology, Dana-Farber Cancer Institute, Boston, Massachusetts

H. FRANKLIN BUNN, MD
Professor of Medicine, Harvard Medical School, Division of Hematology, Brigham and Women's Hospital, Boston, Massachusetts

EDITOR

JENNIFER R. BROWN, MD, PhD
Director, CLL Center and Assistant Professor, Department of Medical Oncology, Dana-Farber Cancer Institute, Harvard Medical School, Boston, Massachusetts

AUTHORS

SEBASTIAN BÖTTCHER, MD
Second Department of Medicine, University Hospital of Schleswig-Holstein, Kiel, Germany

RENIER BRENTJENS, MD, PhD
Associate Attending Physician, Leukemia Service, Department of Medicine, Memorial Sloan-Kettering Cancer Center, New York, New York

JENNIFER R. BROWN, MD, PhD
Director, CLL Center and Assistant Professor, Department of Medical Oncology, Dana-Farber Cancer Institute, Harvard Medical School, Boston, Massachusetts

JOHN C. BYRD, MD
D. Warren Brown Chair of Leukemia Research, Professor of Medicine, Medicinal Chemistry, and Veterinary Biosciences, Director, Division of Hematology, Department of Internal Medicine; Division of Medicinal Chemistry and Pharmacology, The Arthur G. James Comprehensive Cancer Center, College of Pharmacy, The Ohio State University, Columbus, Ohio

NIKOS DARZENTAS, PhD
Molecular Medicine Program, Central European Institute of Technology, Masaryk University, Brno, Czech Republic; Institute of Applied Biosciences, Center for Research and Technology Hellas, Thessaloniki, Greece

MATTHEW S. DAVIDS, MD
Attending Physician, Department of Medical Oncology, CLL Center, Dana-Farber Cancer Institute, Instructor in Medicine, Harvard Medical School, Boston, Massachusetts

MARCO L. DAVILA, MD, PhD
Assistant Attending Physician, Leukemia Service, Department of Medicine, Memorial Sloan-Kettering Cancer Center, New York, New York

PETER DREGER, MD
Department of Medicine V, University of Heidelberg, Heidelberg, Germany

CLAUDIA FAZI, PhD
Laboratory of B Cell Neoplasia, Division of Molecular Oncology, San Raffaele Scientific Institute and Università Vita-Salute San Raffaele, Milano, Italy

PAOLO GHIA, MD, PhD
Laboratory of B Cell Neoplasia, Division of Molecular Oncology; Clinical Unit of Lymphoid Malignancies, Department of Onco-Hematology, San Raffaele Scientific Institute and Università Vita-Salute San Raffaele, Milano, Italy

JOHN G. GRIBBEN, MD, DSc
Gordon Hamilton Fairley Chair of Medical Oncology, Department of Haemato-Oncology, Barts Cancer Institute - a CR-UK Centre of Excellence, Queen Mary University of London, London, United Kingdom

MICHAEL HALLEK, MD
Department I of Internal Medicine, Centre of Integrated Oncology and CECAD, Cluster of Excellence Cellular Stress Responses in Aging-Associated Diseases, University of Cologne, Cologne, Germany

YAIR HERISHANU, MD
Hematology, Tel-Aviv Sourasky Medical Center, Tel-Aviv, Israel

MA. REINA IMPROGO, PhD
Research Fellow, Department of Medical Oncology, Dana-Farber Cancer Institute, Harvard Medical School, Boston, Massachusetts

BEN-ZION KATZ, PhD
Hematology, Tel-Aviv Sourasky Medical Center, Tel-Aviv, Israel

MICHAEL KNEBA, MD, PhD
Second Department of Medicine, University Hospital of Schleswig-Holstein, Kiel, Germany

ANDREW LIPSKY, BA
Hematology Branch, NHLBI, National Institutes of Health, Bethesda, Maryland

JOHN C. RICHES, BM BCh, MRCP
Clinical Research Fellow, Department of Haemato-Oncology, Barts Cancer Institute - a CR-UK Centre of Excellence, Queen Mary University of London, London, United Kingdom

MATTHIAS RITGEN, MD
Second Department of Medicine, University Hospital of Schleswig-Holstein, Kiel, Germany

LYDIA SCARFÒ, MD
Laboratory of B Cell Neoplasia, Division of Molecular Oncology; Clinical Unit of Lymphoid Malignancies, Department of Onco-Hematology, San Raffaele Scientific Institute and Università Vita-Salute San Raffaele, Milano, Italy

ANDREA SCHNAITER, MD
Department of Internal Medicine III, Ulm University, Ulm, Germany

KOSTAS STAMATOPOULOS, MD, PhD
Institute of Applied Biosciences, Center for Research and Technology Hellas; HCT Unit, Hematology Department, G. Papanicolaou Hospital, Exohi, Thessaloniki, Greece

DEBORAH M. STEPHENS, DO
Clinical Fellow, Division of Hematology, Department of Internal Medicine, The Arthur G. James Comprehensive Cancer Center, The Ohio State University, Columbus, Ohio

STEPHAN STILGENBAUER, MD
Department of Internal Medicine III, Ulm University, Ulm, Germany

ADRIAN WIESTNER, MD, PhD
Hematology Branch, NHLBI, National Institutes of Health, Bethesda, Maryland

Contents

This article discusses recent advances in genomic approaches used to understand chronic lymphocytic leukemia. Tools for analyzing DNA-level lesions are described, data obtained from these various platforms summarized, and the clinical relevance of these findings discussed.

Chronic lymphocytic leukemia (CLL) is characterized by the accumulation of mature monoclonal B cells in peripheral blood, bone marrow, spleen, and lymph nodes. The trafficking, survival, and proliferation of CLL cells is tightly regulated by the surrounding tissue microenvironment and is mediated by antigenic stimulation, close interaction with various accessory cells and exposure to different cytokines, chemokines, and extracellular matrix components. In the last decade there have been major advances in the understanding of the reciprocal interactions between CLL cells and the various microenvironmental compartments. This article discusses the role of the microenvironment in the context of efforts to develop novel therapeutics that target the biology of CLL.

Chronic lymphocytic leukemia (CLL) is the most common leukemia in adults. Although significant advances have been made in the treatment of CLL in the last decade, it remains incurable. Treatments may be too toxic for some elderly patients, who constitute most of the individuals with this disease, and there remain subgroups of patients for which this therapy has minimal activity. This article summarizes the current understanding of the immune defects in CLL. It also examines the potential clinical implications of these findings.

Roughly 30% of patients with chronic lymphocytic leukemia (CLL) carry immunoglobulin receptors with highly similar primary sequences. Highly similar, quasi-identical immunoglobulins are termed stereotyped. Patients with CLL can be assigned to different subsets expressing different types of stereotyped immunoglobulin receptors. Reliable identification of stereo-typy may assist in the molecular classification of CLL and thus better-guided, compartmentalized research. In several major subsets, stereotypy extends from shared primary sequences to shared clinicobiological fea-tures and outcome. Reliable identification of stereotypy in CLL may pave the way for tailored treatment strategies applicable to each major stereo-typed subset.

Monoclonal B-cell lymphocytosis (MBL) is defined as a clonal B-cell expansion whereby the B-cell count is less than 5×10^9/L and no symp-toms or signs of lymphoproliferative disorders are detected. Based on B-cell count, MBL is further divided into low-count and clinical MBL. While low-count MBL seems to carry relevance mostly from an immunological perspective, clinical MBL and chronic lymphocytic leukemia appear to be overlapping entities. Only a deeper knowledge of molecular pathways and microenvironmental influences involved in disease evolution will help to solve the main clinical issue, i.e. how to differentiate nonprogressive and progressive cases requiring intensive follow-up.

With the advent of multiple highly effective treatment options, minimal residual disease (MRD) measurements gained interest as a prognostic marker in chronic lymphocytic leukemia. This article provides a model explaining the clinical significance of MRD in different clinical situations and reviews available data to support that model. Factors with a possible impact on the clinical significance of MRD are discussed: technique for MRD quantification, treatment regimen, clinical response, time-point for sampling, and the additional impact of molecular risk features. Also described are data supporting the use of MRD assessments as a surrogate end-point in randomized clinical trials.

Treatment of chronic lymphocytic leukemia has greatly advanced in the past few years since introduction of the fludarabine/cyclosphosphamide/rituximab regimen as first-line therapy. Nevertheless, 17p deletion repre-sents a challenge because conventional treatment does not provide satis-factory results. 17p deletion and *TP53* mutation are the major factors accounting for rapid disease progression, poor response to therapy, early relapse, and short survival. Allogeneic stem cell transplantation harbors curative potential but also considerable morbidity and mortality. Novel agents acting independently of the p53 signaling pathway, with favorable side-effect profiles, are promising. This review summarizes up-to-date knowledge about 17p deletion and the spectrum of treatment options.

Therapy for chronic lymphocytic leukemia (CLL) has evolved dramatically throughout the years. In 1997, rituximab (Rituxan), a CD20 monoclonal antibody (mAb), became the first mAb approved by the Food and Drug Administration for marketing in the treatment of cancer, specifically targeting B-cell malignancies. Over the last 10 years, rituximab or other mAbs including alemtuzumab and ofatumumab have become an integral part of the standard of care for CLL patients as single agents or in combination with chemotherapy or other immunotherapy. This review discusses the currently approved and novel mAbs for the treatment of CLL.

Phosphoinositide 3′-kinase (PI3K) is a key node in the B-cell receptor pathway, which plays a crucial role in the trafficking, survival, and proliferation of chronic lymphocytic leukemia (CLL) cells. This article reviews the biology of PI3K, focusing on its relationship to the CLL microenvironment, and discusses the biological rationale for PI3K inhibition in CLL. Preliminary safety and efficacy data from early phase clinical trials is also discussed. Potential biomarkers for clinical response to PI3K inhibitors such as ZAP-70, IGHV status, and CCL3 are examined. Where PI3K inhibition may fit in the evolving landscape of CLL therapy is also explored.

Chimeric antigen receptor (CAR)-modified T cells targeting CD19 expressed by normal and malignant B cells is a unique therapy for patients with chronic lymphocytic leukemia (CLL); recent results highlight the potential of this therapy for patients with relapsed CLL. Because adoptive transfer of CAR-modified T cells is a novel approach, there are issues for the medical oncologist to consider when evaluating current and future clinical trials for CLL patients. This article reviews the impact of CAR design, T-cell production, T-cell dose, conditioning regimens, and tumor burden at the time of CAR-modified T-cell infusion on the efficacy of this therapy.

This article describes the current role and perspectives of "new" allogeneic stem cell transplantation (alloSCT) in the treatment of chronic lymphocytic leukemia (CLL). Clinical trials and minimal residual disease (MRD) studies provide clear evidence that graft-versus-leukemia activity is working in CLL and can provide long-term MRD-free survival in up to 50% of patients undergoing alloSCT. AlloSCT is effective also in poor-risk

CLL as defined by the European Group for Blood and Marrow Transplantation transplant consensus. Novel forms of (reduced intensity) conditioning have resulted in dramatic reduction of early morbidity and mortality of alloSCT in CLL.

HEMATOLOGY/ONCOLOGY
CLINICS OF NORTH AMERICA

Preface

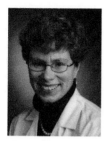

Jennifer R. Brown, MD, PhD
Editor

The last 10 to 15 years have seen an explosion of research in chronic lymphocytic leukemia, perhaps led by the discoveries of the prognostic value of *IGHV* mutational status and of the key recurrent chromosome abnormalities defined by fluorescence in situ hybridization (FISH). Since then, interest in the biology of the disease has continued to expand, leading to the recent explosion of data focused on recurrent somatic mutations in chronic lymphocytic leukemia (CLL), on the impact of the microenvironment in supporting CLL cell survival and proliferation, on the immunodeficiency of CLL, and on the role of B-cell receptor stereotypy in CLL. The identification and characterization of monoclonal B-cell lymphocytosis have led to a redefinition of the diagnostic criteria for CLL in the 2008 update, and now the unusual pattern of lymphocyte redistribution seen with inhibitors of the B-cell receptor (BCR) pathway is leading to further reconsideration of the response criteria. The advent of these inhibitors and many other new therapies currently being tested in the clinic has the potential to transform our treatment paradigms in the coming years. Key areas of focus in the therapeutic arena include the emerging value of minimal residual disease measurements, the still challenging 17p deletion patients, and, of course, the novel agents, particularly the anti-CD20 antibody GA101 and the BCR pathway inhibitors led by the BTK inhibitor ibrutinib (formerly PCI-32765) and the PI3kinase delta inhibitor idelalisib (formerly CAL-101 and GS-1101). Early success with chimeric antigen receptor therapy in CLL holds promise for the future, as does the ever-improving results of allogeneic stem cell transplantation.

This issue of *Hematology/Oncology Clinics of North America* provides a current review of these most exciting new developments in CLL biology and therapy, written by experts who have substantially contributed to the work they discuss. I am grateful to all of them for their willingness to participate and I greatly enjoyed the opportunity to review their thoughtful and scholarly articles. I would also like to thank Patrick Manley and the editorial staff for their gracious efforts to keep everyone on schedule and assure timely completion of the issue. I hope you will enjoy reading the articles, which I think point us toward the rapidly approaching future of CLL, where we will hopefully

Hematol Oncol Clin N Am 27 (2013) xiii–xiv
http://dx.doi.org/10.1016/j.hoc.2013.01.009
0889-8588/13/$ – see front matter © 2013 Published by Elsevier Inc.

hemonc.theclinics.com

have deeper understanding of mechanisms leading us to rationally defined disease subgroups, combined with effective nontoxic targeted therapies based on underlying biology.

Jennifer R. Brown, MD, PhD
Director, CLL Center
Dana-Farber Cancer Institute
450 Brookline Avenue
Boston, MA 02215, USA

E-mail address:
Jennifer_Brown@dfci.harvard.edu

Genomic Approaches to Chronic Lymphocytic Leukemia

Ma. Reina Improgo, PhD, Jennifer R. Brown, MD, PhD*

KEYWORDS

- Chronic lymphocytic leukemia • Genomics • Comparative genomic hybridization
- Single-nucleotide polymorphism arrays • Linkage mapping
- Genome-wide association studies • Whole-exome sequencing
- Whole-genome sequencing

KEY POINTS

- Genomic approaches have led to a recent explosion in knowledge of the spectrum of genetic aberrations in chronic lymphocytic leukemia (CLL).
- Comparative genomic hybridization and high-resolution single-nucleotide polymorphism arrays have been used to detect alterations in copy number, some of which have been associated with prognosis and/or overall survival in CLL.
- Efforts to identify the genetic basis of familial CLL have included genome-wide linkage studies to identify CLL susceptibility genes as well as genome-wide association studies to determine CLL risk loci.
- Within the last couple of years, next-generation sequencing techniques have identified common recurrent somatic mutations in *SF3B1* and *NOTCH1* in CLL. Ongoing work involves the investigation of lower-frequency somatic mutations and clonal evolution over time as well as the identification of germline variants.

Genomics refers to the systematic study of an organism's entire DNA sequence (genome). Molecular information derived from genomic techniques has increased our understanding of many complex diseases, including chronic lymphocytic leukemia (CLL). CLL is the most common form of adult leukemia and is characterized by a highly variable clinical course. Little is known about the molecular correlates underlying the different CLL disease patterns that are clinically evident, and despite epidemiologic evidence showing familial aggregation of CLL, no major predisposing genes have been identified. This article discusses the historical application of genomic techniques to these various problems in CLL: first, the use of comparative genomic hybridization (CGH) and single-nucleotide polymorphism (SNP) arrays to identify somatically

Funded by: NIH, Grant numbers: K23 CA115682.
Conflict of Interest: None.
Department of Medical Oncology, Dana-Farber Cancer Institute, CLL Center, Harvard Medical School, 450 Brookline Avenue, Boston, MA 02215, USA
* Corresponding author.
E-mail address: Jennifer_Brown@dfci.harvard.edu

acquired genetic alterations in CLL, then the use of genome-wide linkage analysis and genome-wide association studies (GWAS) in attempts to determine the cause of heritable predisposition to CLL. Finally, next-generation sequencing technology, which allows detection of both somatic and germline lesions in CLL at unprecedented speeds, is discussed.

TUMOR ANALYSIS BY COMPARATIVE GENOMIC HYBRIDIZATION

The first genome-wide copy-number analyses of CLL were made possible by the development of CGH in the 1990s.[1] CGH allows the detection of chromosomal imbalances using differentially labeled tumor and normal DNA that are cohybridized to normal metaphase chromosomes. Intensities of the fluorescent labels are then used to determine overrepresentation (gain) or underrepresentation (loss) of genomic content in specific chromosomal regions.

In 1995, Bentz and colleagues[2] first applied the CGH method to 28 CLL patients. Copy-number alterations (CNAs) were observed in 68% of the patients, with the most frequent gains found in chromosome 8q and 12 and the most frequent losses in chromosomes 6q, 11q, 13q, and 17p (**Table 1**). A similar study, conducted by Karhu and colleagues[3] using 25 CLL patients, observed chromosomal imbalances in 48% of the cases, with frequent gains in chromosome 12 and frequent losses in chromosome 11q and 13q (see **Table 1**).

To identify chromosomal abnormalities specifically in familial CLL, Summersgill and colleagues[4] used CGH to analyze 24 pedigrees. The investigators detected at least 1 chromosomal imbalance in each patient, with an average of 7 abnormalities per case. The most common gain and loss were observed in the X chromosome (see **Table 1**). The chromosomal imbalances observed in the X chromosome appeared to be more common in familial CLL and were hypothesized to contribute to the differential survival of male and female CLL patients.

Classic CGH used metaphase chromosomes, which have limited resolution. Substitution of the chromosome targets with a matrix or array containing nucleic acids with defined sequences allowed the detection of much smaller gains and losses.[5] This technique, known as matrix-CGH or array-CGH, makes use of sequence pools representative of whole chromosomes or chromosome arms, cloned in bacterial artificial chromosomes (BAC), P1-derived artificial chromosomes (PAC), or other vectors.

An automated matrix-CGH array specific for CLL was developed in 2004 and was validated against 106 CLL cases.[6] Array profiles were compared with cytogenetic data, and showed high specificity and sensitivity. A total of 27 gains and 95 losses were detected using this approach. Novel recurrent genomic imbalances were identified, namely trisomy 19 and a small copy-number gain in the *MYCN* gene on chromosome 2p24 (see **Table 1**). Similarly, Gunn and colleagues[7] analyzed 187 CLL cases using BAC array–based CGH. Copy-number changes were identified in 90% of these cases, with expected frequencies for the common genomic alterations, deletions of 13q, 11q, and 17p with 12 gain. In addition, submicroscopic deletions of chromosome 22q11 were observed in 28 cases (15%).

More recently, the authors' group used high-resolution array-CGH to investigate differences between 37 sporadic and 38 familial cases.[8] Sporadic cases showed significant association with 11q loss, whereas familial cases showed significant association with 14q11 gain. Alterations in 14q11 were also associated with mutated *IGHV* status and homozygous deletions in 13q. Homozygous deletion in 13q was associated with mutated *IGHV*, low expression of ZAP-70, and a significantly longer time to first treatment (TTFT).

Table 1
Chromosomal imbalances in CLL based on CGH and SNP array studies

Chromosome	CGH		SNP Arrays	
	Gains	Losses	Gains	Losses
1	1 (33%)[4]	—	—	1p31 (10%)[14]
2	2p (4%)[3] 2p24 (6%)[6]	2 (25%)[4]	2p14 (28%)[12] 2p16 (6%)[10] 2p22 (28%)[12] 2p (7%)[18]	—
3	3 (19%)[4] 3q (7%)[2]	3p (4%)[2]	3q24 (17%)[12] 3q26 (6%)[13]	—
4	—	4 (25%)[4] 4q (4%)[2]	—	—
5	—	5 (17%)[4]	—	—
6	Trisomy 6 (4%)[3]	6q (11%),[2] (4%)[4] 6q15 (4%)[3]	—	6q (7%)[18]
7	—	7q (4%)[2] 7q31 (4%)[3]	Trisomy 7 (10%)[14]	7q34 (4%)[13]
8	8q (11%)[2]	8p (4%)[2]	8q13 (10%)[14] 8q21 (20%)[14] 8q23 (28%)[12] 8q24 (4%)[13] 8q24.3 (28%)[12] 8q24.13 (28%)[12] 8q24.21 (5%)[18]	8p12 (28%)[12] 8p21 (28%)[12] 8p23 (10%),[14] (28%),[12] (5%)[13] 8q12 (10%)[14]
9	—	—	—	9p21 (10%)[14] 9q21 (22%)[12]
10	—	10q (4%)[2]	—	—
11	11 (38%)[4]	11q (14%),[2] (24%),[3] (17%),[4] (13%)[8]	—	11q22 (13%),[10] (10%),[14] (6%),[13] (27%)[18]
12	Trisomy 12 (16%),[3] (7%)[2] 12p (4%)[2]	12p12 (4%)[3]	Trisomy 12 (13%),[10] (20%),[14] (12%),[13] (11%)[18]	—
13	—	13q (11%),[2] (13%),[4] (53%)[8] 13q13-qter (4%)[3] 13q14-q31 (4%)[3] 13c-q31 (4%)[3]	—	13q14 (51%),[10] (40%),[14] (50%),[12] (51.7%),[17] (57%),[13] (61%)[18]
14	14q (15%)[8]	—	14q32 (28%)[12]	14q31 (3%)[13] 14q32 (33%)[12]
15	Trisomy 15 (4%)[2] 15q (4%)[2]	15q (4%)[2] 15q11 (4%)[3]	15q26 (10%)[14]	15q13 (10%)[14] 15q15.1 (4%)[18]
16	—	16p (4%)[2]	—	—
17	17q (7%)[2]	17p (29%),[2] (4%),[3] (17%)[4]	17q 21.1 (28%)[12] 17q21.31 (33%)[12] 17q21.32 (28%)[12]	17p11 (10%)[14] 17p12 (6%)[13] 17p13 (6%),[10] (20%)[14] 17p (8%)[18]

(continued on next page)

Table 1 (continued)	CGH		SNP Arrays	
Chromosome	Gains	Losses	Gains	Losses
18	18q (4%)[2]	18p (7%)[2]	18q21 (10%)[14]	18q11 (10%)[14] 18q22 (10%)[14]
19	Trisomy 19 (4%),[2] (5%)[6]	—	19p13 (20%)[14]	19p13 (20%)[14] 19q13 (10%)[14]
20	—	—	—	—
21	—	—	—	—
22	22q (4%)[2]	22q11 (15%)[7]	—	22q11 (10%),[14] (33%)[13]
X	X (42%)[4] Xq22 (4%)[3]	X (33%)[4]	—	—

Numbers in parentheses indicate frequencies of gains or losses reported in different studies.
Ref.[4] studied only familial cases.
Abbreviations: CGH, comparative genomic hybridization; CLL, chronic lymphocytic leukemia; SNP, single-nucleotide polymorphism.

TUMOR ANALYSIS BY HIGH-RESOLUTION SINGLE-NUCLEOTIDE POLYMORPHISM ARRAYS

The necessity of overcoming the resolution limits of classic CGH (10–20 Mb) and of array-CGH (0.1 Mb) prompted the use of even higher-resolution platforms. In 2004, Bignell and colleagues[9] demonstrated the utility of using SNP arrays, originally designed for genotyping, to detect CNAs at a genome-wide level. Using the Affymetrix p501 array as a prototype, they showed that simultaneous genotyping and copy-number analysis of cancer cell lines allowed the detection of genomic alterations that would have been missed by array-CGH or genotyping alone, including loss of heterozygosity (LOH) in copy neutral regions as in the case of uniparental disomy (UPD) or as acquired in cancer.

SNP arrays were first applied to CLL samples by Pfeifer and colleagues,[10] using the Affymetrix 10K and 50K arrays. These investigators identified chromosomal imbalances in 65.6% and 81.5% of cases, respectively, indicating greater sensitivity of higher-density arrays. Deletion 13q14 was the most frequent aberration found, followed by trisomy 12, del11q22, and del17p13 (see **Table 1**). In addition, they identified 24 regions with LOH without altered gene dosage.

Kujawski and colleagues[11] subsequently used the 50K Affymetrix SNP array to quantify genome-wide allelic imbalances, including LOH, in 178 CLL patients, to derive a genomic complexity score. The complexity scores correlated well with their clinical end points, TTFT, and time to subsequent therapy (TTST). Specifically, high genomic complexity was found to be an independent risk factor for disease progression and treatment failure.

Forconi and colleagues[12] used a higher-density array (250K Affymetrix) to specifically investigate patients with deletions in 17p, as these show aggressive disease. All cases displayed multiple copy-number changes, with frequent losses in chromosome 8p and frequent gains in chromosome 8q and 2p (see **Table 1**). 8p loss and 2p gain predicted shorter TTFT and poorer overall survival in these 17p patients. The authors subsequently reported a similar association between 8p loss and 17p deletion using the SNP6.0 array.[13]

To determine which platforms allowed reliable detection of CNAs, Gunnarsson and colleagues[14] carried out a comparative study of 4 high-resolution platforms: BAC arrays (32K), oligonucleotide arrays (185K), and 2 SNP arrays (Affymetrix 250K and Illumina 317K). All platforms were able to robustly detect large aberrations, with 29 CNAs concordantly detected, including common alterations. However, small CNAs were detected only by the high-density oligonucleotide and SNP arrays. The oligonucleotide array had lower baseline variation in comparison with the other platforms. The 250K Affymetrix array detected more CNAs than the 317K Illumina array, but the latter detected more LOH events.

To assess the performance of SNP arrays for routine clinical use, Hagenkord and colleagues[15] compared low-density (Affymetrix 10K2.0), medium-density (Affymetrix 250K Nsp), and high-density (Affymetrix SNP6.0) SNP arrays. The 10K2.0 array was found to be unsuitable for use in the clinic because of its relatively poor resolution. The SNP6.0 array was superior in detecting small aberrations but was equivalent to the 250K array for detecting lesions known to be clinically relevant. Furthermore, the 250K array was less costly and easier to manage. The 250K array demonstrated 98.5% concordance with the standard CLL fluorescence in situ hybridization (FISH) panel, but also detected acquired UPD and additional regions of genomic complexity.

Ouillette and colleagues[16] also performed copy-number analysis of 255 CLL patients using Affymetrix 6.0 arrays, and observed at least 2 CNAs in 39% of all cases and 3 or more CNAs in 20% of patients. In addition, they correlated genomic complexity (defined as the total number of CNAs) with clinical outcomes, and found elevated genomic complexity to be an independent marker for aggressive CLL and short overall survival. The same group also analyzed SNP 6.0 arrays to specifically define 13q14 deletions in 255 CLL patients.[17] Large 13q14 deletions encompassing the RB1 gene were detected in 20% of these patients and were associated with decreased survival.

Recently, the authors' group integrated copy-number analysis using Affymetrix 6.0 SNP arrays together with gene-expression profiling in 161 CLL patients.[13] With matched germline controls a median of only 1 somatic CNA per sample was found, suggesting that the CLL genome is relatively stable. The authors identified recurrent CNAs associated with short TTFT: 8q24 amplification, 3q26 amplification, and 8p deletions (see **Table 1**). Amplifications of 3q26 were focused on the PIK3CA gene and amplifications of 8q were focused on MYC and on the regulatory region near MYC, which has been implicated by GWAS in disease risk in CLL and many other cancers.

Similarly, Edelmann and colleagues[18] used the Affymetrix 6.0 array to analyze 353 untreated CLL samples, and identified an average of 1.8 CNAs per case with copy-neutral LOH being found in 6% of cases, most frequently in 13q, 17p, and 11q. Chromosome 13q14 was deleted in 61% of cases, with minimally deleted regions refined to the DLEU1 and DLEU2 genes (see **Table 1**). These investigators also found novel lesions including a frequent deletion at 15q15.1 (4%), with the smallest deletion found in the MAX gene–associated (MGA) gene locus.

Taken together, CGH and SNP array studies of CLL tumors have identified recurrently altered loci that are likely involved in the pathogenesis of CLL and could even potentially be involved in CLL susceptibility. The extent of genomic aberrations, as well as the presence of specific CNAs in addition to those classically identified by FISH, such as 2p gain, 3q gain, 8p deletion, and 8q gain, have been suggested to have clinical relevance and should be tested in prospective clinical trials to evaluate their true usefulness as predictors for clinical outcomes.

GERMLINE GENOME-WIDE LINKAGE MAPPING

Genome-wide linkage mapping, also known as genome scanning, is a high-throughput method that uses genetic markers to assess the likelihood that a marker associated with a disease phenotype is linked to a predisposing gene. These studies are typically done on germline DNA to identify genes involved in heritability, and this field developed in parallel with the early studies on tumor DNAs. The statistical likelihood that a particular genetic marker is linked to the phenotype in question is usually represented by a logarithm of the odds (LOD) score, which is a measure of the probability that an observed linkage is indeed a true linkage. By convention, a LOD of 3.0 or more is required for significance, as this indicates that the odds are 1000 to 1 in favor of genetic linkage. LOD scores of 2.0 or greater are considered suggestive, and LOD scores of at least 1.0 indicate regions that require follow-up studies.

Goldin and colleagues[19] first used genome-wide linkage mapping to genotype 18 CLL families. This study scanned 359 microsatellite markers in 28 panels using a medium-density linkage mapping set. LOD scores of at least 1 were observed for chromosomes 1, 3, 6, 12, 13, and 17, but none of these showed significant or suggestive linkage. A follow-up study was later conducted in 28 families, focusing on markers around the aforementioned regions of interest.[20] Similarly, the data did not support linkage in chromosomes 1, 3, 6, 12, and 17. The investigators argue that chromosome 13q21.33 remained a region of interest because it was significant at the locus level although not at the genome-wide level. Fine mapping of this region using interphase FISH in 6 CLL families revealed a minimally deleted region in 13q21.33-q22.2 shared by 4 families.[21] Two asymptomatic siblings who shared this haplotype had monoclonal B-cell lymphocytosis, which is thought to be a precursor of CLL. Sequencing of the 13 genes found in this region revealed 85 polymorphisms, although none of these were coding or frameshift mutations. An intronic polymorphism in the *PIBF1* gene cosegregated with the haplotype shared by 3 affected members of one family.

In 2005, Sellick and colleagues[22] analyzed a bigger cohort of 115 families using the Affymetrix GeneChip Mapping 10kv1 Xba array. Again, no region of significant linkage was observed in this study. Chromosome 11p11 displayed suggestive linkage and chromosomes 5q22-23, 6p22, 10q25, and 14q32 yielded LOD scores greater than 1.15. Although none of these regions correspond to those commonly found in cytogenetic studies or in earlier studies focused on tumor analysis, this is not necessarily surprising because the regions defined by Sellick and colleagues[22] should be associated with germline disease predisposition rather than the tumor-related somatic alterations described in most previous studies.

To increase detection power, Sellick and colleagues[23] analyzed an additional 101 pedigrees using the GeneChip Mapping 10Kv2.0 Xba array, which scans 10,200 SNP markers. The results of this study were then pooled with the results from the 105 families in their previous cohort. Chromosome 2q21.2 emerged as a major susceptibility locus. This locus contains the gene encoding the chemokine receptor 4 (*CXCR4*). The same group analyzed the genotype frequency of rs2228014, a polymorphic variant in *CXCR4*, in 1058 CLL cases and 1807 controls.[24] No evidence was found that rs2228014 influences CLL risk. However, 3 cases with *CXCR4* mutations were identified, a finding that would be of interest for further investigation.

As shown by these studies, the ability to find a significant LOD score depends on the study power, which is dependent, in turn, on the size of the families and the numbers of affected and unaffected individuals available to be studied. In CLL, study power can be a particular problem because of relatively small families with just a few affected individuals, some of whom may be deceased before the study. Individual genetic events that are likely causative in single families have been described,[25–27] but as yet no recurrent highly penetrant predisposing gene has been identified. These findings suggest that such a gene may not exist, and that CLL risk may more typically arise from the combination of multiple lower-risk alleles.

GENOME-WIDE ASSOCIATION STUDIES

The absence of a major highly penetrant disease-causing locus in CLL identifiable by linkage suggests that genetic predisposition to CLL may lie in the co-inheritance of multiple lower-risk variants. GWAS allows the identification of such variants for particular diseases. The first GWAS conducted for CLL analyzed 299,983 SNPs in a total of 1529 cases and 3115 controls from a European cohort.[28] Seven SNPs representing 6 CLL risk loci were identified in this study, namely rs17483466, rs13397985, rs872071, rs9378805, rs735665, rs7176508, and rs11083846 (**Table 2**). The strongest statistical evidence was obtained for rs872071 and rs9378805, both of which map to a region on chromosome 6p25.3 near the interferon regulatory factor 4 (*IRF4*) gene. In addition, the risk genotype of rs872071 was found to correlate with lower expression of *IRF4* in lymphoblastoid cell lines.[29] Fine-scale mapping of the 6p25.3 locus narrowed the association signal to an 18-kb region containing the 3′-untranslated region (UTR) of *IRF4*.[30] This region is predicted to encode a binding site for the *trans*-acting regulatory element *MZF1*, a growth suppressor in hematopoietic cells, but the biology of how this alteration in *IRF4* may predispose to CLL is not yet understood.[31] Furthermore, *IRF4* has since been shown to be somatically mutated in 1.5% of CLL cases,[32] leading to increased activity, and to be amplified in the germline of a family with Mendelian-type inheritance of CLL, leading to decreased expression.[27] Indeed, although these various lines of evidence implicate *IRF4* in CLL, the underlying biological mechanisms of *IRF4* involvement in CLL remain obscure.

To further verify the association of these risk SNPs with CLL, Crowther-Swanepoel and colleagues[33] genotyped a Spanish cohort consisting of 424 cases and 450 controls as well as a Swedish cohort consisting of 400 cases and 400 controls. The investigators confirmed an association between CLL risk and rs13397985, rs872071, rs735665, rs7176508, and rs11083846 (see **Table 2**). An extension study performed by the same group identified 4 additional susceptibility loci, with 8q24.21 (a GWAS susceptibility region for multiple solid tumors, which likely functions as a *MYC* enhancer) and 16q24.1 (containing *IRF8*) appearing the most interesting (see **Table 2**).[34] Another extension study by the same group, using pooled data from previous work as well as new datasets from Poland, Italy, and the United kingdom, reported additional risk loci at 15q25.2 (near *CPEB1*) and 18q21.1 (near *CXXC1* and *MBD1*).[35]

Slager and colleagues[36] later evaluated risk SNPs in a Caucasian cohort from the United States consisting of 438 cases and 328 controls. Associations were confirmed for the previously described SNPs rs17483466, rs13397985, rs872071, rs735665, rs7176508, and rs9378805 (see **Table 2**). To identify SNPs specifically associated with familial CLL, the same group conducted a GWAS enriched for familial cases.[37] Using a total of 407 CLL patients, 102 of which were familial cases, and 296 controls, they found 4 SNPs with genome-wide significance in the 16q24.1 locus containing the *IRF8* gene (see **Table 2**). All 4 risk alleles were found to be associated with decreased *IRF8* mRNA levels in lymphocytes. SNPs found to be specifically associated with familial CLL include rs615672, rs674313, and rs502771 (near *HLA-DRB5*), and rs9272219 and rs9272535 (near *HLA-DQA1*).

Meta-analysis of the aforementioned GWAS, followed by validation in an independent case-control series, identified a novel risk locus at chromosome 6p21.33.[38]

Table 2
GWAS loci and SNPs associated with CLL risk

Risk Locus	SNP	Risk Allele	Nearest Gene(s)	SNP Location	Population
2q13	rs17483466	G	*ACOXL, BCL2L11*	Intron 10 of *ACOXL*	European (UK)[28] Caucasian (USA)[36,37]
2q37.1	rs13397985	G	*SP140, SP110*	Intron 1 of *SP140*	European (UK)[28] Caucasian (USA)[36,37] Spanish[33] Swedish[33]
2q37.3	rs757978	A	*FARP2*	Exon 9	Combined: European (UK), Spanish, Swedish[34] Caucasian (USA)[37]
6p21.3	rs210134	G	*BAK1*	~100 kb telomeric	Meta-analysis: European (UK), Spanish, Swedish, Caucasian (USA)[38]
	rs210142	C	*BAK1*	Intron 1	Meta-analysis: European (UK), Spanish, Swedish, Caucasian (USA)[38]
6p25.3	rs872071	G	*IRF4*	3′-UTR	European (UK)[28] Caucasian (USA)[36,37] Spanish[33] Swedish[33]
	rs9378805	C	*IRF4*	~10 kb from 3′-UTR	European (UK)[28] Caucasian (USA)[36,37]
8q24.21	rs2456449	G	*MYC* (enhancer element)	—	Combined: European (UK), Spanish, Swedish[34] Caucasian (USA)[37]
11q24.1	rs735665	A	*GRAMD1B*	~50 kb centromeric	European (UK)[28] Caucasian (USA)[36,37] Spanish[33] Swedish[33]
15q21.3	rs7169431	A	*NEDD4, RFX7*	—	Combined: European (UK), Spanish, Swedish[34] Caucasian (USA)[37]

(continued on next page)

Table 2 (continued)					
Risk Locus	SNP	Risk Allele	Nearest Gene(s)	SNP Location	Population
15q23	rs7176508	A	—	—	European (UK)[28] Spanish[33] Swedish[33]
	rs11072110	T	—	—	Caucasian (USA)[36]
	rs10220831	G	—	—	Caucasian (USA)[36]
	rs35707742	G	—	—	Caucasian (USA)[36]
	rs4777184	T	—	—	Caucasian (USA)[36]
15q25.2	rs783540	G	CPEB1	Intron 2	Combined: European (UK), Italian, Polish[35]
16q24.1	rs305061	T	IRF8	~19 kb telomeric	Combined: European (UK), Spanish, Swedish[34] Caucasian (USA)[37]
	rs305077	C	IRF8	Intron 3	Caucasian (USA)[37]
	rs391525	G	IRF8	Intron 3	Caucasian (USA)[37]
	rs2292982	G	IRF8	Intron 3	Caucasian (USA)[37]
	rs2292980	C	IRF8	Intron 3	Caucasian (USA)[37]
18q21.1	rs1036935	T	CXXC1, MBD1	Telomeric	Combined: European (UK), Italian, Polish[35]
19q13.32	rs11083846	A	PRKD2, STRN4	Intron 3 of PRKD2	European (UK)[28] Spanish[33] Swedish[33]

— indicates that no known genes, transcripts, or microRNAs lie within a 250-kb region flanking the marker.

Abbreviations: GWAS, genome-wide association studies; SNP, single-nucleotide polymorphism; UTR, untranslated region.

The 2 risk SNPs in this locus are rs210134, which lies 100 kb telomeric to the BCL2 antagonist killer (*BAK1*) gene, and rs210142, which lies in intron 1 of *BAK1*. A strong relationship between the risk allele of rs210134 and reduced *BAK1* expression was also found in lymphoblastoid cell lines. BAK1 is known to promote apoptosis by antagonizing BCL2 and other antiapoptotic proteins.[39]

Most risk SNPs identified by GWAS are located in noncoding or intergenic regions, prompting the hypothesis that their function lies in regulating gene expression. To identify SNPs that alter gene expression in CLL, Sille and colleagues[40] performed expression quantitative trait loci analysis, an approach involving integration of genome-wide SNP data with gene-expression profiles, in an attempt to identify genes that are differentially expressed based on the genotype of GWAS SNPs. Using publicly available databases, they found a total of 19 SNPs associated with differential gene expression in lymphoblastoid cell lines: 16 SNPs associated with expression of *SP140*, a putative tumor-suppressor gene; and 3 SNPs linked to expression of *DACT3*, a member of the WNT/β-catenin pathway, and of *GNG8*, a gene involved in G-protein–coupled receptor signaling. Of these, 14 were found to lie in predicted regulatory elements, several of which have been implicated in CLL or other hematologic malignancies. These results suggest that these genes may be involved in CLL pathogenesis, but further validation will be required.

MOVING TO SEQUENCE-LEVEL ANALYSIS

Direct Sanger sequencing (first generation) has enabled the identification of key mutations in CLL, including somatic mutations in TP53[41–44] and ATM,[45–47] which appear to play important roles in the pathogenesis of CLL. However, somatic mutations in TP53 and ATM are present in only 10% to 40% of CLL cases depending on prior therapy. Furthermore, systematic sequencing of tyrosine kinases in CLL also revealed no somatic mutations,[48] and sequencing of the entire kinome did not identify recurrently mutated kinase genes in CLL.[49] These experiments reveal the limitations of Sanger sequencing, which is slow, labor-intensive, and not high-throughput.

Next-generation sequencing (NGS) technologies have therefore been used in an effort to determine the full spectrum of genetic lesions in CLL. Also known as second-generation sequencing, NGS refers to methods that involve simultaneous detection of nucleotides from multiple amplified DNA clones.[50] NGS allows more rapid sequencing of entire exomes, genomes, and transcriptomes at lower cost, and can facilitate the discovery of novel chromosomal rearrangements and copy-number alterations. NGS is also able to identify genetic lesions occurring at low frequency in clinical samples by sequencing at higher or deeper coverage, that is, by sequencing more amplified clones per region.

Whole-exome sequencing (WES) was first performed in CLL by Fabbri and colleagues,[51] in combination with SNP array analysis. From 5 CLL patients, 40 somatic nonsilent mutations were observed, involving 39 distinct genes. Direct Sanger sequencing of coding and splice-site regions of all mutated genes were then performed in an independent panel of 48 CLL cases. From the results of the combined analyses, 5 recurrently mutated genes emerged, namely NOTCH1, TP53, PLEKHG5, TGM7, and BIRC3 (**Table 3**). NOTCH1 mutations were detected at significantly higher frequency in chemorefractory CLL and during disease progression to Richter syndrome. Integration of WES and copy-number data revealed a total of 52 genetic lesions (range of 7–13 lesions per case), with 40 somatic mutations (ranging from 6–10 mutations per case) and 12 copy-number alterations (ranging from 1–5 alterations per case).

Around the same time, Puente and colleagues[52] reported results of their whole-genome sequencing of 4 CLL cases, composed of 2 IGHV unmutated and 2 IGHV mutated cases. These investigators identified 46 somatic mutations in 45 genes. To validate mutations in 26 expressed genes, they used a combination of polymerase chain reaction amplification and Illumina sequencing of pooled samples from a set of 169 additional patients. Four recurrently mutated genes were identified: NOTCH1, XPO1, MYD88, and KLH6. MYD88 and KLH6 were associated with mutated IGHV status, whereas NOTCH1 and XPO1 were associated with unmutated IGHV status. The recurrent mutation in MYD88 was associated with younger age and clinically advanced stage at diagnosis. This same mutation has been identified by the authors' group in their CLL cohort[53] as well as in diffuse large B-cell lymphoma, where it has been shown to confer survival of cancer cells.[54]

The authors' group recently conducted whole-exome and whole-genome sequencing in 88 and 3 CLL patients, respectively.[53] The patients were selected to reflect the full cytogenetic spectrum of CLL including 17p and 11q deletions. Nine significantly mutated genes were identified, namely TP53, ATM, MYD88, and NOTCH1 (all previously implicated in CLL) as well as SF3B1, ZMYM3, MAPK1, FBXW7, and DDX3X. SF3B1 was the second most frequently mutated gene in this cohort, and occurred in association with deletions in chromosome 11q, which is associated with poor CLL prognosis. SF3B1 had been previously found to be mutated in

Table 3
Genes with recurrent mutations in CLL identified in whole-genome/whole-exome sequencing studies

Gene	Frequency (%)	Reference
TP53	16.5	[53]
	7.5	[51]
SF3B1	15.4	[53]
	9.7	[57]
NOTCH1	15.1	[51]
	12.2	[52]
	12.1	[57]
	4.4	[53]
ATM	9.9	[53]
MYD88	9.8	[53]
	2.9	[52]
CHD2	4.8	[57]
LRP1B	4.8	[57]
POT1	4.8	[57]
FBXW7	4.4	[53]
ZMYM3	4.4	[53]
PLEKHG5	3.8	[51]
BIRC3	3.8	[51]
TGM7	3.8	[51]
DDX3X	3.3	[53]
MAPK1	3.3	[53]
XPO1	2.4	[52]
KLHL6	1.8	[52]

myelodysplastic syndromes.[55] Tumor samples with mutations in SF3B1 were found to have alterations in premessenger RNA splicing, consistent with SF3B1 being a component of the core spliceosome. The presence of an SF3B1 mutation was an independent predictor of short TTFT in multivariable analysis in this cohort. Mutations in FBXW7 may also be interesting, as FBXW7 is important for proteosomal degradation of NOTCH.[56] The authors also found novel, nonsynonymous mutations in WNT pathway members DKK2 and BCL9, although no individual recurrent driver mutations were found. Somatic mutations in CLL clustered in pathways involved in cell-cycle regulation, DNA repair, NOTCH signaling, inflammation, RNA processing, and WNT signaling.

In the context of the International Cancer Genome Consortium, Quesada and colleagues[57] performed large-scale sequencing involving 105 CLL patients and also identified SF3B1 among 78 genes recurrently mutated in CLL. Clinical analysis showed that patients with SF3B1 mutations presented with advanced disease at diagnosis, and were characterized by adverse features such as elevated β2-microglobulin levels and unmutated IGHV status. In addition, patients with SF3B1 mutations had significantly shorter time to disease progression and lower 10-year survival rates. Other genes found to be recurrently mutated in this study include NOTCH1, POT1, CHD2, and LRP1B. TP53 and ATM mutations were rare in this study, likely because these patients represented an untreated cohort.

Thus, sequencing efforts to date have identified SF3B1 and NOTCH1 as somatically mutated in 10% to 15% of CLLs, with other mutations, apart from the previously identified *TP53* and *ATM*, generally occurring in 5% or fewer patients. The latter mutations are likely still significant, but their relatively low frequency and diversity will make understanding and targeting them more complicated. Data to date suggest that *SF3B1* and *NOTCH1* are both associated with poor prognosis, but these findings remain to be confirmed in prospective clinical trials.

SUMMARY

Genomic approaches have provided a comprehensive understanding of genomic alterations in CLL and, most recently, of the somatic mutational landscape in CLL. Significant prognostic associations have been suggested for particular chromosomal gains and losses such as 8p deletion and 8q24 gain; for the total number of copy-number alterations; and for particular somatic mutations such as *SF3B1* and *NOTCH1*. New recurrently mutated genes have been identified (eg, *SF3B1*) whose role in cancer was previously unknown and is still poorly understood, but is currently under active investigation.

To date, efforts to use genomics to elucidate germline predisposition to CLL either through linkage mapping or GWAS have found associated markers, but the underlying causative pathogenesis has remained elusive. Ongoing efforts applying NGS to the germline of familial CLL cases will be more challenging than the somatic analysis completed so far but will lead, it is hoped, to meaningful insights in the years to come.

While the advances are encouraging, many avenues of investigation remain. As a community we are now in a position to form a fully integrated model of genomic and biological prognostic factors and to start to incorporate this into clinical practice. We are also poised to begin targeting specific mutational events with therapies in the clinic. Drugs that target *NOTCH1* are already in the clinic for other disease indications, which may facilitate their evaluation in CLL. Targeting may also become possible for *SF3B1*, as we learn more about its role in the pathogenesis of CLL and as better inhibitory drugs advance into the clinic. It is expected that advances in the understanding of germline predisposition to CLL, though remaining slow, will start to benefit from NGS. The explosion of genomic knowledge in CLL has just begun and is just starting to expand into the clinic, but in the coming years as our understanding expands and ongoing technological innovation fuels new discoveries, the impact of genomic discovery on prognosis and treatment of CLL is expected to come to fruition.

REFERENCES

1. Kallioniemi A, Kallioniemi OP, Sudar D, et al. Comparative genomic hybridization for molecular cytogenetic analysis of solid tumors. Science 1992;258(5083): 818–21.
2. Bentz M, Huck K, du Manoir S, et al. Comparative genomic hybridization in chronic B-cell leukemias shows a high incidence of chromosomal gains and losses. Blood 1995;85(12):3610–8.
3. Karhu R, Knuutila S, Kallioniemi OP, et al. Frequent loss of the 11q14-24 region in chronic lymphocytic leukemia: a study by comparative genomic hybridization. Tampere CLL Group. Genes Chromosomes Cancer 1997;19(4):286–90.
4. Summersgill B, Thornton P, Atkinson S, et al. Chromosomal imbalances in familial chronic lymphocytic leukaemia: a comparative genomic hybridisation analysis. Leukemia 2002;16(7):1229–32.
5. Solinas-Toldo S, Lampel S, Stilgenbauer S, et al. Matrix-based comparative genomic hybridization: biochips to screen for genomic imbalances. Genes Chromosomes Cancer 1997;20(4):399–407.

6. Schwaenen C, Nessling M, Wessendorf S, et al. Automated array-based genomic profiling in chronic lymphocytic leukemia: development of a clinical tool and discovery of recurrent genomic alterations. Proc Natl Acad Sci U S A 2004; 101(4):1039–44.

7. Gunn SR, Bolla AR, Barron LL, et al. Array CGH analysis of chronic lymphocytic leukemia reveals frequent cryptic monoallelic and biallelic deletions of chromosome 22q11 that include the PRAME gene. Leuk Res 2009;33(9): 1276–81.

8. Setlur SR, Ihm C, Tchinda J, et al. Comparison of familial and sporadic chronic lymphocytic leukaemia using high resolution array comparative genomic hybridization. Br J Haematol 2010;151(4):336–45.

9. Bignell GR, Huang J, Greshock J, et al. High-resolution analysis of DNA copy number using oligonucleotide microarrays. Genome Res 2004;14(2):287–95.

10. Pfeifer D, Pantic M, Skatulla I, et al. Genome-wide analysis of DNA copy number changes and LOH in CLL using high-density SNP arrays. Blood 2007;109(3): 1202–10.

11. Kujawski L, Ouillette P, Erba H, et al. Genomic complexity identifies patients with aggressive chronic lymphocytic leukemia. Blood 2008;112(5):1993–2003.

12. Forconi F, Rinaldi A, Kwee I, et al. Genome-wide DNA analysis identifies recurrent imbalances predicting outcome in chronic lymphocytic leukaemia with 17p deletion. Br J Haematol 2008;143(4):532–6.

13. Brown JR, Hanna M, Tesar B, et al. Integrative genomic analysis implicates gain of PIK3CA at 3q26 and MYC at 8q24 in chronic lymphocytic leukemia. Clin Cancer Res 2012;18(14):3791–802.

14. Gunnarsson R, Staaf J, Jansson M, et al. Screening for copy-number alterations and loss of heterozygosity in chronic lymphocytic leukemia—a comparative study of four differently designed, high resolution microarray platforms. Genes Chromosomes Cancer 2008;47(8):697–711.

15. Hagenkord JM, Monzon FA, Kash SF, et al. Array-based karyotyping for prognostic assessment in chronic lymphocytic leukemia: performance comparison of Affymetrix 10K2.0, 250K Nsp, and SNP6.0 arrays. J Mol Diagn 2010;12(2): 184–96.

16. Ouillette P, Collins R, Shakhan S, et al. Acquired genomic copy number aberrations and survival in chronic lymphocytic leukemia. Blood 2011;118(11):3051–61.

17. Ouillette P, Collins R, Shakhan S, et al. The prognostic significance of various 13q14 deletions in chronic lymphocytic leukemia. Clin Cancer Res 2011; 17(21):6778–90.

18. Edelmann J, Holzmann K, Miller F, et al. High-resolution genomic profiling of chronic lymphocytic leukemia reveals new recurrent genomic alterations. Blood 2012;120(24):4783–94.

19. Goldin LR, Ishibe N, Sgambati M, et al. A genome scan of 18 families with chronic lymphocytic leukaemia. Br J Haematol 2003;121(6):866–73.

20. Ng D, Marti GE, Fontaine L, et al. High-density mapping and follow-up studies on chromosomal regions 1, 3, 6, 12, 13 and 17 in 28 families with chronic lymphocytic leukaemia. Br J Haematol 2006;133(1):59–61.

21. Ng D, Toure O, Wei MH, et al. Identification of a novel chromosome region, 13q21.33-q22.2, for susceptibility genes in familial chronic lymphocytic leukemia. Blood 2007;109(3):916–25.

22. Sellick GS, Webb EL, Allinson R, et al. A high-density SNP genomewide linkage scan for chronic lymphocytic leukemia-susceptibility loci. Am J Hum Genet 2005; 77(3):420–9.

23. Sellick GS, Goldin LR, Wild RW, et al. A high-density SNP genome-wide linkage search of 206 families identifies susceptibility loci for chronic lymphocytic leukemia. Blood 2007;110(9):3326–33.
24. Crowther-Swanepoel D, Qureshi M, Dyer MJ, et al. Genetic variation in CXCR4 and risk of chronic lymphocytic leukemia. Blood 2009;114(23):4843–6.
25. Calin GA, Trapasso F, Shimizu M, et al. Familial cancer associated with a polymorphism in ARLTS1. N Engl J Med 2005;352(16):1667–76.
26. Raval A, Tanner SM, Byrd JC, et al. Downregulation of death-associated protein kinase 1 (DAPK1) in chronic lymphocytic leukemia. Cell 2007;129(5):879–90.
27. Brown JR, Hanna M, Tesar B, et al. Germline copy number variation associated with Mendelian inheritance of CLL in two families. Leukemia 2012;26(7):1710–3.
28. Di Bernardo MC, Crowther-Swanepoel D, Broderick P, et al. A genome-wide association study identifies six susceptibility loci for chronic lymphocytic leukemia. Nat Genet 2008;40(10):1204–10.
29. Stranger BE, Forrest MS, Clark AG, et al. Genome-wide associations of gene expression variation in humans. PLoS Genet 2005;1(6):e78.
30. Crowther-Swanepoel D, Broderick P, Ma Y, et al. Fine-scale mapping of the 6p25.3 chronic lymphocytic leukaemia susceptibility locus. Hum Mol Genet 2010;19(9):1840–5.
31. Gaboli M, Kotsi PA, Gurrieri C, et al. Mzf1 controls cell proliferation and tumorigenesis. Genes Dev 2001;15(13):1625–30.
32. Havelange V, Pekarsky Y, Nakamura T, et al. IRF4 mutations in chronic lymphocytic leukemia. Blood 2011;118(10):2827–9.
33. Crowther-Swanepoel D, Mansouri M, Enjuanes A, et al. Verification that common variation at 2q37.1, 6p25.3, 11q24.1, 15q23, and 19q13.32 influences chronic lymphocytic leukaemia risk. Br J Haematol 2010;150(4):473–9.
34. Crowther-Swanepoel D, Broderick P, Di Bernardo MC, et al. Common variants at 2q37.3, 8q24.21, 15q21.3 and 16q24.1 influence chronic lymphocytic leukemia risk. Nat Genet 2010;42(2):132–6.
35. Crowther-Swanepoel D, Di Bernardo MC, Jamroziak K, et al. Common genetic variation at 15q25.2 impacts on chronic lymphocytic leukaemia risk. Br J Haematol 2011;154(2):229–33.
36. Slager SL, Goldin LR, Strom SS, et al. Genetic susceptibility variants for chronic lymphocytic leukemia. Cancer Epidemiol Biomarkers Prev 2010;19(4):1098–102.
37. Slager SL, Rabe KG, Achenbach SJ, et al. Genome-wide association study identifies a novel susceptibility locus at 6p21.3 among familial CLL. Blood 2011;117(6):1911–6.
38. Slager SL, Skibola CF, Di Bernardo MC, et al. Common variation at 6p21.31 (BAK1) influences the risk of chronic lymphocytic leukemia. Blood 2012;120(4):843–6.
39. Chittenden T, Harrington EA, O'Connor R, et al. Induction of apoptosis by the Bcl-2 homologue Bak. Nature 1995;374(6524):733–6.
40. Sille FC, Thomas R, Smith MT, et al. Post-GWAS functional characterization of susceptibility variants for chronic lymphocytic leukemia. PLoS One 2012;7(1):e29632.
41. Gaidano G, Ballerini P, Gong JZ, et al. p53 mutations in human lymphoid malignancies: association with Burkitt lymphoma and chronic lymphocytic leukemia. Proc Natl Acad Sci U S A 1991;88(12):5413–7.
42. Wattel E, Preudhomme C, Hecquet B, et al. p53 mutations are associated with resistance to chemotherapy and short survival in hematologic malignancies. Blood 1994;84(9):3148–57.

43. Zenz T, Krober A, Scherer K, et al. Monoallelic TP53 inactivation is associated with poor prognosis in chronic lymphocytic leukemia: results from a detailed genetic characterization with long-term follow-up. Blood 2008;112(8):3322–9.

44. Zenz T, Eichhorst B, Busch R, et al. TP53 mutation and survival in chronic lymphocytic leukemia. J Clin Oncol 2010;28(29):4473–9.

45. Bullrich F, Rasio D, Kitada S, et al. ATM mutations in B-cell chronic lymphocytic leukemia. Cancer Res 1999;59(1):24–7.

46. Schaffner C, Stilgenbauer S, Rappold GA, et al. Somatic ATM mutations indicate a pathogenic role of ATM in B-cell chronic lymphocytic leukemia. Blood 1999; 94(2):748–53.

47. Austen B, Skowronska A, Baker C, et al. Mutation status of the residual ATM allele is an important determinant of the cellular response to chemotherapy and survival in patients with chronic lymphocytic leukemia containing an 11q deletion. J Clin Oncol 2007;25(34):5448–57.

48. Brown JR, Levine RL, Thompson C, et al. Systematic genomic screen for tyrosine kinase mutations in CLL. Leukemia 2008;22(10):1966–9.

49. Zhang X, Reis M, Khoriaty R, et al. Sequence analysis of 515 kinase genes in chronic lymphocytic leukemia. Leukemia 2011;25(12):1908–10.

50. Meyerson M, Gabriel S, Getz G. Advances in understanding cancer genomes through second-generation sequencing. Nat Rev Genet 2010;11(10):685–96.

51. Fabbri G, Rasi S, Rossi D, et al. Analysis of the chronic lymphocytic leukemia coding genome: role of NOTCH1 mutational activation. J Exp Med 2011; 208(7):1389–401.

52. Puente XS, Pinyol M, Quesada V, et al. Whole-genome sequencing identifies recurrent mutations in chronic lymphocytic leukaemia. Nature 2011;475(7354): 101–5.

53. Wang L, Lawrence MS, Wan Y, et al. SF3B1 and other novel cancer genes in chronic lymphocytic leukemia. N Engl J Med 2011;365(26):2497–506.

54. Ngo VN, Young RM, Schmitz R, et al. Oncogenically active MYD88 mutations in human lymphoma. Nature 2011;470(7332):115–9.

55. Yoshida K, Sanada M, Shiraishi Y, et al. Frequent pathway mutations of splicing machinery in myelodysplasia. Nature 2011;478(7367):64–9.

56. Welcker M, Clurman BE. FBW7 ubiquitin ligase: a tumour suppressor at the crossroads of cell division, growth and differentiation. Nat Rev Cancer 2008; 8(2):83–93.

57. Quesada V, Conde L, Villamor N, et al. Exome sequencing identifies recurrent mutations of the splicing factor SF3B1 gene in chronic lymphocytic leukemia. Nat Genet 2012;44(1):47–52.

Biology of Chronic Lymphocytic Leukemia in Different Microenvironments

Clinical and Therapeutic Implications

Yair Herishanu, MD[a], Ben-Zion Katz, PhD[a], Andrew Lipsky, BA[b], Adrian Wiestner, MD, PhD[b,*]

KEYWORDS

- Chronic lymphocytic leukemia • Microenvironment • B-cell receptor signaling
- Targeted therapy

KEY POINTS

- CLL is characterized by the accumulation of mature monoclonal B cells in peripheral blood, bone marrow, spleen, and lymph nodes.
- Signals from the B-cell receptor (BCR) and the tissue microenvironment converge on several key intracellular signaling pathways, including the phosphatidylinositide 3-kinase/protein kinase B, mitogen-activated protein kinase/extracellular signal-regulated kinase, and nuclear factor-kappa B pathways, and promote leukemic cell proliferation, survival, and resistance to chemotherapy.
- Tissue sites provide a supportive microenvironment composed of T cells, stromal cells, cytokines, chemokines, and extracellular matrix components.
- The lymph node is a pivotal site of CLL cell activation and proliferation through antigenic stimulation.
- The dependence of CLL cells on signals from the BCR and tissue microenvironment presents opportunities for targeted therapy. Inhibitors of BCR signaling and therapeutic approaches to chemically dissect CLL cells from the supportive microenvironment have shown encouraging clinical results.

INTRODUCTION

Chronic lymphocytic leukemia (CLL) is the most common leukemia in the Western world. An often indolent lymphoproliferative disorder, CLL is characterized by

Research Support: A.W. is supported by the Intramural Research Program of the National, Heart, Lung and Blood Institute, NIH.

[a] Hematology Institute, Tel-Aviv Sourasky Medical Center, 6 Weizman Street, Tel-Aviv 64239, Israel; [b] Hematology Branch, NHLBI, National Institutes of Health, Building 10, CRC 3-5140, 10 Center Drive, Bethesda, MD 20892-1202, USA
* Corresponding author.
E-mail address: wiestnera@mail.nih.gov

Hematol Oncol Clin N Am 27 (2013) 173–206
http://dx.doi.org/10.1016/j.hoc.2013.01.002
0889-8588/13/$ – see front matter Published by Elsevier Inc.

progressive accumulation of monoclonal, small, mature-appearing CD5[+] B cells in peripheral blood, bone marrow, and secondary lymphoid organs.[1] With the notable exception of allogeneic stem cell transplantation, CLL is currently an incurable disease, despite good initial responses to chemoimmunotherapy, which prolong overall survival.[2] Current treatment modalities seem to eradicate malignant CLL cells less efficiently in bone marrow and lymph nodes than in peripheral blood. Thus, patients who initially achieve remission eventually develop recurrent disease. Moreover, the differential response of the disease in different anatomic locations indicates a significant role of the tissue microenvironment in supporting CLL cell survival, enabling them to evade the toxic effects of chemotherapy.

Recent work has demonstrated that the trafficking, survival, and proliferation of CLL cells is tightly regulated by the surrounding tissue microenvironment (**Fig. 1**). This conclusion is bolstered by several lines of evidence. When cultured in vitro, CLL cells rapidly undergo apoptosis, but they can be temporarily rescued from programmed cell death by contact with stromal cells. Stromal cells are also known to confer a protective effect against chemotherapy-induced apoptosis.[3,4] In addition, there are differences in the characteristics of CLL cells in the various tissue compartments. CLL cells in the peripheral blood are arrested in the G0/G1 phase of the cell cycle[5] and display features

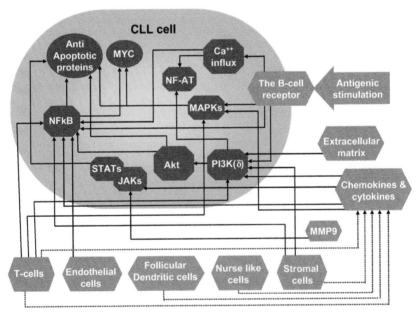

Fig. 1. The CLL microenvironmental signalosome: the convergence of microenvironment-induced signaling responses into biochemical pathways within CLL cells. Microenvironmental elements (◼) including cells (eg, T cells, nurselike cells), the extracellular matrix, and enzymes (eg, MMP9) stimulate CLL cells either directly (*arrows*) or via mediators such as cytokines and chemokines (*dashed arrows*). These extracellular triggers converge into an array of intracellular biochemical responses (◼), resulting in the upregulation of MYC and antiapoptotic proteins (●), as well as additional cellular responses. JAK, Janus kinase; MAPK, mitogen-activated protein kinase; MMP-9, metalloprotinse-9; NF-AT, nuclear factor of activated T-cells; NF-κB, nuclear factor-kappa B; PI3K, phosphatidylinositide 3-kinase; STAT, signal transducer and activator of transcription.

that are consistent with a defect in programmed cell death and prolonged survival in vivo.[1] Previously, this observation was thought to suggest that CLL is a malignancy of quiescent nonproliferating cells. However, recent data on telomere length[6] and in vivo measurement of CLL cell kinetics demonstrated that CLL cells exhibit a more prominent turnover than previously appreciated.[7] Patients with a higher proliferation rate are more likely to have active disease and clinical progression.[7,8] This apparent discrepancy is because proliferation of CLL cells takes place primarily in the secondary lymphoid tissues, although it also occurs to a lesser extent in bone marrow, in areas with a vaguely nodular architecture termed pseudofollicles or proliferation centers.[8,9]

The significant differences in the properties of the cells in peripheral blood and lymphoid tissues are, at least in part, explained by antigenic stimulation and close interaction with various accessory cells as well as by exposure to different cytokines, chemokines, and extracellular matrix components (see **Fig. 1**). In the last decade there have been major advances in the understanding of the reciprocal interactions between CLL cells and the various microenvironmental compartments. This article discusses the role of the microenvironment in the context of efforts to develop novel therapeutics that target the biology of CLL.

CLL CELLS IN THE CONTEXT OF THE NORMAL IMMUNE SYSTEM

Normal B cells are programmed to rapidly respond to the environment, while causing little damage to normal tissues. They have the ability to recognize, process, and present foreign antigens to other components of the immune system, and to undergo maturation and eventually secrete antibodies directed at a specific antigen. They can undergo programmed cell death when their role is over. The reciprocal interaction of B cells with the surrounding environment leads to recruitment of cellular elements into specific tissue compartments. Furthermore, B cells migrate to various compartments that regulate their differentiation, proliferation, and survival or apoptosis. This normal immune response is achieved via multiple proteins that are produced by the B cell and the surrounding microenvironmental cells, leading to a well-orchestrated and tightly regulated sequence of events.

It is not surprising that CLL cells, the malignant counterpart of normal B cells, retain the ability to interact with their surrounding environment. However, the finely tuned orchestration and normal compartmentalization of the immune response is altered. The cause of this malignant transformation is most likely a combination of genetic predisposition and environmental triggers, leading to genetic and epigenetic changes resulting in exaggeration of positive signals and attenuation of inhibitory and pro-apoptotic mechanisms.

INTERPLAY BETWEEN TUMOR BIOLOGY AND THE LOCAL MICROENVIRONMENT

Invasion of the primary and second lymphoid tissues by CLL cells disrupts the normal tissue architecture and physiology. The spleen and lymph nodes are diffusely infiltrated by CLL cells, whereas the bone marrow is involved in an interstitial, nodular, and/or diffuse pattern. CLL cells retain the capacity to react to a variety of external stimuli and the tissue microenvironment provides supporting signals that may differ within the various anatomic sites.

CLL cells respond to the surrounding microenvironment in vivo as demonstrated by the activation of specific signaling pathways in the tumor cells in the tissue microenvironment resulting in changes in gene expression, cellular activation, proliferation, and apoptotic threshold.[8,10] In a genome wide microarray study the authors found that purified CLL cells isolated concomitantly from peripheral blood, bone marrow, and lymph nodes show characteristic gene expression profiles that reflect differential activation of signaling pathways in the various anatomic compartments.[8] In particular, CLL cells in the lymph node upregulated more than 100 genes responsive to B-cell receptor (BCR) activation and nuclear factor-kappa B (NF-κB) signaling and are involved in proliferation. Several studies reported on comparative measurements of activation markers expressed on CLL cells and their proliferation rates in different anatomic compartments.[8,11–14] The expression of activation markers such as CD38 and CD69 as well as proliferation are increased in CLL cells in the lymph node and bone marrow compared with circulating cells.[8,11–13] Likewise, the antiapoptotic regulators B-cell lymphoma extra large (BCL-XL), survivin, and myeloid cell leukemia sequence 1 (MCL1) are expressed at higher levels in CLL cells in lymph nodes compared with their counterparts in peripheral blood.[15] In addition, apoptotic priming, which describes the proximity of a cell to the apoptotic threshold, is reduced in bone marrow–resident CLL cells.[10]

THE MICROENVIRONMENT
Antigenic Stimulation and BCR Signaling

BCR signaling is a crucial component of normal B-cell development and plays an important role in differentiation, survival, proliferation, and antibody secretion. Conclusive experimental evidence established the importance of BCR signaling in the pathogenesis of activated B-celllike diffuse large B-cell lymphoma.[16,17] Although the evidence is somewhat more circumstantial, BCR activation is now also emerging as a central stimulus in the pathogenesis of CLL.[18–22] This view is based on several lines of evidence including specific BCR structures indicating a restricted antigen specificity of CLL cells,[23,24] immunophenotypic characteristics shared with antigen-experienced B cells,[25–27] as well as phenotypic characteristics of anergic B cells,[28,29] the demonstration of ongoing BCR signaling in vivo,[8] and a correlation of increased BCR activation or reactivity with clinical outcome.[30]

Based on the presence or absence of somatic mutations in the immunoglobulin heavy chain variable (IGHV) gene expressed by clonal cells, CLL can be divided into 2 main subgroups.[31,32] Expression of a mutated IGHV identifies a subtype that follows a stable or slowly progressive course, whereas expression of an unmutated IGHV gene is associated with progressive disease and inferior survival.[31,32] In addition, CLL cells use a restricted repertoire of IGHV genes, which encode part of the antigen interacting domains of the BCR. Thus, preferential usage of certain IGHV genes indicates a role for antigen selection in the development of the disease.[23,24] Furthermore, some cases express virtually identical BCRs, so-called stereotyped BCRs, that recognize shared antigens.[33–35] These antigens remain incompletely defined but in many cases may be the target antigens of so-called polyreactive or natural antibodies, including microbial antigens and autoantigens expressed by dying cells.[36–38] In the case of unmutated CLL, it is believed that the particular molecular motifs involved in tumor development are autoantigens; this view is supported by the observation that most of the CLL clones exhibiting stereotyped BCRs also demonstrate unmutated IGHV genes, as well as several studies of soluble immunoglobulins (Igs) demonstrating polyautoreactivity in unmutated CLL.[39–42] In contrast, stimulation via foreign antigen is likely to underlie the pathogenesis of mutated CLL, which exhibits less structural restriction of the BCR.[41] At present, our understanding of where B cells encounter antigen is incomplete. However, the secondary lymphoid tissues are likely to be the major anatomic site for BCR-antigen interaction. Antigens arriving through the lymph flow are sequestered and immobilized by cellular elements in the lymph nodes,[43] thus providing an optimal setting for BCR stimulation. This is consistent with our observation of stronger BCR activation on CLL cells on the lymph nodes compared with blood or bone marrow.[8]

BCR signaling can be broadly divided into 2 main types; one that is antigen independent or tonic[44] and another that is antigen-mediated (**Fig. 2**). Tonic signaling is mediated via phosphatidylinositide 3-kinase (PI3K)α and PI3Kδ, whereas antigen-dependent signaling involves activation of PI3Kδ in addition to several tyrosine kinases and adapter molecules. Antigen-dependent signaling is initiated by the tyrosine kinases LYN and spleen tyrosine kinase (SYK). In vitro studies have shown that BCR engagement on CLL cells triggers an intracellular signaling cascade leading to calcium mobilization, activation of the mitogen-activated protein kinase kinase/extracellular-signal regulated kinase (MEK/ERK), AKT/mammalian target of rapamycin (mTOR), and NF-κB pathways, and upregulation of the antiapoptotic proteins MCL1, BCL-XL, and X-linked inhibitor of apoptosis (XIAP) (see **Fig. 1**).[45–49]

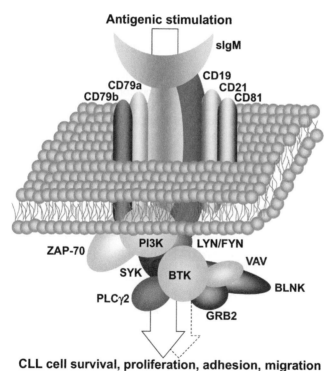

Fig. 2. The BCR, a signaling complex that delivers microenvironment-derived information into the CLL cell. The sIgM serves as the backbone of the BCR, and is associated with other transmembrane molecules (eg, CD19, CD21). The transmembrane components of the BCR associate with a variety of enzymes (eg, SYK, BTK) and scaffold proteins (eg, BLNK) to form a signaling complex. This complex translates extracellular cues, predominantly antigenic stimulation, into CLL cellular responses including survival, proliferation, adhesion, and migration (*arrow*). Tonic or cell-autonomous activation (*dashed arrow*) does not require extracellular stimuli. BLNK, B-cell linker; BTK, Bruton tyrosine kinase; GRB2, growth factor receptor-bound protein 2; PLCγ2, Phospholipase Cγ2; sIg, surface immunoglobulin; SYK, spleen tyrosine kinase; zap-70, zeta-associated protein of 70-kDa.

Recently, a type of BCR signaling that seems to be unique to CLL cells has been described. Specifically, Duhren-von Minden and colleagues[50] showed that epitopes in the framework region of surface immunoglobulins (sIg) expressed on CLL cells serve as autoantigens, raising the possibility of autostimulation of the leukemic cells. Building on previous work demonstrating that the pre-BCR is able to induce ligand-independent cell-autonomous signaling by binding to an intrinsic pre-BCR glycosylation site,[51] the group found that the BCRs of CLL cells constitutively signal even in the absence of any added antigen. This type of signaling was equally demonstrated for BCRs derived from mutated and unmutated CLLs, and seemed to be cell autonomous in that it was demonstrable on isolated individual cells.[50] Such autonomous activation was not found with BCRs derived from multiple myeloma or other lymphoma cells. The heavy-chain complementarity-determining region (HCDR3) of the BCR was identified as the crucial interacting unit, because its insertion into a nonautonomously active BCR resulted in autonomously driven signaling. The investigators then showed that the HCDR3 interacts with an intrinsic motif in the framework region 2 (FR2) of the sIg's VH region.[50] Mutations in this internal FR2 epitope abrogated any autonomous signaling, demonstrating that this epitope acts as an autoantigen binding to CLL BCRs. This finding does not negate the important role of the classic model of extrinsic antigen in the pathogenesis of CLL. Further study is warranted to define the respective roles of the 2 modes of BCR signaling in CLL.

The responsiveness of CLL cells to BCR activation in vitro is heterogeneous.[52] *IGHV* unmutated CLL cells are typically BCR signaling competent, whereas *IGHV* mutated CLL cells respond weakly or not at all to BCR crosslinking induced by anti-IgM antibodies.[30] The Zeta-associated protein of 70-kDa (ZAP-70), a transducing signaling kinase downstream of the T-cell receptor, is expressed in most cases of *IGHV* unmutated CLL but less frequently in *IGHV* mutated CLL.[25,53–55] Expression of ZAP-70, akin to *IGHV* mutation status, serves as a powerful prognostic marker and correlates with a more aggressive disease course.[54–57] ZAP-70 expression is associated with increased BCR signaling in vitro.[46] The nonresponsiveness to BCR activation in some CLL cells is reminiscent of anergized B cells and suggests that these CLL cells are chronically stimulated by antigen in vivo.[29,30] Consistent with this view is the low expression of surface IgM in CLL compared with normal B cells and the recovery of BCR responsiveness after prolonged culture in vitro.[28] Furthermore, CLL cells that do not respond to surface IgM crosslinking respond to anti-IgD or anti-CD79a antibodies, indicating that the intracellular signaling pathway is functional.[30] Nevertheless, it has become clear that the presence of ZAP-70 enhances BCR responsiveness.[58] This effect of ZAP-70 is independent of the kinase domain, but requires recruitment of ZAP-70 to the BCR.[59,60] The demonstration of decreased internalization of an activated BCR in a B-cell line that was engineered to express ZAP-70 provides a link between decreased IgM expression that correlates with the absence of ZAP-70 and an anergic phenotype.[60] Thus, one effect of ZAP-70 might be to interfere with anergy by maintaining higher IgM expression.

In vitro, BCR crosslinking protects CLL cells from apoptosis primarily through the PI3K/AKT pathway and increased expression of MCL1.[45,48,61] BCR triggering also upregulates adhesion and costimulatory molecules, and increases CLL cell migration in response to the chemokines CXCL12 and CXCL13.[62] Moreover, BCR signaling likely plays a central role in promoting CLL cell proliferation. In vitro engagement of the BCR in CLL cells induces expression of MYC, cyclin D2, and cyclin-dependent kinase 4 (CDK4). Although BCR activation promotes G1 cell cycle progression, cell division is not induced.[49,63] Presumably additional costimulatory signals such as CD40L and interleukin (IL)-4, provided in the tissue microenvironment, are required.

Cell-Cell Interactions

Most studies exploring the cellular interactions in CLL have been performed using peripheral blood cells. Experimental methods relying on the investigation of circulating CLL cells in isolation lack the ability to appropriately mimic the complex cellular interactions occurring in the lymphatic niche. Despite this limitation, many in vitro observations have elucidated the in vivo crosstalk between CLL cells and nonmalignant cells.[64,65] In the tissue microenvironment, CLL cells reside in close contact with T lymphocytes, stromal cells, endothelial cells, follicular dendritic cells, and macrophages. Interactions between these components regulate CLL cell trafficking, survival, and proliferation in a manner that may be partly dependent on direct physical cell-to-cell contact or mediated through the exchange of soluble factors (see **Fig. 1**).

T Cells

The interaction between CLL cells and T cells is an important component of the malignant process. First, T cells are important for CLL cell proliferation.[66,67] This has been directly demonstrated in a xenograft murine model of CLL in which activated CD4$^+$ T cells were required for CLL cell proliferation.[66] In patients with CLL, T cells, predominantly of the CD4$^+$ type, often make up a substantial fraction of the lymphoid infiltrate in the bone marrow and lymph nodes,[68] where they are located both around and within proliferation centers.[11,69] CD40, a key regulator of B-cell–T-cell interaction, is stimulated by CD4$^+$ T cells expressing CD154,[70] the ligand for CD40, that are preferentially colocalized with CLL cells in pseudofollicular proliferation centers.[9] CLL cells activated in vitro via CD40, alone or in combination with IL-4, enter the cell cycle[71,72] and are rescued from both spontaneous[73] and drug-induced apoptosis.[74] CD40 signaling in CLL cells induces antiapoptotic molecules such as MCL1, BCL-XL, BFL1, and survivin.[9,75,76] Promotion of CLL cell survival and proliferation by CD40 signaling is mediated through the PI3K/AKT, MEK/ERK,[72,76] and NF-κB pathways.[72–74] Survivin, a member of the family of inhibitor of apoptosis proteins (IAPs), which is preferentially expressed in the large proliferating CLL cells interspersed with T cells in lymph node pseudofollicles, integrates apoptosis resistance and proliferation.[9,77]

In addition to interactions mediated through direct cell-cell contact, T cells also secrete soluble factors that may contribute to CLL cell growth and survival. IL-4 inhibits spontaneous and drug-induced apoptosis in CLL cells via a mechanism involving BCL-2 upregulation.[78] Both IL-2[79] and tumor necrosis factor (TNF)α[80,81] variably induce CLL cell proliferation. Similarly, interferon (IFN)γ,[82] IFNα,[83] and IL-13[84] were also shown to support CLL cell survival.

Second, CLL cells can modify the cellular immune system to evade immune surveillance. Mechanisms are most likely multifactorial including production of immune-suppressing cytokines such as tumor growth factor-β[85] and IL-10,[86] and expression of reduced levels of adhesion and costimulatory molecules,[87] as well as increased numbers and altered function of regulatory T cells.[88,89] Gene expression profiling of purified T cells from patients with CLL revealed changes in genes involved mainly in cell differentiation, cytoskeleton and vesicle formation, trafficking, and cytotoxicity that contribute to decreased immune response.[90] Accordingly, CD4$^+$ and CD8$^+$ T cells in CLL show impaired ability to form immunologic synapses, which is induced by direct cell contact with CLL cells[91] and is mediated through tumoral expression of CD200, CD270, CD274, and CD276.[92]

Stromal Cells

Mesenchymal stromal cells (MSC) are another important cellular component of the tissue microenvironment. Early studies exploring CLL-stromal cell interactions relied on bone marrow-derived stromal cells.[3,93] These cells consist of a heterogeneous population of cells that provide structural and functional support for normal hematopoiesis. Since then, other types of human and murine MSCs have been shown to exhibit similar effects on CLL cells.[94] Stromal cells produce and secrete various cytokines, chemokines, proangiogenic factors, and extracellular matrix components, and express surface receptors that predominantly regulate CLL cell migration and survival. The CLL-MSC crosstalk is bidirectional; thus, tumor cells are not only being supported by stromal cells but also are capable of activating and inducing stromal cell proliferation and secretion of mediators that sustain and intensify the malignant process.[95–98] In the lymphoid tissues of patients with CLL, stromal cells are diffusely located throughout the tissue and in perivascular areas where they admix with CLL cells.[99] The stromal cells are highly productive of CXCL12[100] and are markedly positive for α-smooth muscle actin (αSMA), a marker induced in myofibroblasts that have been activated by tumor stromal-specific growth factors.[99] CLL cells cocultured with bone marrow stromal cells are rescued from both spontaneous[3,93,101] and drug-induced apoptosis,[3,101] in a mechanism dependent on direct cell-cell contact.[3,4] Murine fibroblast cell lines have been shown to protect CLL cells from apoptosis by maintaining expression of the antiapoptotic proteins BCL-XL, XIAP and flice inhibitory protein long (FLIP$_L$) in the leukemic cells. Furthermore, cell-cell interactions activate the NF-κB pathway in a PI3K-dependent manner.[72] CXCL12, secreted from stromal cells, guides CLL cell migration toward the stromal layer and promotes penetration beneath it, a phenomenon called pseudoemperipolesis.[101]

Both cell surface receptors and extracellular matrix elements were reported to be responsible for the enhanced survival of CLL cells that are in contact with the stroma layer. Adherence of CLL cells to stromal cells is mediated simultaneously through integrins β1 and β2.[93] MSCs highly express vascular cell adhesion molecule 1 (VCAM-1).[102] Binding of α4β1 integrin (CD49d/CD29 or VLA-4) to either VCAM-1 or to the extracellular matrix component fibronectin rescues CLL cells from both spontaneous apoptosis and fludarabine-induced apoptosis,[93,103] through PI3K/AKT signaling and BCL-X$_L$ upregulation.[104]

Another aspect of CLL cell interaction with the stroma layer involves metalloproteinase (MMP)-9, vascular endothelial growth factor (VEGF), and endothelial cells. MMP-9, the major MMP produced by CLL cells, promotes their extravasation and lymphoid tissue infiltration through proteolytic degradation of basement membranes and extracellular matrix components.[105] Independently of its proteolytic activity, MMP-9 also partially mediates CLL cell survival in bone marrow–derived stromal cell coculture.[106] Binding of MMP9 to α4β1 and CD44v in CLL cells results in LYN and signal transducer and activator of transcription (STAT) 3 activation and induction of MCL1.[104] Expression of MMP9 in CLL cells is regulated through α4β1 integrins and CXCL12.[105] In this respect, CLL cells in the bone marrow and lymph nodes acquire and express higher levels of surface MMP-9 than could be attributed to tumor cell activation in the tissue microenvironment or derived from their adjacent accessory cells.[104] The proangiogenic molecule VEGF also decreases spontaneous or drug-induced apoptosis of CLL cells through upregulation of MCL1, XIAP, and STAT3 signaling.[107,108] In cocultures of CLL cells with bone marrow–derived stromal cells, vast amounts of VEGF seem to be secreted from the stromal cells and VEGF blockade results in decreased CLL cell survival.[109] CLL cells cocultured with human vascular endothelial cells are also protected from apoptosis in a mechanism involving NF-κB–mediated upregulation of B-cell CLL/lymphoma 2 (BCL2), MCL1, and BCL-XL.[110] Endothelial cells further increase expression of CD38 and CD49 in CLL cells in an NF-κB–dependent mechanism.[110] In addition, activation of CD44 on CLL cells by extracellular matrix components such as hyaluronic acid can promote CLL cell survival through activation of the PI3K pathway.[111]

Follicular Dendritic Cells

The literature on the role of follicular dendritic cells (FDCs) in CLL is limited. FDCs are accessory cells within normal germinal centers that retain intact antigen-antibody complexes on their cell surface and present these antigens to B cells.[112] Normal germinal center B cells that bind to the immune complexes survive and differentiate into either memory B cells or plasma cells.[112] FDCs are normally detected in secondary lymphoid tissue but not in bone marrow.[113] In CLL, FDCs are seen in the lymph nodes, pseudofollicles,[69,114,115] and in bone marrow of patients with nodular involvement.[116] FDCs secrete several important prosurvival factors and growth factors (eg, B cell-activating factor (BAFF) and IL-15) and express other important adhesion molecules such as VCAM-1, intercellular adhesion molecule 1 (ICAM-1), plexin B1, and CD44.[69,112] The effect of FDCs on CLL cells was studied using an FDC cell line (HK cells); the HK cells were shown to rescue CLL cells from spontaneous and drug-induced apoptosis in a manner that was dependent on direct cell-cell contact and associated with an increase in MCL1.[117]

Tissue Macrophages, Monocytes, and Nurselike Cells

An intriguing example of the distinct ability of CLL cells to affect normal cellular elements, leading to the loss of normal compartmentalization and spatial control of the immune response, is the recently described phenomenon of the interaction between CLL cells and nurselike cells (NLCs). NLCs are an in vitro model believed to represent a counterpart of tissue-associated macrophages in vivo. In long-term cultures of peripheral blood mononuclear cells from patients with CLL, large, round, occasionally binucleated CD68-expressing cells grow out.[118,119] NLCs were so named because CLL cells surround these cells, giving them a survival advantage. Cells with similar phenotype are also detected in vivo in secondary lymphoid tissues of patients with CLL,[119] thus strengthening their biological relevance; yet, their numbers in the tissues are probably low.[99] NLCs actually differentiate from monocytes and their differentiation is dependent on cell-cell contact with CLL cells.[119] Monocytes obtained from normal donors cocultured with purified CLL cells also differentiate into NLCs[119] but normal B cells do not induce differentiation of monocytes into NLCs.[119] Coculturing CLL cells with NLCs protects CLL cells from spontaneous and drug-induced apoptosis[101,118] in a mechanism that is partially mediated through an increase in MCL1 expression.[120] NLCs produce and secrete chemokines and growth factors including CXCL12 and CXCL13 as well as BAFF and a proliferation-inducing ligand (APRIL), which attract CLL cells into the tissue compartment and support their survival and proliferation.

BAFF and APRIL are TNF superfamily members that are important for B-cell differentiation and survival.[121–123] CLL cells themselves also express BAFF and APRIL and their receptors.[124,125] However, NLCs express higher levels of BAFF and APRIL than CLL cells.[120] BAFF binds to BAFF receptor (BAFF-R), B-cell maturation antigen (BCMA), and transmembrane activator calcium modulator and cyclophilin ligand interactor (TACI), whereas APRIL binds only to the latter 2 receptors. BAFF and/or APRIL decrease both spontaneous and drug-induced apoptosis of CLL cells.[120,124,125]

Coculturing CLL cells with NLCs in the presence of a decoy receptor that binds both BAFF and APRIL partially abolishes the protective effect of the NLCs on the viability of the CLL cells.[120] Recently, it has been shown that BAFF, in cooperation with MYC, can lead to the development of a CLL like lymphoproliferation in mice.[126] MYC and its target genes are upregulated in CLL cells in the lymph node[8] and MYC is upregulated by BAFF[126] and by BCR engagement in vitro.[127] CLL cells that highly express MYC are more susceptible to apoptosis and can be rescued by BAFF.[126]

Additional interactions between CLL cells and accessory cells in the tissue microenvironment involve the ligation of CD38 to CD31 and of CD100 to plexin B1. CD38 levels on the surface of CLL cells are variable and high CD38 expression is a poor prognostic factor in CLL.[31] In proliferation centers, CD38 is upregulated in CLL cells exposed to activated T cells expressing CD40L.[11] CD31, the ligand for CD38, is expressed on endothelial cells and NLCs. CD31 induces proliferation and prolongs the survival of CD38$^+$ CLL cells.[128] CD100, a transmembrane protein that belongs to the semaphorin family, is expressed on CLL cells.[129] The high affinity receptor for CD100, plexin B1, is expressed on bone marrow stromal cells, FDCs, NLCs, and activated T cells.[129] It has been demonstrated that engagement of CD100 by plexin B1 increases CLL cell proliferation and prolongs survival.[128,129]

TRAFFICKING AND HOMING OF CLL CELLS INTO LYMPHOID TISSUES

Chemokines consist of 2 major subgroups. One group of homeostatic chemokines is constitutively produced and secreted within the tissue microenvironment and serves to maintain physiologic trafficking. The second group includes inflammatory chemokines, which are primarily induced in inflamed tissues to recruit effector cells.[130] Serum levels of some of the chemokines or their cognate receptors are highly increased in patients with CLL and a more effective chemotactic response is a characteristic of more aggressive subtypes of CLL cells. The responsiveness of circulating CLL cells to chemokine stimulation might facilitate the trafficking, homing, and invasion of leukemic cells into the nourishing tissue microenvironment.

An example of a chemokine that critically regulates CLL cell migration is CXCL12, a homeostatic chemokine that plays a critical role in normal trafficking and homing. CXCL12 is constitutively secreted at high levels by stromal cells and in vitro by NLCs.[118] CXCR4 (CD184), the receptor for CXCL12, is highly expressed on circulating CLL cells,[131–133] which migrate more efficiently toward CXCL12 than normal B lymphocytes.[131,132] CLL cells expressing CD38 and/or ZAP-70 show stronger intracellular signaling and better chemotaxis in response to CXCL12 than cells with no CD38 or ZAP-70 expression.[133–135]

CXCL13 is another homeostatic chemokine, which, along with its cognate receptor, CXCR5, plays a central role in the recruitment of B cells into the B-cell zone of secondary lymphoid organs.[136] CXCL13 is constitutively secreted by stromal cells in the B-cell areas of the secondary lymphoid tissues.[137] CXCL13 is expressed in vitro by NLCs as well as in vivo in the CD68$^+$ macrophages present in CLL lymph nodes.[112,137] Serum CXCL13 levels are higher in patients with CLL compared with healthy individuals[137] and CXCR5 is also highly expressed in CLL cells.[137,138]

CCL19 and CCL21 are chemokines that regulate the recruitment of lymphocytes into the T-cell zone areas of the secondary lymphoid tissues through ligation to their cognate receptor CCR7.[139] CCL19 and CCL21 are detected in the stroma and in the high endothelial venules of lymph nodes in CLL, and the latter are an important route of lymphocyte entry into secondary lymphoid tissue.[140] Circulating CLL cells express high levels of CCR7,[133,141] which are higher in ZAP-70$^+$ CLL cells and in patients with prominent lymphadenopathy.[133,140] CLL cells that are ZAP-70[+] or from patients with marked lymphadenopathy migrate more efficiently toward these chemokines.[133,140,142]

CLL cells are not only capable of responding to cellular elements in the tissue microenvironment but also actively recruit cells from the microenvironment to their immediate vicinity. This involves CLL cell secretion of chemokines such as CCL17, CCL22, CCL3, and CCL4. CCL22 and CCL17 are T-cell attracting chemokines induced in CD40-activated CLL cells in the lymph nodes and bone marrow.[70] Thus, CLL cells can attract CD4[+] T cells to the bone marrow and lymph nodes that augment tumor cell proliferation and survival and further induce release of CCL22, creating a positive feedback loop that further promotes the malignant process.[70]

CCL3 and CCL4 are proinflammatory chemokines crucial for the response to infection, the mediation of inflammation and the recruitment of monocytes and T cells from the blood into the tissue compartments.[143] CLL cells secrete these 2 chemokines in response to activation of BCR and CD38 as well as during coculture with NLCs. Expression of CCL3 and CCL4 in CLL cells during coculture with NLCs positively correlates with ZAP-70 positivity.[144] CCL3 and CCL4 are also overexpressed in CD38[+]CD49d[+] CLL cells more than tin CD38[−]/CD49d[−] cells.[145] Both CCR1 and CCR5, which are the cognate receptors for CCL3 and CCL4, are expressed on monocytes and macrophages and induce their migration.[145] Consistently, higher numbers of tumor-infiltrating CD68[+] macrophages were detected in the bone marrow of patients with CD38[+]CD49d[+] CLL.[145] CCL3 may also indirectly protect CLL cells from apoptosis via induction of VCAM-1 in endothelial cells.[145] Plasma levels of CCL3 and CCL4 are increased in patients with CLL compared with healthy individuals[144] and high CCL3 levels correlate with poor prognosis in CLL.[146]

SIGNALING PATHWAYS ACTIVATED IN THE TISSUE MICROENVIRONMENT

Given that CLL cells respond in vitro to a wide variety of external stimuli (see **Fig. 1**), it is a great challenge to determine which signaling pathways are the most relevant in vivo. Clearly, engagement of the BCR, via either autonomous or extrinsic mechanisms provides a signal. The PI3K/AKT, MAPK/ERK, NF-κB, WNT, Janus kinase (JAK)/STAT, and NOTCH signaling pathways have been reported to mediate survival and/or proliferation of CLL in vitro. In particular, the PI3K/AKT, MEK/ERK, and NF-κB pathways have been shown to be activated in the tissue microenvironment. Because the composition of the microenvironment can vary between tissues, different signaling pathways may be engaged in different locations. This may be particularly the case for the lymph nodes and for the so-called proliferation centers. The activity of many intracellular signals seems to be stronger and/or more sustained in patients with more aggressive subtypes of the disease and correlates with enhanced tumor proliferation and more rapid disease progression.[8,147] In particular, PI3K/AKT signaling regulates CLL cell survival and trafficking.[148] The PI3K/AKT pathway mediates the chemotactic response of CLL cells toward CXCL12,[131,132,135] CXCL13,[137] CCL19, and CCL21[133,140,149] and promotes CLL cell survival in response to a variety of external stimuli including BCR activation,[45] CD40L,[72] VCAM-1,[104] CCL19, CCL21, and many others. The inhibition of apoptosis in CLL cells through PI3K/AKT signaling is partially dependent on activation of NF-κB and upregulation of antiapoptotic genes (eg, BCL-XL and BFL-1). The classic NF-κB pathway has been shown to be activated in CLL cells in the lymph node more than in those derived from peripheral blood. A variety of in vitro stimuli induce NF-κB activity in CLL cells including engagement of the BCR[48] or CD40,[72–74] exposure to cytokines such as BAFF or APRIL,[120] and coculture with stromal cells[72] or endothelial cells.[110] Compared with normal B cells, CLL cells overexpress antiapoptotic proteins such as BCL-2 and MCL1[150,151] and the resistance to apoptosis is further enhanced in the lymphoid tissues via upregulation of BCL-2 family molecules including MCL1 BCL-XL and survivin.[10,15] MCL1 expression in CLL cells is commonly regulated through PI3K/AKT signaling.[45] BCL-XL can be upregulated in CLL cells through BCR[45] and CD40 signaling[75] or through VCAM-1,[104] stromal cells,[72] and endothelial cells.[110] The MAPK/ERK pathway also transmits prosurvival signals in CLL cells, as demonstrated in response to stimulation with CXCL12, CXCL13, CCL19, and CCL21. In addition, the MEK/ERK pathway is an important regulator of cell cycle progression and proliferation. MEK1/2 activity is important for MYC expression and S-phase entry of CLL cells. MEK/ERK mediates MYC expression in response to engagement of the BCR and Toll like receptor (TLR) 9 (induced in vitro by CpG oligonucleotide) and with BAFF stimulation.[126,127] Accordingly, both phosphorylated ERK and MYC are mostly expressed in large proliferating CLL cells confined to the proliferation centers within the lymph nodes.[127] MYC can contribute to genomic instability by selecting cells with defective DNA damage response, and its expression may be a driver of clonal evolution.[152]

Cell proliferation is regulated by D-type cyclins that bind to CDK4 and CDK6, resulting in the phosphorylation of the retinoblastoma protein and the G1-S phase transition of the cell cycle. Cyclin D2 is overexpressed in CLL cells,[153] especially in cells residing in the lymph nodes.[8] IgM ligation induces cyclin D2 and CDK4 in CLL cells.[63] The downregulation of the cell cycle inhibitor p27 and progression of CLL cells into the S phase are probably dependent on additional costimulatory signals, such as CD40 ligand and IL-4, that are provided mainly by T-helper (Th) lymphocytes in the proliferation centers of the lymph node.[154] Accordingly, within CLL cells in the proliferation centers, cyclin D2 is highly expressed and p27 is downregulated.[155] Cyclin D2 expression is regulated either directly through NF-κB or indirectly by MYC. Consistent with this finding is the observation that NF-κB activity is increased in the lymph nodes and particularly enhanced in CLL cells within the proliferation centers.[8,155]

MODELS OF THE CLL MICROENVIRONMENT

Modeling tumor-host interactions is an area of intensive investigation. Such models are of particular interest given that tissue-resident CLL cells are not readily available. Currently, the most widely used in vivo model for CLL is the transgenic TCL1 mouse, in which the human *TCL1* gene is expressed under the control of the Ig heavy chain variable region promoter and enhancer.[156] TCL1 is an oncogene commonly activated in mature T-cell lymphomas that enhances AKT signaling. Onset of disease occurs late in life and the tumor cells in TCL1 transgenic mice are relatively large lymphoid cells, expressing unmutated *IGHV* genes.[156] There is evidence for a role of BCR signaling in this model and a dysregulation of the T-cell compartment similar to what has been described in human CLL.[157] The TCL1 transgenic model has also been used successfully to study novel therapeutic approaches (discussed later). In contrast to the transgenic model, New Zealand Black (NZB) mice spontaneously develop autoimmunity and B-cell hyperactivity early in life, and a CLL like disease manifests later in life. The late-onset clonal disease is of the *IGVH* unmutated type, which is also ZAP-70 positive.[158] NZB mice were found to harbor a point mutation in the 3'-flanking sequence of pre–mir-16-1, which results in decreased levels of miR-16 in lymphoid tissues.[159] This is reminiscent of the most common chromosomal lesion in human CLL: a deletion of the 13q14 chromosomal region containing the *mir-15a/16-1* and *DLEU2* genes.[160] Recently, Klein and colleagues[161] showed that deletion of the 13q14-minimal deleted region (MDR) harboring the DLEU2/miR-15a/16-1 cluster in mice results in the development of a condition that resembles human CLL. The leukemic cells of these mice express unmutated *IGHV* genes and some of them even present with BCRs showing stereotypical antigen-binding regions.[161] Other transgenic mice models of CLL include (NZB × NZW)F1 mice programmed to express IL5,[162] mice overexpressing both BCL2 and a TNF receptor-associated factor,[163] and MYC/BAFF transgenic mice.[126]

A complementary approach has been to xenograft the Mec-1 cell line or primary CLL cells[66,164–168] into immune-compromised mice. Recently, Bagnara and colleagues[66] reported that peripheral blood mononuclear cells (PBMCs) from patients with CLL xenografted into NOD/scid/γc [null] (NSG) mice localized and proliferated primarily in the murine spleen. These investigators found that proliferation of CLL cells in vivo was dependent on coengrafted human T cells. Furthermore, by comparing CLL cells isolated from spleens of xenografted mice to CLL cells from human blood and lymph nodes, Sun and colleagues[165] showed that the murine spleen microenvironment supports CLL cell proliferation and activation to a similar degree as the human lymph node, which notably includes activation of BCR and NF-κB signaling in the xenografted cells. The model was then used to test the in vivo effects of ibrutinib, a Bruton tyrosine kinase (BTK) inhibitor in clinical development. Ibrutinib inhibited BCR and NF-κB signaling induced by the microenvironment, decreased proliferation, induced apoptosis, and reduced the tumor burden in vivo.[167] Thus, these data indicate that the spleen of xenografted NSG mice can sufficiently model the role of the human microenvironment on CLL cells to make this a valid model for investigations of tumor microenvironment interactions and the evaluation of possible novel treatment approaches.

TARGETING THE MICROENVIRONMENT IN CLL

The increasing appreciation of the role of the microenvironment in supporting CLL cell proliferation and survival as well as its contribution to chemoresistance has informed novel therapeutic approaches. Accordingly, a major effort is underway to find efficient ways to chemically dissect CLL cells from the microenvironmental signals, by either blocking extracellular triggers or abrogating intracellular signaling (**Fig. 3**). In recent years, different compounds have been developed that are able to antagonize surface receptors or cytokines including small molecules that target signaling kinases and antiapoptotic proteins. Clinically, impressive responses characterized by diminished lymphadenopathy and splenomegaly have been observed with some of these novel agents.

CXCR4 Receptor Antagonists

CLL cells in the peripheral blood express high levels of the surface receptor CXCR4, which signals for chemotaxis, polymerization of actin, and migration through the vascular endothelium.[131] Blockade of the CXCR4-CXCL12 axis using CXCR4 receptor antagonists such as plerixafor (AMD3100) or T140 can efficiently antagonize CXCL12-mediated signaling and chemotaxis as well as stroma-mediated protection from both spontaneous and drug-induced apoptosis.[101,169] The clinical use of plerixafor in CLL is investigated in combination with rituximab. Preliminary results showed that this agent induces dose-dependent mobilization of CLL cells to the peripheral blood.[170]

Targeting BAFF and APRIL

As previously mentioned, BAFF and APRIL signaling through their cognate receptors BAFF-R, TACI, and BCMA are important for normal B-cell survival and may play a role

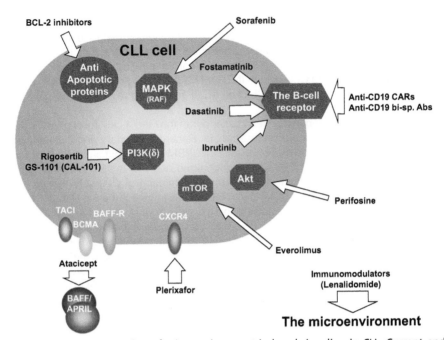

Fig. 3. Therapeutic targeting of microenvironment-induced signaling in CLL. Current and experimental CLL therapeutics (*arrows*) target the various components of the microenvironment-CLL milieu and its associated signaling network. Thus, the BCR and its associated components are targeted by antibodies (anti-CD19) or small molecules (eg, SYK [eg, fostamatinib] or BTK inhibitors [eg, ibrutinib]). Small molecules are also used to inhibit mTOR, Akt, PI3Kδ, and the MAPK cascades. Extracellular inhibitors such as plerixafor or atacicept can block the association of CXCL12 or BAFF/APRIL, respectively, with their receptors on the CLL cell. Both the microenvironment (eg, the immune system) and the outcome of its signaling responses in the CLL cells (eg, upregulation of BCL-2) are avenues for therapeutic targeting. bi-sp. Abs, bi-specific antibodies; CARs, chimeric antibody receptors.

in CLL. Atacicept is a recombinant soluble form of the extracellular binding domain of TACI. By acting as a molecular decoy, it neutralizes the effects of BAFF and APRIL, blocking the activation of TACI, BCMA, and the BAFF receptor. A phase Ib study of atacicept demonstrated that intravenous doses of up to 27 mg/kg were well tolerated in 21 patients with refractory or relapsed CLL with 1 partial response (PR) (overall response rate [ORR] 5%) in the highest dose cohort.[171]

Targeting BCR Signaling

The pivotal role of BCR signaling in CLL pathogenesis points to this pathway as an ideal target for novel anti-CLL therapy (see **Fig. 3**). Small-molecule drugs targeting SYK, BTK, or PI3K isoform p110delta (PI3Kδ) show impressive results in patients with relapsed/refractory CLL as well as in treatment-naive CLL (reviewed in[20,21]). In the first few weeks of treatment with these agents, responses typically manifest with a substantial regression in lymphadenopathy that is frequently paralleled by transient lymphocytosis.[172–174] The early increase in the circulating lymphocytes is assumed to reflect redistribution of the CLL cells from the lymphatic tissues into the circulation, as a consequence of disruption of mechanisms involved in migration and retention of the tumor cells in their protective tissue microenvironments.[175,176]

Continued treatment over the course of months results in a gradual decrease in lymphocytosis and a deepening of responses with a high rate of remission achieved with increasing duration of treatment.[172] The clinical responses seen with these kinase inhibitors are attributed to the combined effects of direct cell cytotoxicity, inhibition of survival pathways, and impairment of CLL cell trafficking and tissue retention.

LYN Inhibitors

LYN, an SRC family nonreceptor tyrosine kinase, plays an important role in initiation as well as in the termination of BCR signaling. This dual role of LYN is due to its propagation of the BCR signal via phosphorylation of SYK and its concurrent activation of inhibitory phosphatases that terminate the response. Dasatinib, which was originally approved for treatment of chronic myeloid leukemia, is an oral kinase inhibitor primarily targeting ABL and SRC kinases but it also inhibits other kinases, including BTK.[177] In preclinical studies, dasatinib has been shown to induce apoptosis of CLL cells that was associated with reduction in MCL1 and BCL-XL expression.[178–180] In a phase II trial in 15 patients with relapsed or refractory CLL, treatment with dasatinib (140 mg/d) achieved an overall response of 20% with progression-free survival of 7.5 months. The major adverse reaction of the treatment was myelosuppression.[181]

SYK Inhibitors

SYK is a key protein kinase of proximal BCR signal transduction that is also involved in B-cell migration and adhesion independently of BCR activity.[182] After BCR engagement, SYK is phosphorylated by LYN and amplifies the BCR signal through activation of downstream signaling pathways. SYK phosphorylation on the activating Y352 residue has been demonstrated in peripheral blood CLL cells.[183] In addition, CLL cells in the lymph node show increased phosphorylation of SYK compared with peripheral blood CLL cells, indicating activation of the kinase in the tissue microenvironment.[8]

To date, several SYK inhibitors have been studied in CLL in vitro and in vivo, including fostamatinib (R788, the oral prodrug of R406, the active metabolite), PRT318, and P505-15. In preclinical studies, treatment with SYK inhibitors resulted in inhibition of BCR activation, moderate apoptosis of CLL cells, reduced basal kinase activity of SYK, AKT, and ERK, and decreased MCL1 levels.[183] Furthermore, SYK inhibitors have been shown to antagonize exogenous prosurvival signals provided by stromal cell or NLC coculture,[62,183,184] secretion of BCR-regulated chemokines CCL3 and CCL4,[62,183,184] and migration toward CXCL12 and CXCL13.[62,184] In an Eµ-TCL1 transgenic mouse model, treatment with fostamatinib inhibited BCR signaling, reduced the proliferation and survival of the leukemic clone, and extended the life of the treated mice.[185]

Fostamatinib was the first SYK inhibitor introduced into clinical study.[174] In a phase I/II trial in patients with relapsed/refractory B-cell malignancy, fostamatinib was shown to be well tolerated with the most common adverse reactions being myelosuppression, fatigue, and diarrhea. The highest ORR was achieved in patients with CLL/small lymphocytic lymphoma (SLL) (55%, 6 of 11, with a median progression-free survival of 6.4 months), compared with only 10% to 22% in other non-Hodgkin lymphomas (NHLs).[174] The on-target effect of fostamatinib in CLL has been demonstrated by downregulation of BCR-regulated target genes in tumor cells of patients with CLL on fostamatinib.[186] Furthermore, fostamatinib inhibited CLL cell activation and proliferation. However, there was no correlation between the degree of inhibition of BCR signaling and clinical response suggesting that pathways bypassing BCR activation might play a role in shaping the response to such kinase inhibitors.[186] Fostamatinib is being tested in late-stage clinical trials for rheumatoid arthritis[187] and in patients with diffuse large B-cell lymphoma. Some novel SYK inhibitors have shown promising preclinical activity, and may have increased potency and specificity.[184]

BTK Inhibitors

BTK is a member of the TEC family of kinases that is critical for BCR signaling.[188] Mutations in BTK result in X-linked agammaglobulinemia, an inherited disorder manifesting with profound decrease in antibody production and a severe defect in B-cell development.[189] BTK mRNA and protein expression levels are increased in CLL cells.[190] Ibrutinib (PCI-32765) is an orally administered irreversible and specific inhibitor of BTK that induces modest apoptosis in CLL cells irrespective of *IGHV* mutational status or interphase cytogenetics, and overcomes prosurvival and proliferation signals provided by various tissue microenvironmental elements (such as CD40L, BAFF, IL-4, IL-6, TNFα, fibronectin and stromal cells coculture, and CpG oligonucleotide).[176,190] Ibrutinib abrogates CLL cell signaling, migration, and adhesion in response to tissue homing chemokines (such as CXCL12, CXCL13, and CCL19) and abrogates integrin $\alpha 4\beta 1$-mediated adhesion to fibronectin and VCAM-1.[175,176,190] Both in vitro and in vivo, ibrutinib has been reported to inhibit CLL cell secretion of CLL3 and CCL4.[176] At the molecular level, this agent inhibits BTK tyrosine phosphorylation after BCR or CD40 stimulation and abrogates activation of downstream signaling pathways including ERK, PI3K, and NF-κB in CLL cells.[190] Treatment with ibrutinib in the TCL1 mice model of CLL resulted in inhibition of disease progression.[176]

A phase I open-label dose-escalation study evaluated the efficacy and tolerability of ibrutinib in patients with relapsed or refractory B-cell NHL and B-cell CLL.[191] Dose escalation proceeded to 12.5 mg/kg without dose-limiting side effects and with pharmacodynamic evidence for complete inhibition of BTK. Sixty percent of all patients achieved an overall response (OR), with 16% achieving a complete response (CR); 16 patients with CLL/SLL were evaluated, with an objective response reported in 11 of these patients (69%). The observed responses were of marked duration, as the median progression-free survival for all patients reported at the time of data cutoff was 13.6 months. A subsequent phase Ib/II study of ibrutinib in patients with CLL who were either greater than 65 years of age and previously untreated or diagnosed with relapsed or refractory disease, further demonstrated that ibrutinib was well tolerated; the most common side effects included diarrhea, fatigue, and nausea. The ORR was 71% for treatment-naive patients, 67% for relapsed or refractory patients, and 50% for high-risk patients.[172] The estimated progression-free survival at 26 months was 75% for the relapsed/refractory cohort and 96% for treatment-naive patients demonstrating a remarkable duration of response.

Targeting the PI3K/AKT/mTOR Signaling Pathway

The PI3K/AKT/mTOR signaling pathway is a critical intracellular signaling cascade controlling cell survival and proliferation in both malignant and nonmalignant cells. PI3K is a pivotal hub connecting multiple extracellular signals to cellular responses. PI3K acts to convert phosphatidylinositol 4,5-bisphosphate (PI(4,5)P2) to (PI(3,4,5) P3), which in turn forms a functional signaling complex with BTK and AKT. Several isoforms of PI3K have been characterized; the δ isoform of PI3K is selectively expressed in hematopoietic cells and functions to relay BCR, BAFF, CD30, and TLR signaling. CLL cells express PI3Kδ and display increased PI3K activity.[192] Given the selective expression of PI3Kδ, in contrast to the more pervasive α and β isoforms, specific inhibition of the δ isoform is not expected to be toxic to normal tissues. Many PI3K inhibitors are currently being investigated in both preclinical and clinical settings. ON 01910.Na (rigosertib), a multikinase PI3K inhibitor in phase III trials for myelodysplastic syndrome, has demonstrated promising preclinical in vitro activity, inducing apoptosis in CLL cells that are cultured in contact with stromal cells via a dual mechanism of action involving both PI3K/AKT inhibition and induction of oxidative stress.[193]

GS-1101 (CAL-101)

GS-1101 is an orally available, highly selective PI3Kδ inhibitor that induces apoptosis in CLL cells.[194] The cytotoxic effect of GS-1101 is maintained despite the presence of various microenviromental components that normally support malignant CLL cells (including stromal cells, NLCs, fibronectin, CD145 or TNFα BAFF and BCR stimulation). GS-1101 also inhibits the secretion of both antiapoptotic and proinflammatory cytokines.[192,195] GS-1101 sensitizes CLL cells to drug-induced apoptosis in the presence of stromal coculture[195] and inhibits CLL cell chemotaxis toward CXCL12 and CXCL13.[195] The drug abrogates constitutive PI3K signaling in CLL cells as well as AKT and/or ERK activation by anti-IgM, soluble CD40 ligand, and chemokines.[195,196] In patients with CLL treated with GS-1101, the serum levels of CCL3, CCL4, and CXCL13 were markedly reduced.[195] A phase I study in 54 patients with previously treated CLL demonstrated the acceptable safety and promising clinical activity of GS-1101, with 26% of patients achieving an OR.[173] A greater than 50% reduction in lymphadenopathy was observed in 80% of patients. Adverse events grade 3 or higher were minimal and included pneumonia and neutropenia; they were observed in less than a quarter of patients. Phase II/III clinical trials of GS-1101 are currently underway.

AKT Inhibitors

The serine/threonine kinase AKT is a key nodal regulator of cellular survival known to phosphorylate several cellular substrates including caspase 8,[197] caspase 9,[198] BAD,[199] mTor,[200] and the Forkhead family of transcription factors.[201] Furthermore, AKT activation is associated with resistance to chemotherapy. Early-phase clinical trials are underway investigating the use of AKT inhibitors in several malignancies including chronic myelocytic leukemia, although experience with these agents in CLL is limited. MK-2206, an orally active allosteric AKT inhibitor, has been shown to enhance the antitumor efficacy of other chemotherapeutic agents in vitro in several malignancies, although clinical use in CLL has not been reported.[202] Perifosine, another oral inhibitor of AKT, is undergoing phase II evaluation in patients with refractory and relapsed leukemia.[203] Pending the outcome of these and other clinical trials, further investigation is warranted to determine the usefulness of AKT inhibitors in CLL.

mTOR Inhibitors

mTOR, a serine/threonine kinase of the PI3K/AKT/mTOR signaling network, is involved in cell growth, metabolism, and proliferation and is commonly activated in B-cell neoplasms. Rapamycin (sirolimus, rapamune, Wyeth) is an immunosuppressive drug used to prevent rejection in organ transplantation. The drug profoundly blocks BCR-mediated proliferation.[204] Preclinical studies in CLL have shown that rapamycin or its analogue RAD001 blocks cell cycle progression by interfering with expression of critical cell cycle molecules.[205] Everolimus (RAD001, afinitor, Novartis), an orally available derivative of sirolimus, was evaluated in a phase II pilot trial in previously treated patients with CLL. The study was stopped early because of increased toxicity, although the drug showed modest clinical activity.[206] In another phase II study, everolimus (10 mg/d) administered to patients with recurrent/refractory CLL achieved PR in 18% of patients.[207] In a subset of these patients, treatment with everolimus was accompanied by an increase in lymphocytosis in parallel with a reduction in lymphadenopathy.

Targeting the RAF/MEK/ERK Signaling Pathway

Sorafenib (BAY43-9006; nexavar) is an oral, small-molecule, multikinase inhibitor approved for the treatment of advanced renal cell carcinoma[208] and unresectable hepatocellular carcinoma.[209] Sorafenib is a potent RAF serine/threonine kinase inhibitor targeting the RAF/MEK/ERK pathway and inhibits other receptor tyrosine kinases involved in tumor progression and angiogenesis.[210] Sorafenib induces CLL cell death that is mediated via caspase activation and a decrease in MCL1.[211–213] It overcomes apoptosis protection induced by NLC or stromal cell coculture and stromal-mediated chemoresistance.[211–214] The drug has been shown to block RAF/MEK/ERK signaling and the chemotaxis response induced by CXCL12 in CLL cells.[211,214] It has also been shown to inhibit RAF and ERK activation by NLCs or stromal cells[213,214] and to interfere with VEFGR/STAT3 signaling induced by stromal cell coculture.[213] Sorafenib also abrogates BCR-mediated signaling and survival in CLL cells. CLL cells derived from the lymph nodes are more sensitive to sorafenib than the cells found in peripheral blood.[214] The clinical efficacy and tolerability of sorafenib in relapsed CLL is currently being evaluated in a phase II clinical trial.

Targeting Antiapoptotic Proteins

The resistance of CLL cells to apoptosis is related to high expression of the BCL-2 family antiapoptotic proteins. The overexpression of these antiapoptotic proteins in CLL is endogenous as well as extrinsic and is in part regulated by signals derived from the tissue microenvironment.[151] Therefore, in recent years, several therapeutic strategies have been developed to target antiapoptotic proteins in CLL, including antisense BCL-2 oligonucleotide, BH3 mimetics, and others.

Oblimersen sodium is a synthetic BCL-2 antisense oligonucleotide that induces a decrease in BCL-2 mRNA and protein levels and apoptosis in CLL cells.[215] Oblimersen sodium, when combined with different cytotoxic drugs, increases CLL cell apoptosis. In a phase I/II trial, oblimersen sodium as a single agent, showed minimal activity in patients with relapsed/refractory CLL. Dosing was limited by development of a cytokine release syndrome. At a dosage of 3 mg/kg/d, 2 (8%) of 26 patients achieved PR.[216] A phase III study in patients with relapsed/refractory CLL showed that addition of oblimersen to fludarabine plus cyclophosphamide (FC) increased the CR/nodular PR (nPR) rate compared with FC alone.[217] Accordingly, CR/nPR was achieved in 20 (17%) of 120 patients in the oblimersen group and 8 (7%) of 121 patients in the FC-only group.[217] The combination of oblimersen-FC further resulted in increased survival in subsets of patients who achieved a least a PR and in those who had fludarabine-sensitive disease.[217,218]

Obatoclax mesylate (GX15-070) is a small-molecule pan-BCL-2 antagonist. This compound belongs to a class of BH3 mimetic agents that inhibit the activity of the antiapoptotic BCL-2 members that antagonize the proapoptotic proteins BAX and BAK.[219] The BH3-only proteins BAX and BAK are directly sequestered and repressed by the antiapoptotic BCL-2 proteins. BH3 mimetic drugs BAX and BAK induce their release allowing them to oligomerize and trigger apoptosis via the formation of pores in the outer mitochondrial membrane. In a phase I trial, administration of obatoclax to patients heavily pretreated with advanced CLL resulted in a PR in 1 out of 26 patients. The major toxicities were neurologic including somnolence, ataxia, and euphoria.[220]

BH3 Mimetics

The BH3 mimetics, ABT-737 and its orally active analogue navitoclax, inhibit BCL-2, BCL-XL, and BCL-W. In preclinical studies, ABT-737 has been shown to induce rapid and potent proapoptotic activity in CLL cells independently of the common clinical and prognostic parameters in CLL.[221,222] Addition of cytotoxic agents sensitizes CLL cells in vitro to ABT-737.[222] In a phase I study of 29 patients with relapsed/refractory CLL, a navitoclax dosage of at least 100 mg/d achieved durable PRs in 35% of patients.[223] Navitoclax was also active in high-risk patients with fludarabine-refractory disease, bulky lymphadenopathy, and deletion of 17p.[223] The major dose-limiting toxicity was thrombocytopenia related to inhibition of BCL-XL.[223]

AT-101 (gossypol isomer) is a small-molecule pan-BCL-2 antagonist. In preclinical studies, AT101 was shown to both induce CLL cell apoptosis and to overcome resistance mediated by stromal cell coculture, while sparing normal stromal cells.[224] A phase I trial of AT-101 in treatment-naive patients with CLL with high-risk disease demonstrated that the drug was well tolerated.[225] Furthermore, 5 of 6 patients in this trial exhibited a decrease in lymphocyte count, whereas all patients demonstrated a reduction in lymphadenopathy.

XIAP

XIAP, which inhibits the proteolytic activity of caspase-3 via direct binding, is highly expressed in CLL cells, and plays an important role in TNF-related apoptosis-inducing ligand (TRAIL)-induced apoptosis.[226] Because CLL cells have previously exhibited resistance to TRAIL-based treatments, novel inhibitors of XIAP have been developed in the hope of overcoming TRAIL resistance in CLL.[227] One such novel small-molecule inhibitor, compound A (CA), has been shown to render tumor cells from patients with 17p deletion, *IGVH* unmutated type CLL, susceptible to TRAIL in vitro.

Immunomodulatory Drugs

Lenalidomide, a derivative of thalidomide, is an immunomodulatory agent that has significant activity in 5q− myelodysplastic syndrome, multiple myeloma, and other B-cell malignancies. In relapsed or refractory CLL, intermittent lenalidomide at 25 mg/d (3 weeks on/1 week off drug) was associated with acceptable toxicity, and achieved an ORR of 47%, with 9% of patients demonstrating CR.[228] Another trial of relapsed/refractory patients with CLL treated with daily lenalidomide at a dose of 10 mg produced an ORR of 32%, with 7% CR.[229] In a treatment-naive setting, elderly patients with CLL treated with lenalidomide achieved an ORR of 65%, including 10% CR and an additional 5% CR with residual cytopenias.[230] The activity of lenalidomide is irrespective of unfavorable genomic abnormalities such as unmutated *IGHV* or fludarabine-refractory disease status. However, at least 6 to 9 months of treatment may be needed to achieve the best possible response.[229] The most common toxicity of lenalidomide is myelosuppression.[228,229] Lenalidomide is frequently associated with a cytokine release syndrome and tumor flare reaction (observed in 30% to 58% of patients) or tumor lysis syndrome.[228,231,232] Tumor flare is a unique immune-mediated response to lenalidomide therapy characterized by painful lymph node enlargement that may be accompanied by fever and/or bone pain. It is generally managed with corticosteroids, although in more severe cases narcotics and hospitalization may be necessary.[229,231] Tumor flare may be predictive of clinical response to treatment with lenalidomide.[233] The optimal dosing schedule of lenalidomide is not well defined; and a dose of 25 mg once daily in cases of relapsed CLL may be associated with unacceptable toxicity in some patients.[231] Furthermore, lenalidomide may be associated with an increased frequency of venous thromboembolism that may be related to endothelial dysfunction in the context of inflammatory cytokine secretion. Continuous low-dose lenalidomide (10 mg) is generally well tolerated and effective.[229] The treatment is accompanied by increased serum Ig levels and typically reduces

CCL3 and CCL4 plasma levels, which might indicate an inhibitory effect on intracellular signaling in CLL cells.[230]

The mechanism of action of lenalidomide is not completely understood. In contrast to thalidomide, lenalidomide has weak antiangiogenic effects.[229] Lenalidomide induces transient immune activation including expression of costimulatory molecules such as CD40, CD80, and CD86 on CLL cells,[231,232] which may be mediated through PI3Kδ.[194] It also increases the levels of IL-6, IL-10, IL-2R, IFNγ, and TNFα in serum.[229,232] Lenalidomide in part restores T-cell function by enhancing the formation of immunologic synapses and promoting intracellular signaling.[91,157,234] In lymph node biopsies from patients with CLL treated with lenalidomide, a shift toward a Th-1 type immune reaction with production of IFNγ was documented, suggesting that lenalidomide might be able to restore antitumor immunity and immune surveillance in vivo.[235] Furthermore, lenalidomide enhances NK cell activity[236] and improves antibody-mediated cellular cytotoxicity directed by rituximab.[237]

SUMMARY AND OUTLOOK

Interactions of CLL cells with the surrounding microenvironment play a central role in the pathogenesis and progression of the disease. The nature of these interactions depends on the properties of the CLL cell itself but also likely depends on the properties of the microenvironment specific to the patient, which may be shaped by the baseline expression levels of cytokines, the composition of various T-cell subsets, stromal cell populations, and responses to antigenic stimulation. Major progress in the last decade has led to a much better understanding of both direct and indirect cellular interactions involved in CLL oncogenesis, and to the development of multiple new and promising therapies (see **Fig. 3**). Although there is still much to learn, it seems possible that, within a few years, improved understanding of key aspects of tumor biology and the development of novel therapeutic approaches will combine to change the natural history of CLL.

REFERENCES

1. Caligaris-Cappio F, Hamblin TJ. B-cell chronic lymphocytic leukemia: a bird of a different feather. J Clin Oncol 1999;17(1):399–408.
2. Hallek M, Fischer K, Fingerle-Rowson G, et al. Addition of rituximab to fludarabine and cyclophosphamide in patients with chronic lymphocytic leukaemia: a randomised, open-label, phase 3 trial. Lancet 2010;376(9747):1164–74.
3. Panayiotidis P, Jones D, Ganeshaguru K, et al. Human bone marrow stromal cells prevent apoptosis and support the survival of chronic lymphocytic leukaemia cells in vitro. Br J Haematol 1996;92(1):97–103.
4. Lagneaux L, Delforge A, De Bruyn C, et al. Adhesion to bone marrow stroma inhibits apoptosis of chronic lymphocytic leukemia cells. Leuk Lymphoma 1999;35(5–6):445–53.
5. Andreeff M, Darzynkiewicz Z, Sharpless TK, et al. Discrimination of human leukemia subtypes by flow cytometric analysis of cellular DNA and RNA. Blood 1980;55(2):282–93.
6. Damle RN, Temburni S, Calissano C, et al. CD38 expression labels an activated subset within chronic lymphocytic leukemia clones enriched in proliferating B cells. Blood 2007;110(9):3352–9.
7. Messmer BT, Messmer D, Allen SL, et al. In vivo measurements document the dynamic cellular kinetics of chronic lymphocytic leukemia B cells. J Clin Invest 2005;115(3):755–64.

8. Herishanu Y, Perez-Galan P, Liu D, et al. The lymph node microenvironment promotes B-cell receptor signaling, NF-kappaB activation, and tumor proliferation in chronic lymphocytic leukemia. Blood 2011;117(2):563–74.

9. Granziero L, Ghia P, Circosta P, et al. Survivin is expressed on CD40 stimulation and interfaces proliferation and apoptosis in B-cell chronic lymphocytic leukemia. Blood 2001;97(9):2777–83.

10. Davids MS, Deng J, Wiestner A, et al. Decreased mitochondrial apoptotic priming underlies stroma-mediated treatment resistance in chronic lymphocytic leukemia. Blood 2012;120(17):3501–9.

11. Patten PE, Buggins AG, Richards J, et al. CD38 expression in chronic lymphocytic leukemia is regulated by the tumor microenvironment. Blood 2008;111(10):5173–81.

12. Ghia P, Guida G, Stella S, et al. The pattern of CD38 expression defines a distinct subset of chronic lymphocytic leukemia (CLL) patients at risk of disease progression. Blood 2003;101(4):1262–9.

13. Jaksic O, Paro MM, Kardum Skelin I, et al. CD38 on B-cell chronic lymphocytic leukemia cells has higher expression in lymph nodes than in peripheral blood or bone marrow. Blood 2004;103(5):1968–9.

14. Quijano S, Lopez A, Rasillo A, et al. Association between the proliferative rate of neoplastic B cells, their maturation stage, and underlying cytogenetic abnormalities in B-cell chronic lymphoproliferative disorders: analysis of a series of 432 patients. Blood 2008;111(10):5130–41.

15. Smit LA, Hallaert DY, Spijker R, et al. Differential Noxa/Mcl-1 balance in peripheral versus lymph node chronic lymphocytic leukemia cells correlates with survival capacity. Blood 2007;109(4):1660–8.

16. Rui L, Schmitz R, Ceribelli M, et al. Malignant pirates of the immune system. Nat Immunol 2011;12(10):933–40.

17. Davis RE, Ngo VN, Lenz G, et al. Chronic active B-cell-receptor signalling in diffuse large B-cell lymphoma. Nature 2010;463(7277):88–92.

18. Ghia P, Chiorazzi N, Stamatopoulos K. Microenvironmental influences in chronic lymphocytic leukaemia: the role of antigen stimulation. J Intern Med 2008; 264(6):549–62.

19. Stevenson FK, Krysov S, Davies AJ, et al. B-cell receptor signaling in chronic lymphocytic leukemia. Blood 2011;118(16):4313–20.

20. Wiestner A. Emerging role of kinase-targeted strategies in chronic lymphocytic leukemia. Blood 2012;120(24):4684–91.

21. Woyach JA, Johnson AJ, Byrd JC. The B-cell receptor signaling pathway as a therapeutic target in CLL. Blood 2012;120(6):1175–84.

22. Davids MS, Brown JR. Targeting the B cell receptor pathway in chronic lymphocytic leukemia. Leuk Lymphoma 2012;53(12):2362–70.

23. Fais F, Ghiotto F, Hashimoto S, et al. Chronic lymphocytic leukemia B cells express restricted sets of mutated and unmutated antigen receptors. J Clin Invest 1998;102(8):1515–25.

24. Tobin G, Thunberg U, Karlsson K, et al. Subsets with restricted immunoglobulin gene rearrangement features indicate a role for antigen selection in the development of chronic lymphocytic leukemia. Blood 2004;104(9):2879–85.

25. Rosenwald A, Alizadeh AA, Widhopf G, et al. Relation of gene expression phenotype to immunoglobulin mutation genotype in B cell chronic lymphocytic leukemia. J Exp Med 2001;194(11):1639–47.

26. Klein U, Tu Y, Stolovitzky GA, et al. Gene expression profiling of B cell chronic lymphocytic leukemia reveals a homogeneous phenotype related to memory B cells. J Exp Med 2001;194(11):1625–38.

27. Damle RN, Ghiotto F, Valetto A, et al. B-cell chronic lymphocytic leukemia cells express a surface membrane phenotype of activated, antigen-experienced B lymphocytes. Blood 2002;99(11):4087–93.

28. Mockridge CI, Potter KN, Wheatley I, et al. Reversible anergy of sIgM-mediated signaling in the two subsets of CLL defined by VH-gene mutational status. Blood 2007;109(10):4424–31.

29. Muzio M, Apollonio B, Scielzo C, et al. Constitutive activation of distinct BCR-signaling pathways in a subset of CLL patients: a molecular signature of anergy. Blood 2008;112(1):188–95.

30. Lanham S, Hamblin T, Oscier D, et al. Differential signaling via surface IgM is associated with VH gene mutational status and CD38 expression in chronic lymphocytic leukemia. Blood 2003;101(3):1087–93.

31. Damle RN, Wasil T, Fais F, et al. Ig V gene mutation status and CD38 expression as novel prognostic indicators in chronic lymphocytic leukemia. Blood 1999; 94(6):1840–7.

32. Hamblin TJ, Davis Z, Gardiner A, et al. Unmutated Ig V(H) genes are associated with a more aggressive form of chronic lymphocytic leukemia. Blood 1999;94(6): 1848–54.

33. Agathangelidis A, Darzentas N, Hadzidimitriou A, et al. Stereotyped B-cell receptors in one-third of chronic lymphocytic leukemia: a molecular classification with implications for targeted therapies. Blood 2012;119(19): 4467–75.

34. Messmer BT, Albesiano E, Efremov DG, et al. Multiple distinct sets of stereotyped antigen receptors indicate a role for antigen in promoting chronic lymphocytic leukemia. J Exp Med 2004;200(4):519–25.

35. Stamatopoulos K, Belessi C, Moreno C, et al. Over 20% of patients with chronic lymphocytic leukemia carry stereotyped receptors: pathogenetic implications and clinical correlations. Blood 2007;109(1):259–70.

36. Chu CC, Catera R, Hatzi K, et al. Chronic lymphocytic leukemia antibodies with a common stereotypic rearrangement recognize nonmuscle myosin heavy chain IIA. Blood 2008;112(13):5122–9.

37. Binder M, Lechenne B, Ummanni R, et al. Stereotypical chronic lymphocytic leukemia B-cell receptors recognize survival promoting antigens on stromal cells. PLoS One 2010;5(12):e15992.

38. Herve M, Xu K, Ng YS, et al. Unmutated and mutated chronic lymphocytic leukemias derive from self-reactive B cell precursors despite expressing different antibody reactivity. J Clin Invest 2005;115(6):1636–43.

39. Lanemo Myhrinder A, Hellqvist E, Sidorova E, et al. A new perspective: molecular motifs on oxidized LDL, apoptotic cells, and bacteria are targets for chronic lymphocytic leukemia antibodies. Blood 2008;111(7):3838–48.

40. Catera R, Silverman GJ, Hatzi K, et al. Chronic lymphocytic leukemia cells recognize conserved epitopes associated with apoptosis and oxidation. Mol Med 2008; 14(11–12):665–74.

41. Chiorazzi N, Efremov DG. Chronic lymphocytic leukemia: a tale of one or two signals? Cell Res 2012. http://dx.doi.org/10.1038/cr.2012.152.

42. Chu CC, Catera R, Zhang L, et al. Many chronic lymphocytic leukemia antibodies recognize apoptotic cells with exposed nonmuscle myosin heavy chain IIA: implications for patient outcome and cell of origin. Blood 2010;115(19): 3907–15.

43. Clark EA, Ledbetter JA. How B and T cells talk to each other. Nature 1994; 367(6462):425–8.

44. Contri A, Brunati AM, Trentin L, et al. Chronic lymphocytic leukemia B cells contain anomalous Lyn tyrosine kinase, a putative contribution to defective apoptosis. J Clin Invest 2005;115(2):369–78.

45. Longo PG, Laurenti L, Gobessi S, et al. The Akt/Mcl-1 pathway plays a prominent role in mediating antiapoptotic signals downstream of the B-cell receptor in chronic lymphocytic leukemia B cells. Blood 2008;111(2):846–55.

46. Chen L, Widhopf G, Huynh L, et al. Expression of ZAP-70 is associated with increased B-cell receptor signaling in chronic lymphocytic leukemia. Blood 2002;100(13):4609–14.

47. Hivroz C, Geny B, Brouet JC, et al. Altered signal transduction secondary to surface IgM cross-linking on B-chronic lymphocytic leukemia cells. Differential activation of the phosphatidylinositol-specific phospholipase C. J Immunol 1990;144(6):2351–8.

48. Petlickovski A, Laurenti L, Li X, et al. Sustained signaling through the B-cell receptor induces Mcl-1 and promotes survival of chronic lymphocytic leukemia B cells. Blood 2005;105(12):4820–7.

49. Krysov S, Potter KN, Mockridge CI, et al. Surface IgM of CLL cells displays unusual glycans indicative of engagement of antigen in vivo. Blood 2010; 115(21):4198–205.

50. Duhren-von Minden M, Ubelhart R, Schneider D, et al. Chronic lymphocytic leukaemia is driven by antigen-independent cell-autonomous signalling. Nature 2012;489(7415):309–12.

51. Ubelhart R, Bach MP, Eschbach C, et al. N-linked glycosylation selectively regulates autonomous precursor BCR function. Nat Immunol 2010;11(8):759–65.

52. Zupo S, Isnardi L, Megna M, et al. CD38 expression distinguishes two groups of B-cell chronic lymphocytic leukemias with different responses to anti-IgM antibodies and propensity to apoptosis. Blood 1996;88(4):1365–74.

53. Wiestner A, Rosenwald A, Barry TS, et al. ZAP-70 expression identifies a chronic lymphocytic leukemia subtype with unmutated immunoglobulin genes, inferior clinical outcome, and distinct gene expression profile. Blood 2003;101(12): 4944–51.

54. Crespo M, Bosch F, Villamor N, et al. ZAP-70 expression as a surrogate for immunoglobulin-variable-region mutations in chronic lymphocytic leukemia. N Engl J Med 2003;348(18):1764–75.

55. Rassenti LZ, Huynh L, Toy TL, et al. ZAP-70 compared with immunoglobulin heavy-chain gene mutation status as a predictor of disease progression in chronic lymphocytic leukemia. N Engl J Med 2004;351(9):893–901.

56. Orchard JA, Ibbotson RE, Davis Z, et al. ZAP-70 expression and prognosis in chronic lymphocytic leukaemia. Lancet 2004;363(9403):105–11.

57. Rassenti LZ, Jain S, Keating MJ, et al. Relative value of ZAP-70, CD38, and immunoglobulin mutation status in predicting aggressive disease in chronic lymphocytic leukemia. Blood 2008;112(5):1923–30.

58. Chen L, Apgar J, Huynh L, et al. ZAP-70 directly enhances IgM signaling in chronic lymphocytic leukemia. Blood 2005;105(5):2036–41.

59. Chen L, Huynh L, Apgar J, et al. ZAP-70 enhances IgM signaling independent of its kinase activity in chronic lymphocytic leukemia. Blood 2008;111(5):2685–92.

60. Gobessi S, Laurenti L, Longo PG, et al. ZAP-70 enhances B-cell-receptor signaling despite absent or inefficient tyrosine kinase activation in chronic lymphocytic leukemia and lymphoma B cells. Blood 2007;109(5):2032–9.

61. Bernal A, Pastore RD, Asgary Z, et al. Survival of leukemic B cells promoted by engagement of the antigen receptor. Blood 2001;98(10):3050–7.

62. Quiroga MP, Balakrishnan K, Kurtova AV, et al. B cell antigen receptor signaling enhances chronic lymphocytic leukemia cell migration and survival: specific targeting with a novel Syk inhibitor, R406. Blood 2009;114(5):1029–37.

63. Deglesne PA, Chevallier N, Letestu R, et al. Survival response to B-cell receptor ligation is restricted to progressive chronic lymphocytic leukemia cells irrespective of Zap70 expression. Cancer Res 2006;66(14):7158–66.

64. Burger JA. Nurture versus nature: the microenvironment in chronic lymphocytic leukemia. Hematology Am Soc Hematol Educ Program 2011;2011:96–103.

65. Dal Bo M, Bomben R, Zucchetto A, et al. Microenvironmental interactions in chronic lymphocytic leukemia: hints for pathogenesis and identification of targets for rational therapy. Curr Pharm Des 2012;18(23):3323–34.

66. Bagnara D, Kaufman MS, Calissano C, et al. A novel adoptive transfer model of chronic lymphocytic leukemia suggests a key role for T lymphocytes in the disease. Blood 2011;117(20):5463–72.

67. Devereux S. Two-faced T cells in CLL. Blood 2011;117(20):5273–4.

68. Pizzolo G, Chilosi M, Ambrosetti A, et al. Immunohistologic study of bone marrow involvement in B-chronic lymphocytic leukemia. Blood 1983;62(6):1289–96.

69. Stevenson FK, Caligaris-Cappio F. Chronic lymphocytic leukemia: revelations from the B-cell receptor. Blood 2004;103(12):4389–95.

70. Ghia P, Strola G, Granziero L, et al. Chronic lymphocytic leukemia B cells are endowed with the capacity to attract CD4+, CD40L+ T cells by producing CCL22. Eur J Immunol 2002;32(5):1403–13.

71. Fluckiger AC, Rossi JF, Bussel A, et al. Responsiveness of chronic lymphocytic leukemia B cells activated via surface Igs or CD40 to B-cell tropic factors. Blood 1992;80(12):3173–81.

72. Cuni S, Perez-Aciego P, Perez-Chacon G, et al. A sustained activation of PI3K/NF-kappaB pathway is critical for the survival of chronic lymphocytic leukemia B cells. Leukemia 2004;18(8):1391–400.

73. Furman RR, Asgary Z, Mascarenhas JO, et al. Modulation of NF-kappa B activity and apoptosis in chronic lymphocytic leukemia B cells. J Immunol 2000;164(4):2200–6.

74. Romano MF, Lamberti A, Tassone P, et al. Triggering of CD40 antigen inhibits fludarabine-induced apoptosis in B chronic lymphocytic leukemia cells. Blood 1998;92(3):990–5.

75. Kitada S, Zapata JM, Andreeff M, et al. Bryostatin and CD40-ligand enhance apoptosis resistance and induce expression of cell survival genes in B-cell chronic lymphocytic leukaemia. Br J Haematol 1999;106(4):995–1004.

76. Hallaert DY, Jaspers A, van Noesel CJ, et al. c-Abl kinase inhibitors overcome CD40-mediated drug resistance in CLL: implications for therapeutic targeting of chemoresistant niches. Blood 2008;112(13):5141–9.

77. Li F, Ambrosini G, Chu EY, et al. Control of apoptosis and mitotic spindle checkpoint by survivin. Nature 1998;396(6711):580–4.

78. Dancescu M, Rubio-Trujillo M, Biron G, et al. Interleukin 4 protects chronic lymphocytic leukemic B cells from death by apoptosis and upregulates Bcl-2 expression. J Exp Med 1992;176(5):1319–26.

79. Trentin L, Cerutti A, Zambello R, et al. Interleukin-15 promotes the growth of leukemic cells of patients with B-cell chronic lymphoproliferative disorders. Blood 1996;87(8):3327–35.

80. Foa R, Massaia M, Cardona S, et al. Production of tumor necrosis factor-alpha by B-cell chronic lymphocytic leukemia cells: a possible regulatory role of TNF in the progression of the disease. Blood 1990;76(2):393–400.

81. Reittie JE, Yong KL, Panayiotidis P, et al. Interleukin-6 inhibits apoptosis and tumour necrosis factor induced proliferation of B-chronic lymphocytic leukaemia. Leuk Lymphoma 1996;22(1–2):83–90 follow 186, color plate VI.

82. Buschle M, Campana D, Carding SR, et al. Interferon gamma inhibits apoptotic cell death in B cell chronic lymphocytic leukemia. J Exp Med 1993;177(1):213–8.

83. Panayiotidis P, Ganeshaguru K, Jabbar SA, et al. Alpha-interferon (alpha-IFN) protects B-chronic lymphocytic leukaemia cells from apoptotic cell death in vitro. Br J Haematol 1994;86(1):169–73.

84. Chaouchi N, Wallon C, Goujard C, et al. Interleukin-13 inhibits interleukin-2-induced proliferation and protects chronic lymphocytic leukemia B cells from in vitro apoptosis. Blood 1996;87(3):1022–9.

85. Lotz M, Ranheim E, Kipps TJ. Transforming growth factor beta as endogenous growth inhibitor of chronic lymphocytic leukemia B cells. J Exp Med 1994; 179(3):999–1004.

86. Fayad L, Keating MJ, Reuben JM, et al. Interleukin-6 and interleukin-10 levels in chronic lymphocytic leukemia: correlation with phenotypic characteristics and outcome. Blood 2001;97(1):256–63.

87. Ranheim EA, Kipps TJ. Activated T cells induce expression of B7/BB1 on normal or leukemic B cells through a CD40-dependent signal. J Exp Med 1993;177(4): 925–35.

88. Beyer M, Kochanek M, Darabi K, et al. Reduced frequencies and suppressive function of CD4+CD25hi regulatory T cells in patients with chronic lymphocytic leukemia after therapy with fludarabine. Blood 2005;106(6):2018–25.

89. Biancotto A, Dagur PK, Fuchs JC, et al. Phenotypic complexity of T regulatory subsets in patients with B-chronic lymphocytic leukemia. Mod Pathol 2012; 25(2):246–59.

90. Gorgun G, Holderried TA, Zahrieh D, et al. Chronic lymphocytic leukemia cells induce changes in gene expression of CD4 and CD8 T cells. J Clin Invest 2005; 115(7):1797–805.

91. Ramsay AG, Johnson AJ, Lee AM, et al. Chronic lymphocytic leukemia T cells show impaired immunological synapse formation that can be reversed with an immunomodulating drug. J Clin Invest 2008;118(7):2427–37.

92. Ramsay AG, Gribben JG. The 3 Rs in CLL immune dysfunction. Blood 2010; 115(13):2563–4.

93. Lagneaux L, Delforge A, Bron D, et al. Chronic lymphocytic leukemic B cells but not normal B cells are rescued from apoptosis by contact with normal bone marrow stromal cells. Blood 1998;91(7):2387–96.

94. Kurtova AV, Balakrishnan K, Chen R, et al. Diverse marrow stromal cells protect CLL cells from spontaneous and drug-induced apoptosis: development of a reliable and reproducible system to assess stromal cell adhesion-mediated drug resistance. Blood 2009;114(20):4441–50.

95. Ding W, Knox TR, Tschumper RC, et al. Platelet-derived growth factor (PDGF)-PDGF receptor interaction activates bone marrow-derived mesenchymal stromal cells derived from chronic lymphocytic leukemia: implications for an angiogenic switch. Blood 2010;116(16):2984–93.

96. Ding W, Nowakowski GS, Knox TR, et al. Bi-directional activation between mesenchymal stem cells and CLL B-cells: implication for CLL disease progression. Br J Haematol 2009;147(4):471–83.

97. Ghosh AK, Secreto CR, Knox TR, et al. Circulating microvesicles in B-cell chronic lymphocytic leukemia can stimulate marrow stromal cells: implications for disease progression. Blood 2010;115(9):1755–64.

98. Schulz A, Toedt G, Zenz T, et al. Inflammatory cytokines and signaling pathways are associated with survival of primary chronic lymphocytic leukemia cells in vitro: a dominant role of CCL2. Haematologica 2011;96(3):408–16.

99. Ruan J, Hyjek E, Kermani P, et al. Magnitude of stromal hemangiogenesis correlates with histologic subtype of non-Hodgkin's lymphoma. Clin Cancer Res 2006;12(19):5622–31.

100. Orimo A, Gupta PB, Sgroi DC, et al. Stromal fibroblasts present in invasive human breast carcinomas promote tumor growth and angiogenesis through elevated SDF-1/CXCL12 secretion. Cell 2005;121(3):335–48.

101. Burger M, Hartmann T, Krome M, et al. Small peptide inhibitors of the CXCR4 chemokine receptor (CD184) antagonize the activation, migration, and antiapoptotic responses of CXCL12 in chronic lymphocytic leukemia B cells. Blood 2005;106(5):1824–30.

102. Pittenger MF, Mackay AM, Beck SC, et al. Multilineage potential of adult human mesenchymal stem cells. Science 1999;284(5411):143–7.

103. de la Fuente MT, Casanova B, Moyano JV, et al. Engagement of alpha4beta1 integrin by fibronectin induces in vitro resistance of B chronic lymphocytic leukemia cells to fludarabine. J Leukoc Biol 2002;71(3):495–502.

104. Redondo-Munoz J, Ugarte-Berzal E, Terol MJ, et al. Matrix metalloproteinase-9 promotes chronic lymphocytic leukemia b cell survival through its hemopexin domain. Cancer Cell 2010;17(2):160–72.

105. Redondo-Munoz J, Escobar-Diaz E, Samaniego R, et al. MMP-9 in B-cell chronic lymphocytic leukemia is up-regulated by alpha4beta1 integrin or CXCR4 engagement via distinct signaling pathways, localizes to podosomes, and is involved in cell invasion and migration. Blood 2006;108(9):3143–51.

106. Ringshausen I, Dechow T, Schneller F, et al. Constitutive activation of the MAP-kinase p38 is critical for MMP-9 production and survival of B-CLL cells on bone marrow stromal cells. Leukemia 2004;18(12):1964–70.

107. Lee YK, Bone ND, Strege AK, et al. VEGF receptor phosphorylation status and apoptosis is modulated by a green tea component, epigallocatechin-3-gallate (EGCG), in B-cell chronic lymphocytic leukemia. Blood 2004;104(3):788–94.

108. Lee YK, Shanafelt TD, Bone ND, et al. VEGF receptors on chronic lymphocytic leukemia (CLL) B cells interact with STAT 1 and 3: implication for apoptosis resistance. Leukemia 2005;19(4):513–23.

109. Gehrke I, Gandhirajan RK, Poll-Wolbeck SJ, et al. Bone marrow stromal cell-derived vascular endothelial growth factor (VEGF) rather than chronic lymphocytic leukemia (CLL) cell-derived VEGF is essential for the apoptotic resistance of cultured CLL cells. Mol Med 2011;17(7–8):619–27.

110. Buggins AG, Pepper C, Patten PE, et al. Interaction with vascular endothelium enhances survival in primary chronic lymphocytic leukemia cells via NF-kappaB activation and de novo gene transcription. Cancer Res 2010;70(19):7523–33.

111. Herishanu Y, Gibellini F, Njuguna N, et al. Activation of CD44, a receptor for extracellular matrix components, protects chronic lymphocytic leukemia cells from spontaneous and drug induced apoptosis through MCL-1. Leuk Lymphoma 2011;52(9):1758–69.

112. Park CS, Choi YS. How do follicular dendritic cells interact intimately with B cells in the germinal centre? Immunology 2005;114(1):2–10.

113. Chilosi M, Pizzolo G, Fiore-Donati L, et al. Routine immunofluorescent and histochemical analysis of bone marrow involvement of lymphoma/leukaemia: the use of cryostat sections. Br J Cancer 1983;48(6):763–75.

114. Ratech H, Sheibani K, Nathwani BN, et al. Immunoarchitecture of the "pseudo-follicles" of well-differentiated (small) lymphocytic lymphoma: a comparison with true follicles. Hum Pathol 1988;19(1):89–94.

115. Schmid C, Isaacson PG. Proliferation centres in B-cell malignant lymphoma, lymphocytic (B-CLL): an immunophenotypic study. Histopathology 1994;24(5):445–51.

116. Chilosi M, Pizzolo G, Caligaris-Cappio F, et al. Immunohistochemical demonstration of follicular dendritic cells in bone marrow involvement of B-cell chronic lymphocytic leukemia. Cancer 1985;56(2):328–32.

117. Pedersen IM, Kitada S, Leoni LM, et al. Protection of CLL B cells by a follicular dendritic cell line is dependent on induction of Mcl-1. Blood 2002;100(5):1795–801.

118. Burger JA, Tsukada N, Burger M, et al. Blood-derived nurse-like cells protect chronic lymphocytic leukemia B cells from spontaneous apoptosis through stromal cell-derived factor-1. Blood 2000;96(8):2655–63.

119. Tsukada N, Burger JA, Zvaifler NJ, et al. Distinctive features of "nurselike" cells that differentiate in the context of chronic lymphocytic leukemia. Blood 2002;99(3):1030–7.

120. Nishio M, Endo T, Tsukada N, et al. Nurselike cells express BAFF and APRIL, which can promote survival of chronic lymphocytic leukemia cells via a paracrine pathway distinct from that of SDF-1alpha. Blood 2005;106(3):1012–20.

121. Schiemann B, Gommerman JL, Vora K, et al. An essential role for BAFF in the normal development of B cells through a BCMA-independent pathway. Science 2001;293(5537):2111–4.

122. Schneider P, Takatsuka H, Wilson A, et al. Maturation of marginal zone and follicular B cells requires B cell activating factor of the tumor necrosis factor family and is independent of B cell maturation antigen. J Exp Med 2001;194(11):1691–7.

123. Mackay F, Schneider P, Rennert P, et al. BAFF AND APRIL: a tutorial on B cell survival. Annu Rev Immunol 2003;21:231–64.

124. Kern C, Cornuel JF, Billard C, et al. Involvement of BAFF and APRIL in the resistance to apoptosis of B-CLL through an autocrine pathway. Blood 2004;103(2):679–88.

125. Novak AJ, Bram RJ, Kay NE, et al. Aberrant expression of B-lymphocyte stimulator by B chronic lymphocytic leukemia cells: a mechanism for survival. Blood 2002;100(8):2973–9.

126. Zhang W, Kater AP, Widhopf GF, et al. B-cell activating factor and v-Myc myelocytomatosis viral oncogene homolog (c-Myc) influence progression of chronic lymphocytic leukemia. Proc Natl Acad Sci U S A 2010;107(44):18956–60.

127. Krysov S, Dias S, Paterson A, et al. Surface IgM stimulation induces MEK1/2-dependent MYC expression in chronic lymphocytic leukemia cells. Blood 2012;119(1):170–9.

128. Deaglio S, Vaisitti T, Bergui L, et al. CD38 and CD100 lead a network of surface receptors relaying positive signals for B-CLL growth and survival. Blood 2005;105(8):3042–50.

129. Granziero L, Circosta P, Scielzo C, et al. CD100/Plexin-B1 interactions sustain proliferation and survival of normal and leukemic CD5+ B lymphocytes. Blood 2003;101(5):1962–9.

130. Moser B, Loetscher P. Lymphocyte traffic control by chemokines. Nat Immunol 2001;2(2):123–8.

131. Burger JA, Burger M, Kipps TJ. Chronic lymphocytic leukemia B cells express functional CXCR4 chemokine receptors that mediate spontaneous migration beneath bone marrow stromal cells. Blood 1999;94(11):3658–67.

132. Mohle R, Failenschmid C, Bautz F, et al. Overexpression of the chemokine receptor CXCR4 in B cell chronic lymphocytic leukemia is associated with increased functional response to stromal cell-derived factor-1 (SDF-1). Leukemia 1999;13(12):1954–9.

133. Richardson SJ, Matthews C, Catherwood MA, et al. ZAP-70 expression is associated with enhanced ability to respond to migratory and survival signals in B-cell chronic lymphocytic leukemia (B-CLL). Blood 2006;107(9):3584–92.

134. Vaisitti T, Aydin S, Rossi D, et al. CD38 increases CXCL12-mediated signals and homing of chronic lymphocytic leukemia cells. Leukemia 2010;24(5):958–69.

135. Deaglio S, Vaisitti T, Aydin S, et al. CD38 and ZAP-70 are functionally linked and mark CLL cells with high migratory potential. Blood 2007;110(12):4012–21.

136. Gunn MD, Ngo VN, Ansel KM, et al. A B-cell-homing chemokine made in lymphoid follicles activates Burkitt's lymphoma receptor-1. Nature 1998;391(6669):799–803.

137. Burkle A, Niedermeier M, Schmitt-Graff A, et al. Overexpression of the CXCR5 chemokine receptor, and its ligand, CXCL13 in B cell chronic lymphocytic leukemia. Blood 2007;110(9):3316–25.

138. Ticchioni M, Essafi M, Jeandel PY, et al. Homeostatic chemokines increase survival of B-chronic lymphocytic leukemia cells through inactivation of transcription factor FOXO3a. Oncogene 2007;26(50):7081–91.

139. Reif K, Ekland EH, Ohl L, et al. Balanced responsiveness to chemoattractants from adjacent zones determines B-cell position. Nature 2002;416(6876):94–9.

140. Till KJ, Lin K, Zuzel M, et al. The chemokine receptor CCR7 and alpha4 integrin are important for migration of chronic lymphocytic leukemia cells into lymph nodes. Blood 2002;99(8):2977–84.

141. Chunsong H, Yuling H, Li W, et al. CXC chemokine ligand 13 and CC chemokine ligand 19 cooperatively render resistance to apoptosis in B cell lineage acute and chronic lymphocytic leukemia CD23+CD5+ B cells. J Immunol 2006;177(10):6713–22.

142. Lopez-Giral S, Quintana NE, Cabrerizo M, et al. Chemokine receptors that mediate B cell homing to secondary lymphoid tissues are highly expressed in B cell chronic lymphocytic leukemia and non-Hodgkin lymphomas with widespread nodular dissemination. J Leukoc Biol 2004;76(2):462–71.

143. Menten P, Wuyts A, Van Damme J. Macrophage inflammatory protein-1. Cytokine Growth Factor Rev 2002;13(6):455–81.

144. Burger JA, Quiroga MP, Hartmann E, et al. High-level expression of the T-cell chemokines CCL3 and CCL4 by chronic lymphocytic leukemia B cells in nurselike cell cocultures and after BCR stimulation. Blood 2009;113(13):3050–8.

145. Zucchetto A, Benedetti D, Tripodo C, et al. CD38/CD31, the CCL3 and CCL4 chemokines, and CD49d/vascular cell adhesion molecule-1 are interchained by sequential events sustaining chronic lymphocytic leukemia cell survival. Cancer Res 2009;69(9):4001–9.

146. Sivina M, Hartmann E, Kipps TJ, et al. CCL3 (MIP-1alpha) plasma levels and the risk for disease progression in chronic lymphocytic leukemia. Blood 2011;117(5):1662–9.

147. Hewamana S, Lin TT, Rowntree C, et al. Rel a is an independent biomarker of clinical outcome in chronic lymphocytic leukemia. J Clin Oncol 2009;27(5):763–9.

148. Fruman DA, Bismuth G. Fine tuning the immune response with PI3K. Immunol Rev 2009;228(1):253–72.

149. Cuesta-Mateos C, Lopez-Giral S, Alfonso-Perez M, et al. Analysis of migratory and prosurvival pathways induced by the homeostatic chemokines CCL19 and CCL21 in B-cell chronic lymphocytic leukemia. Exp Hematol 2010;38(9): 756–64, 764.e1–4.

150. Hanada M, Delia D, Aiello A, et al. bcl-2 gene hypomethylation and high-level expression in B-cell chronic lymphocytic leukemia. Blood 1993;82(6):1820–8.

151. Kitada S, Andersen J, Akar S, et al. Expression of apoptosis-regulating proteins in chronic lymphocytic leukemia: correlations with In vitro and In vivo chemoresponses. Blood 1998;91(9):3379–89.

152. Balogh Z, Reiniger L, Rajnai H, et al. High rate of neoplastic cells with genetic abnormalities in proliferation centers of chronic lymphocytic leukemia. Leuk Lymphoma 2011;52(6):1080–4.

153. Delmer A, Ajchenbaum-Cymbalista F, Tang R, et al. Overexpression of cyclin D2 in chronic B-cell malignancies. Blood 1995;85(10):2870–6.

154. Solvason N, Wu WW, Kabra N, et al. Induction of cell cycle regulatory proteins in anti-immunoglobulin-stimulated mature B lymphocytes. J Exp Med 1996;184(2): 407–17.

155. Igawa T, Sato Y, Takata K, et al. Cyclin D2 is overexpressed in proliferation centers of chronic lymphocytic leukemia/small lymphocytic lymphoma. Cancer Sci 2011;102(11):2103–7.

156. Bichi R, Shinton SA, Martin ES, et al. Human chronic lymphocytic leukemia modeled in mouse by targeted TCL1 expression. Proc Natl Acad Sci U S A 2002;99(10):6955–60.

157. Gorgun G, Ramsay AG, Holderried TA, et al. E(mu)-TCL1 mice represent a model for immunotherapeutic reversal of chronic lymphocytic leukemia-induced T-cell dysfunction. Proc Natl Acad Sci U S A 2009;106(15):6250–5.

158. Phillips JA, Mehta K, Fernandez C, et al. The NZB mouse as a model for chronic lymphocytic leukemia. Cancer Res 1992;52(2):437–43.

159. Raveche ES, Salerno E, Scaglione BJ, et al. Abnormal microRNA-16 locus with synteny to human 13q14 linked to CLL in NZB mice. Blood 2007;109(12):5079–86.

160. Calin GA, Dumitru CD, Shimizu M, et al. Frequent deletions and down-regulation of micro- RNA genes miR15 and miR16 at 13q14 in chronic lymphocytic leukemia. Proc Natl Acad Sci U S A 2002;99(24):15524–9.

161. Klein U, Lia M, Crespo M, et al. The DLEU2/miR-15a/16-1 cluster controls B cell proliferation and its deletion leads to chronic lymphocytic leukemia. Cancer Cell 2010;17(1):28–40.

162. Wen X, Zhang D, Kikuchi Y, et al. Transgene-mediated hyper-expression of IL-5 inhibits autoimmune disease but increases the risk of B cell chronic lymphocytic leukemia in a model of murine lupus. Eur J Immunol 2004;34(10):2740–9.

163. Zapata JM, Krajewska M, Morse HC 3rd, et al. TNF receptor-associated factor (TRAF) domain and Bcl-2 cooperate to induce small B cell lymphoma/chronic lymphocytic leukemia in transgenic mice. Proc Natl Acad Sci U S A 2004; 101(47):16600–5.

164. Bertilaccio MT, Scielzo C, Simonetti G, et al. A novel Rag2-/-gammac-/-xenograft model of human CLL. Blood 2010;115(8):1605–9.

165. Sun X, Herman SEM, Hsieh MM, et al. The NSG - human CLL xenograft model recapitulates the human lymph node microenvironment in regards to B-cell activation and tumor proliferation. ASH Annual Meeting Abstracts [abstract no. 973]. Blood 2011;118(21).

166. Durig J, Ebeling P, Grabellus F, et al. A novel nonobese diabetic/severe combined immunodeficient xenograft model for chronic lymphocytic leukemia

reflects important clinical characteristics of the disease. Cancer Res 2007; 67(18):8653–61.

167. Herman SE, Sun X, Buggy JJ, et al. The Bruton tyrosine kinase inhibitor, PCI-32765, inhibits activation and proliferation of human chronic lymphocytic leukemia cells in the NSG xenograph mouse model of the tissue microenvironment. ASH Annual Meeting Abstracts [abstract no. 596]. Blood 2011;118(21).

168. Aydin S, Grabellus F, Eisele L, et al. Investigating the role of CD38 and functionally related molecular risk factors in the CLL NOD/SCID xenograft model. Eur J Haematol 2011;87(1):10–9.

169. Buchner M, Brantner P, Stickel N, et al. The microenvironment differentially impairs passive and active immunotherapy in chronic lymphocytic leukaemia - CXCR4 antagonists as potential adjuvants for monoclonal antibodies. Br J Haematol 2010;151(2):167–78.

170. Andritsos L, Byrd JC, Jones JA, et al. Preliminary results from a phase I dose escalation study to determine the maximum tolerated dose of plerixafor in combination with rituximab in patients with relapsed chronic lymphocytic leukemia. ASH Annual Meeting Abstracts [abstract no. 2450]. Blood 2010; 116(21).

171. Kofler DM, Gawlik BB, Elter T, et al. Phase 1b trial of atacicept, a recombinant protein binding BLyS and APRIL, in patients with chronic lymphocytic leukemia. Leukemia 2012;26(4):841–4.

172. Byrd JC, Furman RR, Coutre S, et al. The Bruton's tyrosine kinase (BTK) inhibitor ibrutinib (PCI-32765) promotes high response rate, durable remissions, and is tolerable in treatment naive (TN) and relapsed or refractory (RR) chronic lymphocytic leukemia (CLL) or small lymphocytic lymphoma (SLL) patients including patients with high-risk (HR) disease: new and updated results of 116 patients in a phase Ib/II study. ASH Annual Meeting Abstracts [abstract no. 189]. Blood 2012;120(21).

173. Coutre SE, Byrd JC, Furman RR, et al. Phase I study of CAL-101, an isoform-selective inhibitor of phosphatidylinositol 3-kinase P110d, in patients with previously treated chronic lymphocytic leukemia [abstract no. 6631]. J Clin Oncol 2011;29(Suppl).

174. Friedberg JW, Sharman J, Sweetenham J, et al. Inhibition of Syk with fostamatinib disodium has significant clinical activity in non-Hodgkin lymphoma and chronic lymphocytic leukemia. Blood 2010;115(13):2578–85.

175. de Rooij MF, Kuil A, Geest CR, et al. The clinically active BTK inhibitor PCI-32765 targets B-cell receptor- and chemokine-controlled adhesion and migration in chronic lymphocytic leukemia. Blood 2012;119(11):2590–4.

176. Ponader S, Chen SS, Buggy JJ, et al. The Bruton tyrosine kinase inhibitor PCI-32765 thwarts chronic lymphocytic leukemia cell survival and tissue homing in vitro and in vivo. Blood 2012;119(5):1182–9.

177. Hantschel O, Rix U, Schmidt U, et al. The Btk tyrosine kinase is a major target of the Bcr-Abl inhibitor dasatinib. Proc Natl Acad Sci U S A 2007;104(33):13283–8.

178. Amrein L, Hernandez TA, Ferrario C, et al. Dasatinib sensitizes primary chronic lymphocytic leukaemia lymphocytes to chlorambucil and fludarabine in vitro. Br J Haematol 2008;143(5):698–706.

179. Veldurthy A, Patz M, Hagist S, et al. The kinase inhibitor dasatinib induces apoptosis in chronic lymphocytic leukemia cells in vitro with preference for a subgroup of patients with unmutated IgVH genes. Blood 2008;112(4):1443–52.

180. McCaig AM, Cosimo E, Leach MT, et al. Dasatinib inhibits B cell receptor signalling in chronic lymphocytic leukaemia but novel combination approaches are

required to overcome additional pro-survival microenvironmental signals. Br J Haematol 2011;153(2):199–211.

181. Amrein PC, Attar EC, Takvorian T, et al. Phase II study of dasatinib in relapsed or refractory chronic lymphocytic leukemia. Clin Cancer Res 2011;17(9): 2977–86.

182. Mocsai A, Ruland J, Tybulewicz VL. The SYK tyrosine kinase: a crucial player in diverse biological functions. Nat Rev Immunol 2010;10(6):387–402.

183. Gobessi S, Laurenti L, Longo PG, et al. Inhibition of constitutive and BCR-induced Syk activation downregulates Mcl-1 and induces apoptosis in chronic lymphocytic leukemia B cells. Leukemia 2009;23(4):686–97.

184. Hoellenriegel J, Coffey GP, Sinha U, et al. Selective, novel spleen tyrosine kinase (Syk) inhibitors suppress chronic lymphocytic leukemia B-cell activation and migration. Leukemia 2012;26(7):1576–83.

185. Suljagic M, Longo PG, Bennardo S, et al. The Syk inhibitor fostamatinib disodium (R788) inhibits tumor growth in the Emu- TCL1 transgenic mouse model of CLL by blocking antigen-dependent B-cell receptor signaling. Blood 2010;116(23):4894–905.

186. Herman SE, Barr PM, McAuley EM, et al. Fostamatinib inhibits BCR signaling, and reduces tumor cell activation and proliferation in patients with relapsed refractory chronic lymphocytic leukemia. ASH Annual Meeting Abstracts [abstract no. 2882]. Blood 2012;120(21).

187. Kyttaris VC. Kinase inhibitors: a new class of antirheumatic drugs. Drug Des Devel Ther 2012;6:245–50.

188. Buggy JJ, Elias L. Bruton tyrosine kinase (BTK) and its role in B-cell malignancy. Int Rev Immunol 2012;31(2):119–32.

189. Tsukada S, Saffran DC, Rawlings DJ, et al. Deficient expression of a B cell cytoplasmic tyrosine kinase in human X-linked agammaglobulinemia. Cell 1993; 72(2):279–90.

190. Herman SE, Gordon AL, Hertlein E, et al. Bruton tyrosine kinase represents a promising therapeutic target for treatment of chronic lymphocytic leukemia and is effectively targeted by PCI-32765. Blood 2011;117(23):6287–96.

191. Advani RH, Buggy JJ, Sharman JP, et al. Bruton tyrosine kinase inhibitor ibrutinib (PCI-32765) has significant activity in patients with relapsed/refractory B-cell malignancies. J Clin Oncol 2012;31(1):88–94.

192. Herman SE, Gordon AL, Wagner AJ, et al. Phosphatidylinositol 3-kinase-delta inhibitor CAL-101 shows promising preclinical activity in chronic lymphocytic leukemia by antagonizing intrinsic and extrinsic cellular survival signals. Blood 2010;116(12):2078–88.

193. Chapman CM, Sun X, Roschewski M, et al. ON 01910.Na is selectively cytotoxic for chronic lymphocytic leukemia cells through a dual mechanism of action involving PI3K/AKT inhibition and induction of oxidative stress. Clin Cancer Res 2012;18(7):1979–91.

194. Herman SE, Lapalombella R, Gordon AL, et al. The role of phosphatidylinositol 3-kinase-delta in the immunomodulatory effects of lenalidomide in chronic lymphocytic leukemia. Blood 2011;117(16):4323–7.

195. Hoellenriegel J, Meadows SA, Sivina M, et al. The phosphoinositide 3'-kinase delta inhibitor, CAL-101, inhibits B-cell receptor signaling and chemokine networks in chronic lymphocytic leukemia. Blood 2011;118(13):3603–12.

196. Lannutti BJ, Meadows SA, Herman SE, et al. CAL-101, a p110delta selective phosphatidylinositol-3-kinase inhibitor for the treatment of B-cell malignancies, inhibits PI3K signaling and cellular viability. Blood 2011;117(2):591–4.

197. Plate JM. PI3-kinase regulates survival of chronic lymphocytic leukemia B-cells by preventing caspase 8 activation. Leuk Lymphoma 2004;45(8):1519–29.

198. Cardone MH, Roy N, Stennicke HR, et al. Regulation of cell death protease caspase-9 by phosphorylation. Science 1998;282(5392):1318–21.

199. Datta SR, Dudek H, Tao X, et al. Akt phosphorylation of BAD couples survival signals to the cell-intrinsic death machinery. Cell 1997;91(2):231–41.

200. Hahn-Windgassen A, Nogueira V, Chen CC, et al. Akt activates the mammalian target of rapamycin by regulating cellular ATP level and AMPK activity. J Biol Chem 2005;280(37):32081–9.

201. Brunet A, Bonni A, Zigmond MJ, et al. Akt promotes cell survival by phosphorylating and inhibiting a Forkhead transcription factor. Cell 1999;96(6):857–68.

202. Hirai H, Sootome H, Nakatsuru Y, et al. MK-2206, an allosteric Akt inhibitor, enhances antitumor efficacy by standard chemotherapeutic agents or molecular targeted drugs in vitro and in vivo. Mol Cancer Ther 2010;9(7):1956–67.

203. Gills JJ, Dennis PA. Perifosine: update on a novel Akt inhibitor. Curr Oncol Rep 2009;11(2):102–10.

204. Kay JE, Kromwel L, Doe SE, et al. Inhibition of T and B lymphocyte proliferation by rapamycin. Immunology 1991;72(4):544–9.

205. Decker T, Hipp S, Ringshausen I, et al. Rapamycin-induced G1 arrest in cycling B-CLL cells is associated with reduced expression of cyclin D3, cyclin E, cyclin A, and survivin. Blood 2003;101(1):278–85.

206. Decker T, Sandherr M, Goetze K, et al. A pilot trial of the mTOR (mammalian target of rapamycin) inhibitor RAD001 in patients with advanced B-CLL. Ann Hematol 2009;88(3):221–7.

207. Zent CS, LaPlant BR, Johnston PB, et al. The treatment of recurrent/refractory chronic lymphocytic leukemia/small lymphocytic lymphoma (CLL) with everolimus results in clinical responses and mobilization of CLL cells into the circulation. Cancer 2010;116(9):2201–7.

208. Escudier B, Eisen T, Stadler WM, et al. Sorafenib in advanced clear-cell renal-cell carcinoma. N Engl J Med 2007;356(2):125–34.

209. Llovet JM, Ricci S, Mazzaferro V, et al. Sorafenib in advanced hepatocellular carcinoma. N Engl J Med 2008;359(4):378–90.

210. Wilhelm SM, Carter C, Tang L, et al. BAY 43-9006 exhibits broad spectrum oral antitumor activity and targets the RAF/MEK/ERK pathway and receptor tyrosine kinases involved in tumor progression and angiogenesis. Cancer Res 2004;64(19):7099–109.

211. Messmer D, Fecteau JF, O'Hayre M, et al. Chronic lymphocytic leukemia cells receive RAF-dependent survival signals in response to CXCL12 that are sensitive to inhibition by sorafenib. Blood 2011;117(3):882–9.

212. Huber S, Oelsner M, Decker T, et al. Sorafenib induces cell death in chronic lymphocytic leukemia by translational downregulation of Mcl-1. Leukemia 2011;25(5):838–47.

213. Fecteau JF, Bharati IS, O'Hayre M, et al. Sorafenib-induced apoptosis of chronic lymphocytic leukemia cells is associated with downregulation of RAF and myeloid cell leukemia sequence 1 (Mcl-1). Mol Med 2012;18(1):19–28.

214. Lopez-Guerra M, Xargay-Torrent S, Perez-Galan P, et al. Sorafenib targets BCR kinases and blocks migratory and microenvironmental survival signals in CLL cells. Leukemia 2012;26(6):1429–32.

215. Pepper C, Thomas A, Hoy T, et al. Antisense-mediated suppression of Bcl-2 highlights its pivotal role in failed apoptosis in B-cell chronic lymphocytic leukaemia. Br J Haematol 1999;107(3):611–5.

216. O'Brien SM, Cunningham CC, Golenkov AK, et al. Phase I to II multicenter study of oblimersen sodium, a Bcl-2 antisense oligonucleotide, in patients with advanced chronic lymphocytic leukemia. J Clin Oncol 2005;23(30):7697–702.
217. O'Brien S, Moore JO, Boyd TE, et al. Randomized phase III trial of fludarabine plus cyclophosphamide with or without oblimersen sodium (Bcl-2 antisense) in patients with relapsed or refractory chronic lymphocytic leukemia. J Clin Oncol 2007;25(9):1114–20.
218. O'Brien S, Moore JO, Boyd TE, et al. 5-year survival in patients with relapsed or refractory chronic lymphocytic leukemia in a randomized, phase III trial of fludarabine plus cyclophosphamide with or without oblimersen. J Clin Oncol 2009; 27(31):5208–12.
219. Nguyen M, Marcellus RC, Roulston A, et al. Small molecule obatoclax (GX15-070) antagonizes MCL-1 and overcomes MCL-1-mediated resistance to apoptosis. Proc Natl Acad Sci U S A 2007;104(49):19512–7.
220. O'Brien SM, Claxton DF, Crump M, et al. Phase I study of obatoclax mesylate (GX15-070), a small molecule pan-Bcl-2 family antagonist, in patients with advanced chronic lymphocytic leukemia. Blood 2009;113(2):299–305.
221. Vogler M, Butterworth M, Majid A, et al. Concurrent up-regulation of BCL-XL and BCL2A1 induces approximately 1000-fold resistance to ABT-737 in chronic lymphocytic leukemia. Blood 2009;113(18):4403–13.
222. Mason KD, Khaw SL, Rayeroux KC, et al. The BH3 mimetic compound, ABT-737, synergizes with a range of cytotoxic chemotherapy agents in chronic lymphocytic leukemia. Leukemia 2009;23(11):2034–41.
223. Roberts AW, Seymour JF, Brown JR, et al. Substantial susceptibility of chronic lymphocytic leukemia to BCL2 inhibition: results of a phase I study of navitoclax in patients with relapsed or refractory disease. J Clin Oncol 2012;30(5):488–96.
224. Balakrishnan K, Burger JA, Wierda WG, et al. AT-101 induces apoptosis in CLL B cells and overcomes stromal cell-mediated Mcl-1 induction and drug resistance. Blood 2009;113(1):149–53.
225. James DF, Castro JE, Loria O, et al. AT-101, a small molecule Bcl-2 antagonist, in treatment naïve CLL patients (pts) with high risk features; preliminary results from an ongoing phase I trial. 2006 ASCO Annual Meeting Proceedings Part I. J Clin Oncol 2006;24(18S):6605.
226. Eckelman BP, Salvesen GS, Scott FL. Human inhibitor of apoptosis proteins: why XIAP is the black sheep of the family. EMBO Rep 2006;7(10):988–94.
227. Frenzel LP, Patz M, Pallasch CP, et al. Novel X-linked inhibitor of apoptosis inhibiting compound as sensitizer for TRAIL-mediated apoptosis in chronic lymphocytic leukaemia with poor prognosis. Br J Haematol 2011;152(2):191–200.
228. Chanan-Khan A, Miller KC, Musial L, et al. Clinical efficacy of lenalidomide in patients with relapsed or refractory chronic lymphocytic leukemia: results of a phase II study. J Clin Oncol 2006;24(34):5343–9.
229. Ferrajoli A, Lee BN, Schlette EJ, et al. Lenalidomide induces complete and partial remissions in patients with relapsed and refractory chronic lymphocytic leukemia. Blood 2008;111(11):5291–7.
230. Badoux XC, Keating MJ, Wen S, et al. Lenalidomide as initial therapy of elderly patients with chronic lymphocytic leukemia. Blood 2011;118(13):3489–98.
231. Andritsos LA, Johnson AJ, Lozanski G, et al. Higher doses of lenalidomide are associated with unacceptable toxicity including life-threatening tumor flare in patients with chronic lymphocytic leukemia. J Clin Oncol 2008;26(15):2519–25.
232. Aue G, Njuguna N, Tian X, et al. Lenalidomide-induced upregulation of CD80 on tumor cells correlates with T-cell activation, the rapid onset of a cytokine release

syndrome and leukemic cell clearance in chronic lymphocytic leukemia. Haematologica 2009;94(9):1266–73.

233. Chanan-Khan A, Miller KC, Lawrence D, et al. Tumor flare reaction associated with lenalidomide treatment in patients with chronic lymphocytic leukemia predicts clinical response. Cancer 2011;117(10):2127–35.

234. Ramsay AG, Clear AJ, Fatah R, et al. Multiple inhibitory ligands induce impaired T-cell immunologic synapse function in chronic lymphocytic leukemia that can be blocked with lenalidomide: establishing a reversible immune evasion mechanism in human cancer. Blood 2012;120(7):1412–21.

235. Aue G, Pittaluga S, Liu D, et al. Correlates of lenalidomide induced immune stimulation and response in CLL: analysis in patients on treatment. Blood (ASH Annual Meeting Abstracts). Blood 2011;118(21):979.

236. Wu L, Adams M, Carter T, et al. Lenalidomide enhances natural killer cell and monocyte-mediated antibody-dependent cellular cytotoxicity of rituximab-treated CD20+ tumor cells. Clin Cancer Res 2008;14(14):4650–7.

237. Masood A, Chitta K, Paulus A, et al. Downregulation of BCL2 by AT-101 enhances the antileukaemic effect of lenalidomide both by an immune dependant and independent manner. Br J Haematol 2011. http://dx.doi.org/10.1111/j.1365-2141.2011.08984.x.

Understanding the Immunodeficiency in Chronic Lymphocytic Leukemia
Potential Clinical Implications

John C. Riches, BM BCh, MRCP*, John G. Gribben, MD, DSc

KEYWORDS

- Chronic lymphocytic leukemia • Immunodeficiency • T-cell function
- Immunomodulatory drugs • Adoptive T-cell therapies

KEY POINTS

- Chronic lymphocytic leukemia (CLL) is the commonest type of leukemia in adults.
- CLL is associated with a profound immunodeficiency highlighted by the presence of recurrent infections and failure of antitumor immune responses.
- This immunodeficiency is caused by a combination of impaired T-cell and natural killer cell function, and increased numbers of regulatory T cells and nurselike cells.
- Many of the standard treatments for CLL have significant effects on the immune system.
- Immunomodulatory approaches such as lenalidomide, tumor vaccines, and chimeric antigen receptor–modified T cells are showing great promise for the future of CLL treatment.

INTRODUCTION

Chronic lymphocytic leukemia (CLL) is the most common leukemia in adults, with a lifetime risk of 0.49%.[1] It is characterized by the clonal expansion of CD5+IgD+/IgM+ B lymphocytes that accumulate in the peripheral blood (PB), lymph nodes (LNs), bone marrow (BM), liver, and spleen. Although significant advances have been made in the treatment of CLL in the last decade, it remains incurable. Combination chemoimmunotherapy with fludarabine, cyclophosphamide, and rituximab (FCR) is now established as the standard of care, with overall response rates of 95%, and complete remission rates of 44%.[2] However, this treatment is too toxic for many elderly patients, who constitute most of the individuals with this disease, and there remain subgroups of patients for whom this therapy has minimal activity. A critical feature of the inability

Department of Haemato-Oncology, Barts Cancer Institute - a CR-UK Centre of Excellence, Queen Mary University of London, 3rd Floor John Vane Science Centre, Charterhouse Square, London EC1M 6BQ, UK
* Corresponding author.
E-mail address: johnriches@doctors.org.uk

Hematol Oncol Clin N Am 27 (2013) 207–235
http://dx.doi.org/10.1016/j.hoc.2013.01.003
0889-8588/13/$ – see front matter © 2013 Elsevier Inc. All rights reserved.

of patients to tolerate FCR is that it exacerbates the immunodeficiency already present in CLL, which can result in severe infective complications. This article summarizes the current understanding of the immune defects in CLL, with particular emphasis on the role of T cells, natural killer (NK) cells, and nurselike cells (NLCs) in this disease. It also examines the potential clinical implications of these findings, focusing on the immuno-modulatory aspects of current and novel pharmaceutical agents in addition to biologic therapies such as CD40 ligand transduction, vaccination strategies, and chimeric antigen receptor (CAR)–modified T cells.

T-CELL DEFECTS IN CLL
Abnormalities in T-Cell Numbers

Immune dysfunction is a key feature of CLL, highlighted by the hypogammaglobulin-emia, increased susceptibility to infections, and increased incidence of autoimmune anemias that are commonly seen in this disease. As a consequence, attempts to under-stand the role of T cells in CLL have been active areas of investigation. It has been known for some time that the T-cell compartment is highly abnormal in CLL, with one of the earliest studies reporting an increase in absolute numbers of T cells in the PB.[3] This expansion is primarily accounted for by an increase in CD8+ T cells, resulting in a decrease in the CD4/CD8 ratio,[4–7] in contrast with the situation in the LNs and BM, where increased numbers of CD4+ T cells have been reported.[8] The mechanism behind these changes remains unclear, although it has been suggested that the relative reduction in numbers of PB CD4+ T cells is caused by their increased susceptibility to FasL-mediated apoptosis.[9] Several studies have linked changes in the numbers of circulating T-cell numbers to prognosis. Early work showed that there was greater expansion of CD8+ T cells, reflected in decreasing CD4/CD8 ratios, with advancing Rai stage.[4] A more recent study has shown that inverted CD4/CD8 ratios predict shorter time to first treatment and reduced progression-free survival.[10] Furthermore, other investigators have shown that patients with premalignant monoclonal B-cell lymphocy-tosis (MBL) seem to lack any significant expansion in T-cell numbers, in contrast with patients with CLL.[11] However, there may be difficulties trying to prognosticate based on just the PB microenvironment, because another study found that increased numbers of circulating CD8+ T cells correlate with longer median time of survival.[12]

Abnormalities in Cytokine Secretion Profiles

Despite their increased numbers, these T cells show profound defects in function and proliferative capacity, and abnormal cytokine secretion profiles.[13–15] Early studies suggested that CLL was a Th2/Tc2-mediated disease, with increased numbers of CD4+ and CD8+ T cells producing interleukin (IL)-4.[16,17] Further work showed that these IL-4–producing T cells also upregulate CD30 by an IL-4 and OX40L-dependent mechanism.[18,19] Interaction of CD30 with CD30L expressed on the CLL cells results in increased tumor necrosis factor-α (TNF-α) production and CLL cell proliferation. In contrast, ligation of CD30L on the surface of the nonmalignant B cells impairs isotype class switching, and increases their sensitivity to FasL-mediated cell death, potentially contributing to the hypogammaglobulinemia observed in CLL. IL-4 also seems to be able to protect the CLL cells from undergoing apoptosis, by increasing/maintaining BCL-2 protein levels.[20,21] There is evidence to suggest that IL-6 production by CLL cells drives this skew toward IL-4–producing T cells. Healthy T cells stimulated in the presence of tumor supernatant containing high levels of IL-6 have been shown to increase their production of IL-4, findings that could be replicated using recombinant IL-6, or reversed by removal or blockade of this cytokine.[22]

Furthermore, IL-6 has been shown to be increased in the serum of patients with CLL, with higher levels predicting poorer survival.[23,24]

This shift toward a type 2 T-cell response was an attractive hypothesis given that these T cells could be expected to both enhance humoral immunity and help the malignant B cells, while suppressing Th1/Tc1-mediated cellular antitumor immune responses. However, several other reports have described increased production of interferon-γ (IFN-γ) and TNF-α by T cells from patients with CLL, showing correlation with disease stage.[25–29] Furthermore, IFN-γ and TNF-α have been shown to protect CLL cells from apoptosis and induce their proliferation in vitro.[30,31] It is probable that the situation in vivo is more complicated than the traditional Th1/Th2 paradigm, with interplay between a variety of cell types producing a mix of cytokines, chemokines, and cell surface molecules that protect the CLL cells from apoptosis and regulate their proliferation (**Table 1**).

Evidence for Chronic Activation: the Role of Cytomegalovirus?

Another feature of CLL T cells is that they show evidence of chronic activation, with upregulation of activation markers such as CD69, HLA-DR, and CD57, and downregulation of CD28 and CD62L.[42–45] Several reports document expansions of clonal and oligoclonal T cells in CLL, in both CD4+ and CD8+ populations.[46–49] There is also evidence that these oligoclonal expansions are primarily restricted to populations with an activated CD57+ phenotype, suggesting a role for chronic antigen stimulation in their development.[50] However, it remains unclear whether this is directly related to CLL, or whether other factors such as cytomegalovirus (CMV) are involved. CMV is known to have a profound influence on distribution of lymphocyte subsets in healthy individuals, with CMV seropositivity driving the T-cell repertoire toward greater clonality in the elderly.[51,52] Subsequent reports have shown an expansion of CMV-specific CD4+ and CD8+ T cells in patients with CLL, with an effector phenotype.[53–55] It is therefore possible that the earlier reports of clonality and increased expression of activation markers merely reflect an immune response to CMV.

Alterations in Gene Expression: Cytoskeletal Dysfunction and Inhibitory Ligands

An important finding in the immunobiology of CLL was our work showing profound changes in the global gene expression profiles of T cells from patients with CLL

Table 1
Cytokines implicated in the pathogenesis of CLL

Cytokine	Action	Reference
IFN-γ	Protects CLL cells from apoptosis	30
TNF-α	Increases CLL-cell proliferation	31
TGF-β	Inhibits CLL-cell proliferation	32
IL-2	Increases CLL-cell proliferation	33
IL-4	Protects CLL cells from apoptosis	20,21
IL-5	Induces CLL-cell apoptosis	34
IL-6	Protects CLL cells from apoptosis; inhibits CLL-cell proliferation	35,36
IL-7	Increases CLL-cell proliferation; protects CLL cells from apoptosis	37,38
IL-10	Inhibits CLL-cell proliferation; induces CLL-cell apoptosis	39,40
IL-21	Induces CLL-cell apoptosis	41

Abbreviation: TGF, transforming growth factor.

compared with healthy age-matched controls.[56] Despite not being part of the malignant clone, alterations were found in the expression of genes involved in cell differentiation and cytoskeletal formation in patients' CD4+ T cells, and in cytoskeletal formation, vesicle trafficking, and cytotoxicity pathways in patients' CD8+ T cells. Similar defects in gene expression could be induced in healthy T cells by coculturing them with CLL cells. These changes in the expression of cytoskeletal genes translated into a functional defect in filamentous actin (F-actin) polymerization, with T cells from patients with CLL having defective immunologic synapse formation with antigen-presenting cells (APCs).[57] Again, this functional defect could be induced in healthy T cells by coculturing them with CLL cells. In both cases, the induction of the defects relied on direct contact between the CLL cells and the T cells, because the defects were not seen after coculture experiments using the Transwell system.

Similar defects could be observed in T cells taken from the Eμ-TCL1 mouse model of CLL. In this model, the *TCL1* gene is placed under the control of a B cell–specific IgV$_H$ promoter and IgH Eμ enhancer, resulting in mice that develop normally into adulthood, but then subsequently develop lymphadenopathy and hepatosplenomegaly, with increased numbers of circulating CD19+CD5+IgM+ lymphocytes.[58] Despite this model being dependent on a single transgene, T cells from animals that had developed the disease showed alterations in the expression of cytoskeletal genes, and had dysfunctional immunologic synapse formation. Furthermore, infusion of CLL cells into young Eμ-TCL1 mice caused defects comparable with those seen in mice that had clinically apparent leukemia, showing causality of the CLL cells to induce the T-cell defects[59] Another study showed that this model also accurately mimics the shift toward the antigen-experienced phenotype observed in the human disease.[60] This work showed both a skewing of T-cell subsets toward antigen-experienced memory T cells, and development of clonal T-cell populations, consistent with a CLL-dependent antigen-driven skewing of the T cells in these mice.

We have examined the mechanism by which CLL cells induce these defects in the T-cell populations. Using functional screening assays based on actin polymerization responses to APCs, the molecules CD200, CD270 (herpes virus entry mediator [HVEM]), CD274 (programmed death ligand-1 [PD-L1]), and CD276 (B7-H3) induced impaired immunologic synapse formation in both allogeneic and autologous T cells.[61] Higher expression of these molecules was observed on CLL cells compared with healthy B cells, with increased expression of CD200 and CD274 correlating with poor prognosis. Signaling axes involving these inhibitory ligands were also able to induce impaired F-actin polymerization in other cancers, suggesting that both hematologic and solid cancer cells use common immunosuppressive mechanisms to suppress T-cell–mediated antitumor immune responses. There is evidence that some of the receptors for these inhibitory ligands are increased on CLL T cells. Programmed death-1 (PD1; CD279) is an inhibitory T-cell receptor that has been postulated to be important in the maintenance of peripheral tolerance. Engagement of PD-1 by PD-L1 leads to the inhibition of T-cell receptor–mediated lymphocyte proliferation and cytokine secretion.[62] We recently reported that PD-1 expression is increased on CD3+ T cells from patients with CLL and is an indicator of poor prognosis.[61] Another group has reported similar findings, showing that PD-1 expression is increased on CD8+ T cells, with its expression predicting a more aggressive clinical course.[10] However, another report has suggested that PD-1 expression is decreased on effector T cells, which are expanded in CLL.[63] In addition to PD-1, we also have unpublished data showing that expression of a second inhibitory receptor, CD160, is increased on CLL T cells. CD160 interacts with HVEM to inhibit lymphocyte activation, along with B lymphocyte attenuator (BTLA).[64] CD160 is normally expressed on

NK cells, and a subset of CD8+ cytotoxic lymphocytes found in the intestinal epithelium.[65] Circulating cytotoxic T cells from patients with CLL upregulate a range of other inhibitory receptors that are normally found on NK cells, including the killer inhibitory receptors CD158a, CD158b, and CD158e, and the C-type lectin receptor, CD94.[66] The significance of this requires further investigation, but it is possible that pathways normally used in the regulation of NK-cell activity could be coopted to suppress CD8+ cytotoxic lymphocyte function in CLL.

Regulatory T Cells in CLL

In addition to increased expression of inhibitory receptors in CLL, there is also an increase in CD4+CD25^{hi} regulatory T cells (T$_{regs}$) in CLL. T$_{regs}$ have been shown to inhibit proliferation and cytokine release by conventional CD4+CD25− T cells, and increased numbers of T$_{regs}$ are associated with inhibition of antitumor immunity in solid cancers.[67,68] The expansion of T$_{regs}$ in CLL has been postulated to be caused by 2 factors. First, there is evidence of increased formation, facilitated by CD27-CD70 interactions in LN proliferation centers.[69] CD200 expression on the CLL cells may also play a role, because anti-CD200R antibodies promote development of T$_{regs}$, whereas CD200 blockade significantly decreases T$_{reg}$ numbers.[70,71] Second, T$_{regs}$ from patients with CLL have increased resistance to drug-induced apoptosis, compared with T$_{regs}$ from healthy donors, as a consequence of higher expression of BCL-2.[69] The degree of increase correlates with disease stage, with the greatest increases in patients with the most clinically advanced disease.[72–75] T$_{reg}$ numbers were also slightly increased in patients with MBL, although lower than in patients with CLL.[76] The degree of increase in T$_{regs}$ has also been found to be of prognostic significance, with higher numbers of T$_{regs}$ predicting significantly shorter time to first treatment in 2 studies.[77,78] T$_{regs}$ also express CD39, with increased expression of this molecule showing correlation with disease severity and prognosis in CLL.[79,80] Higher frequencies of T$_{regs}$ have also been shown to correlate with decreased T-cell responses against viral and tumor antigens.[73] A further feature of T$_{regs}$ is they express another inhibitory receptor, cytotoxic T lymphocyte–associated antigen-4 (CTLA-4; CD152). CTLA-4 is a homolog of CD28 and acts both directly, by decreasing phosphorylation of signaling proteins proximal to the T-cell receptor, and indirectly, by competing with CD28 for CD80/CD86 binding.[81,82] T cells from patients with CLL have been shown to have significantly increased expression of both surface and cytoplasmic CTLA-4 compared with healthy controls, with expansion of a CD4+CD25+CTLA-4+ subset.[83] Furthermore, although CTLA-4 is normally upregulated on T-cell activation, CLL T cells also showed a greater degree of upregulation of CTLA-4, and prolonged expression.[84] Therefore, it is likely that CTLA-4 signaling is another inhibitory pathway mediating T-cell dysfunction in CLL, in addition to the PD-1:PD-L1, CD160:HVEM, and CD200:CD200R axes (**Fig. 1**).

T Cells as Part of the Protumor Niche

In addition to the role for the CD4+CD25+ subset in the pathogenesis of CLL, evidence is emerging that implicates CD4+ T cells in the development and maintenance of this disease. As mentioned earlier, in contrast with the PB where CD8+ T cells are increased, CD4+ T cells are primarily expanded in the LNs and BM of patients with CLL.[8] It has been suggested that this is caused by production of the chemokine CCL22 by CLL cells, which has been shown to be released into culture supernatants on CLL cell activation. These supernatants were able to induce the migration of activated CD4+CD40L+ T cells expressing the CCL22 receptor, CCR4: migration that could be blocked by antiCCL22 antibodies.[85] A recent article highlighted the

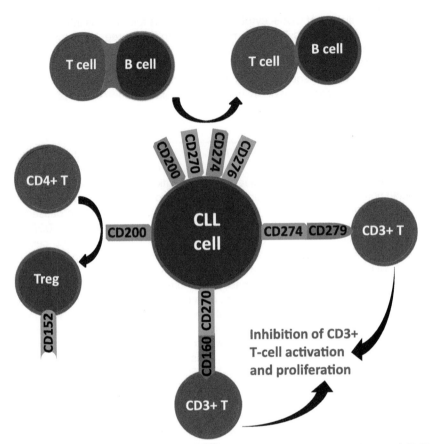

Fig. 1. Inhibitory signaling axes in CLL. Upregulation of CD200, CD270, CD274, and CD276 induces impaired actin polymerization and immunologic synapse formation in CLL T cells. CD200 also promotes the differentiation of CD4+ T cells into T_{regs}, which express CD152 (CTLA-4). CD270 (HVEM) and CD274 (PD-L1) interact with their ligands CD160 and CD279 (PD-1) to inhibit T-cell activation and proliferation.

potential importance of CD4+ T cells in providing a protective niche for engraftment of CLL cells.[86] The ability of primary human CLL cells to engraft and proliferate in a non-obese diabetes/severe combined immunodeficiency/γc^{null} mouse model was assessed. Autologous CD4+ T cells from the patients with CLL were key mediators of CLL-cell growth in these mice, despite representing only a minor component of the transferred lymphocyte population. There was direct correlation between the degree of proliferation of T cells and that of the CLL clone, with selective depletion of CD4+ T cells leading to failure of CLL-cell growth. Further investigation is required to corroborate these findings in patients with CLL, but, taken together, these observations suggest that the expanded CD4+ T cells seen in BM and LNs are a critical part of the protumor microenvironment.

THE ROLE OF OTHER IMMUNE CELLS IN CLL
NLCs and Chemokines

NLCs are another key constituent of the immune microenvironment implicated in providing a protective niche for CLL cells. NLCs are a subset of peripheral blood mononuclear cells (PBMCs) that differentiate into large, round, or fibroblastlike adherent cells in the presence of CLL cells.[87] Although they are thought to originate from CD14+ monocytes, their expression of CD68 is significantly higher than normal monocyte-macrophages, making them more comparable with the CD68+ lymphoma-associated macrophages observed in follicular lymphoma.[88] Further work identified these large CD14+CD68[HI] cells in the spleens of patients with CLL, suggesting that they might also function to promote leukemia cell survival in vivo.[89] An important feature of the biology of CLL cells is that they undergo spontaneous apoptosis when cultured in vitro, in marked contrast with their apparent longevity in vivo.[90] However, when NLCs are present in vitro, the leukemic cells attach to them and are protected from undergoing spontaneous apoptosis. NLCs are thought to promote CLL-cell survival because of a combination of secretion of the chemokine CXCL12, and increased expression of B cell–activating factor of the TNF family (BAFF), and a proliferation-inducing ligand (APRIL).[87,91] In addition, differentiation of monocytes into NLCs is associated with dysregulation of genes involved in antigen presentation and immunity, impairing their antitumor function.[92] The receptor for CXCL12, CXCR4, is expressed at high levels on the surface of CLL B cells, with its expression correlating with Rai stage.[93,94] Therefore, secretion of CXCL12 by both NLCs and stromal cells induces leukemia cell trafficking and homing to protective niches populated by these cells. Furthermore, coculture of CLL cells with NLCs induces the leukemic cells to release 2 T cell–attracting chemokines, CCL3 and CCL4. The production of these chemokines may explain the observation of increased numbers of T cells in CLL pseudo-follicles, where the T cells seem to have been coopted to help B-cell activation and proliferation.[95] Furthermore, increased CCL3 levels correlate with other adverse prognostic markers such as advanced clinical stage and poor-risk cytogenetics, and are predictive of shorter time to first treatment.[96] In addition, CXCL12 acts as a costimulatory factor for CLL CD4+ T cells, resulting in their increased proliferation, cytokine production, and increased expression of activation markers. These activated T cells are then able to enhance the activation and proliferation of the leukemic cells.[97] It is therefore possible that a mix of chemokines including CXCL12, CCL3, and CCL4 results in colocalization of stromal cells, NLCs, and activated CD4+ T cells, which provide sanctuary sites for the tumor cells, protecting them from chemoimmunotherapy and resulting (**Fig. 2**) in drug resistance and disease persistence.[98]

NK Cells

Abnormalities have also been found in other immune cells in CLL. Initial studies revealed that NK cells also have a functional defect in CLL, showing reduced ability to lyse leukemia cell lines associated with a lack of cytoplasmic granules.[99,100] This activity could be restored by the use of IL-2, which also results in increased granularity of the large granular lymphocyte subset.[101] The mechanism by which CLL cells downregulate NK-cell function is not known, although there is some evidence that it may involve soluble factors.[102,103] CLL cells may also inhibit NK cells by direct contact, by their expression of the tolerogenic nonclassic major histocompatibility complex (MHC) class I molecule, HLA-G, or by expression of 4-1BB ligand.[104,105] NK cells from patients with CLL show defective actin polymerization and impaired immunologic synapse formation, comparable with the cytoskeletal dysfunction seen in CLL T cells.[106] The NK-cell defect seems to be of clinical significance, because higher NK-cell numbers were observed in patients with early-stage disease and in those with mutated *IGHV* genes. Furthermore, for patients with a given Rai stage, a higher NK/CLL cell ratio predicted a longer time to treatment, implying a protective effect of NK cells.[107] In support of this, NK cells from patients with MBL have a higher cytolytic

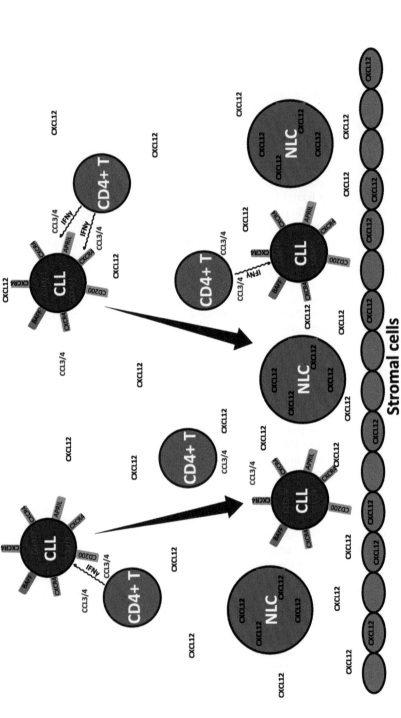

Fig. 2. The CLL niche. CXCL12 produced by stromal cells and NLCs attracts CXCR4-bearing CLL cells into the protective niche. Interaction of CLL cells with NLCs causes: (1) further differentiation of monocytes into NLCs; (2) protection of the CLL cells from apoptosis associated with increased expression of BAFF and APRIL; (3) increased production of CCL3 and CCL4 by CLL cells. CCL3 and CCL4 chemoattract CD4+ T cells, which are activated by CXCL12. These activated T cells produce cytokines including IFN-γ that regulate CLL-cell proliferation and protect them from apoptosis.

capacity than NK cells from patients with CLL.[108] Other studies have shown that numbers of CD3+CD16+CD56+ NK T cells are also important, because a reduction in numbers is associated with disease progression and a higher risk of death in patients with CLL.[109] An understanding of the NK-cell defect may prove to be clinically useful because preclinical studies have shown that NK cells from patients with CLL can be expanded and show cytotoxicity against K562 cells, highlighting their potential as a source of cellular immunotherapy.[110]

There is also evidence suggesting that monocytes and neutrophils are defective in CLL, with the latter having been shown to be deficient in lysozyme and myeloperoxidase, and to modulate CLL B-cell survival through altered secretion of TNF-superfamily proteins.[111,112]

POTENTIAL CLINICAL IMPLICATIONS: IMMUNOTHERAPY FOR CLL
Immunomodulatory Aspects of Cytotoxic Chemotherapy

Virtually all treatment of CLL is immunomodulatory. Treatments that are cytotoxic to the malignant B cells are invariably toxic to other leucocytes, both granulocytes and lymphocytes. One of the most important clinical aspects of cytotoxic chemotherapy is the degree to which it exacerbates the existing immunodeficiency. The ability of a patient to tolerate the treatment is often an important predictor of overall prognosis. In addition to the effects of cytotoxic agents on the tumor cells, there is also the potential for differential toxicity to immune components of the protumoral microenvironment. The purine analogue fludarabine is widely used for the treatment of CLL.[2] Because T-cell depletion is a commonly encountered side effect of this agent, it can be hypothesized that fludarabine treatment has a significant impact on the T-cell microenvironment. Analysis of the composition and function of the T-cell pool in patients with CLL after treatment with fludarabine and cyclophosphamide revealed a rapid and sustained reduction of circulating CD4+ and CD8+ T cells, as expected. T cells surviving this combination had a more mature phenotype, and fludarabine-treated T cells were significantly more responsive to mitogenic stimulation than their untreated counterparts, and showed a shift toward Th1 cytokine secretion.[113] Furthermore, fludarabine therapy seems to have a particularly marked effect on T_{regs}, with both a reduction in the inhibitory function and a decrease in the frequency of this subset after treatment.[72] Both these studies were performed on PB samples, so it would be particularly interesting to examine the impact of fludarabine on CD4+ T cells in LNs and BM.

Improved NK-cell Functionality with Rituximab

Rituximab is a humanized anti-CD20 monoclonal antibody (mAb) widely used in the treatment of B-cell malignancies and autoimmune diseases. The mechanism of action of this agent is not clear, although it seems to be a combination of several factors including antibody-dependent cellular cytotoxicity (ADCC), complement-dependent cytotoxicity (CDC), induction of apoptosis of CD20+ B cells, inhibition of B-cell receptor (BCR) signaling, and regulation of the cell cycle.[114] The efficacy of this agent in CLL is perhaps even more paradoxic, given the low expression of its target antigen on CLL cells compared with normal B cells and other malignant B cells. An important component of the mechanism of action of rituximab in CLL seems to be the enhancement of NK-cell functionality. Opsonization of CLL cells by anti-CD20 antibodies such as rituximab allows binding of the NK-cell Fc receptor, FcγRIII (CD16), to the Fc region of the antibodies. Antibody binding to CD16 results in NK-cell activation, release of cytolytic granules, and consequent target cell apoptosis.[115] Rituximab has been shown to increase NK-cell degranulation as measured by the CD107a assay.[116] There is evidence that FcγR polymorphisms predict response to rituximab in patients with lymphoma.[117] Third-generation monoclonal anti-CD20 antibodies such as obinutuzumab (GA-101) and LFB-R603 that have higher binding affinities for this receptor have been shown to be even more efficient at inducing NK-cell degranulation.[118,119] In vitro experiments have shown that NK-cell functionality can be further enhanced by coculturing the NK cells with cytokines such as IL-21 and IL-15.[120,121] Opsonization of the tumor cells by rituximab may also be important for the activity of other immune cells, because there is evidence that rituximab enhances macrophage killing of CLL cells by increasing phagocytosis-mediated ADCC.[122]

Eviction from the Niche: the Mobilizing Effect of BCR Signaling Inhibitors

There has been a great deal of recent interest in inhibitors of BCR signaling for the treatment of CLL. BCR signaling is known to be crucial for B-cell proliferation and survival, and several major prognostic markers that are clinically useful in CLL are associated with aberrations in BCR signaling. Absence of mutations in immunoglobulin variable (IgV) region genes and expression of zeta-chain–associated protein kinase 70 (ZAP-70) have been shown to correlate with an inferior outcome, and are both associated with increased signaling through the BCR.[123,124] This aberrant BCR signaling was previously thought to be antigen dependent, but a recent publication showed that BCRs from patients with CLL induce antigen-independent cell-autonomous signaling, dependent on the heavy-chain complementarity-determining region (HCDR3) and an internal epitope of the BCR.[125] Several molecules that inhibit kinases downstream of the BCR have been developed and are showing great promise in early-phase clinical trials. An unexpected feature of some of these agents is that there is a transient increase in the circulating lymphocytosis after initiation of treatment, associated with rapid reductions in LN size, consistent with mobilization of the tumor cells from the LNs into the blood. The phosphatidylinositol 3-kinase (PI3K) inhibitor GS1101, the Bruton tyrosine kinase (Btk) inhibitor ibrutinib (PCI-32765), and the mammalian target of rapamycin (mTOR) inhibitor, everolimus, have all been found to induce this lymphocytosis during the first weeks of treatment.[126–128] As discussed earlier, the CXCL12-CXCR4 axis is important for the homing of CLL cells to potential sanctuary sites in the BM and LNs. A small-molecule inhibitor of CXCR4, plerixafor, has also shown clinical activity in patients with CLL, again associated with mobilization of tumor cells into the circulation.[129] It is therefore likely that some of the clinical activity of these novel therapies may be caused by their ability to evict CLL cells from protective microenvironmental niches populated by NLCs, stromal cells, and T cells.[130,131]

CD40L Based Therapies

A key feature of CLL cells is that they have impaired antigen presenting function, caused by reduced expression of costimulatory molecules including CD80 and CD86.[132] CLL-cell activation by ligation of CD40 can upregulate these proteins, along with adhesion molecules such as intercellular adhesion molecule-1 (ICAM-1/CD54).[133–135] Under normal circumstances, this activation signal is provided by T cells, which transiently express CD40L (CD154) after antigen engagement of their T-cell receptors (TCRs).[136] However, this critical axis is impaired in CLL, because the tumor cells seem to be able to directly downmodulate T-cell expression of CD40L.[137] In light of this, several strategies have been developed to reexpress CD40L in the tumor microenvironment, thereby improving CLL-cell antigen-presenting function and overcoming T-cell anergy.

One such strategy has been to use adenoviral vectors to transduce CLL cells to express CD40L. In addition to inducing expression of costimulatory and adhesion molecules on the transduced cells, increased expression of CD40L in the CLL microenvironment can activate other bystander CLL cells, even if they were not transfected. Further preclinical work showed that the transfected CLL cells become effective stimulators of mixed lymphocyte reactions, and induce generation of cytotoxic T cells specific for autologous unmodified CLL cells.[138,139] Similar findings have been reported by culturing CLL cells on CD40L-expressing feeder cells in place of transfection.[140] Use of fibroblasts overexpressing CD40L and OX40L to transfer both these ligands to CLL cells also resulted in the generation of tumor-reactive cytotoxic T lymphocytes.[141] There were some initial concerns that CD40-stimulated CLL cells may become more resistant to apoptosis induced by fludarabine, because of upregulation of the NF-κB/Rel transcription factors.[142] Gene expression profiling performed on CD40-stimulated CLL cells also identified upregulation of several genes involved in the suppression of apoptosis mediated by the TNF family of receptors and NF-κB.[143] However, further investigation showed that, although CD40 stimulation enhanced the constitutive antiapoptotic profile of the CLL cells, and these cells were not sensitive to CD95L, they remained good targets for cytotoxic T cells.[144,145]

An early clinical trial examined the effects of infusions of autologous tumor cells that had been transduced ex vivo with murine CD40L, which was more efficiently expressed than human CD40L. This treatment was well tolerated and the patients showed some PB and LN responses. However, some of the patients developed antibodies against the murine CD40L.[146] In light of this, a recombinant humanized CD40 binding protein, ISF35, was developed, and was tested in a more recent phase I study. The infusions of transduced autologous tumor cells were again well tolerated, and were consistently followed by reductions in circulating lymphocyte counts and lymphadenopathy. The increased levels of this humanized CD40L were associated with induction of a proapoptotic state in the circulating CLL cells, with increased expression of proapoptotic molecules CD95, DR5, p73, and BCL-2 interacting domain (BID), and reduced levels of the antiapoptotic molecule, MCL-1. These findings were also observed in patients with deletion of chromosome 17p.[147] There is a rationale for combining this approach with rituximab, because stimulation of CLL B cells by CD40L sensitizes them to rituximab-induced cell death.[148] However, evidence has emerged that there is significant heterogeneity in the responses of CLL B cells to CD40L stimulation. Patients with CLL B cells that were unresponsive to CD40L showed a poor clinical outcome and shorter time to progression, which was thought to reflect less dependency on the microenvironment and higher autonomous proliferative and survival potential.[149]

Other work has investigated whether there is a role for anti-CD40 mAbs in the treatment of CLL. Two therapeutic antibodies that target the CD40 antigen are in development, dacetuzumab (SGN-40), which acts as a partial agonist, and lucatumumab (HCD122), which blocks CD40-mediated signaling.[150,151] However, phase I trials using these agents have shown minimal single-agent activity, but they warrant further investigation as part of combination therapies.[152,153] Preclinical experiments have suggested that dacetuzumab treatment in combination with the immunomodulatory agent lenalidomide enhanced direct apoptosis and ADCC against primary CLL cells.[154] However, it is possible that this activity represents tumor cell opsonization and the induction of NK-cell responses, as much as a direct biologic effect of CD40 binding.

Vaccine Therapy for CLL

The observation that CLL cells maintain some residual B-cell function, which can be enhanced by appropriate stimulation, has led to attempts to induce an effective autologous immune response by vaccine therapy. A vital component of this approach is identifying a suitable tumor-associated antigen (TAA) with which to induce an immune response. An ideal TAA should be only expressed on the tumor cells to avoid induction of autoimmunity, should be expressed on all of the tumor cells, and should be essential for tumor cell survival to prevent the emergence of antigen-negative variants and immune escape. The major challenge to cancer vaccines is that the tumor cells are derived from self, with the consequence that few TAAs have these characteristics. In light of this, the search for possible TAAs has focused on proteins that are either commonly mutated in the malignant cells or are aberrantly expressed. Serologic identification by recombinant expression cloning (SEREX) has been used to detect such mutated proteins, and cytotoxic T-cell responses could be generated against these antigens.[155] Several other TAAs have been identified in CLL, including survivin, fibromodulin, RHAMM (CD168), FMNL1, MDM2, and CD23.[156–161] Of particular interest is the oncofetal surface antigen receptor tyrosine kinase–like orphan receptor 1 (ROR1), which has the advantage that it is selectively expressed by malignant B cells, although it is also expressed by undifferentiated embryonic stem cells, and at low levels in adipose tissue.[162] When 6 patients with CLL were infused with autologous CLL cells that had undergone adenoviral transfection with CD154, 3 of them (50%) subsequently generated antibodies against ROR1.[163] Furthermore, upregulation of CD154 by lenalidomide has also recently been shown to induce production of ROR1 tumor-specific antibodies, notably in a patient who had not received prior therapy with rituximab.[164]

A particular feature of B-cell malignancies is that there is a further type of TAA in the form of the immunoglobulin idiotype.[165] The surface immunoglobulin expressed by the malignant B cells is unique to each clone, and thus represents an attractive target for vaccine strategies. Using a bioinformatics approach, several human immunoglobulin–derived peptides were identified that were capable of inducing cytotoxic T cells. Furthermore, autologous cytotoxic T cells specific for these peptides were able to kill primary malignant CLL cells. One of the problems with this method is that the uniqueness of the idiotype means that any potential vaccine would have to be individualized to each patient. However, peptides generated from the framework regions of the immunoglobulin molecule, regions that show less variability between patients, were immunogenic, allowing a single such peptide to be used in several patients.[166] A second problem with idiotype vaccination strategies is that the immunoglobulin idiotype is only weakly immunogenic, and often only generating humoral responses.[167,168] A solution to this is the use of heteroclitic peptides, in which MHC-binding amino acid residues are modified to bind MHC more tightly, while leaving the T-cell recognition residues intact, inducing more potent immune responses.[169]

In the normal immune system, the most potent APCs are dendritic cells (DCs). This property can be exploited by manipulating DCs to take up antigen in vitro, before presenting it to T cells, causing their activation and proliferation. There have been several clinical studies that have investigated the use of DCs in CLL. In one such study, DCs were generated from unrelated donors, before being pulsed ex vivo with patient CLL-cell lysate or apoptotic bodies. They were subsequently administered to patients with early-stage CLL, a subset of whom showed clinical responses. These investigators then studied autologous DCs pulsed with CLL-cell lysates, and a subset of patients showed responses associated with an increase in T cells specific for RHAMM/CD168 and fibromodulin.[170,171] A further study used oxidizing radiation to augment the immunogenicity of the CLL cells by improving their antigen-presenting function, resulting in enhanced T-cell antitumor activity and clinical responses.[172]

Lenalidomide

Lenalidomide has recently been shown to have significant clinical activity in CLL.[173] Its mechanism of action is not well understood, but it is thought to act primarily by enhancing antitumor immunity and reducing production of protumoral factors in the CLL microenvironment. Lenalidomide and its analogues thalidomide and pomalidomide, were originally identified for their ability to inhibit production of TNF-α from lipopolysaccharide-stimulated PBMCs in vitro.[174] Lenalidomide has also been shown to have costimulatory effects, causing T-cell activation with increased production of IL-2 and IFN-γ, and triggering tyrosine phosphorylation of CD28 with downstream activation of NF-κB.[174–176] A key part of these agents' mechanism of action seems to be their ability to activate cytoskeletal pathways, which are critical regulators of T-cell activation. In particular, it has been shown that pomalidomide can activate the cytoskeletal regulators Rac1 and RhoA in CD4+ T cells.[177] We have shown that the functional defect of T cells in CLL is associated with alterations in the expression of cytoskeletal genes and defective immunologic synapse formation. We subsequently showed that treatment of both autologous T cells and CLL cells with lenalidomide resulted in repair of this defect, suggesting that this may be a key component of this agent's activity in CLL.[57]

In addition, there is also evidence to suggest that lenalidomide has effects on CLL cells directly, by inducing CD40L expression through a PI3K kinase–dependent pathway. The CD40L-positive CLL cells also upregulate BID, DR5, and p73, sensitizing them to TNF-related apoptosis-inducing ligand (TRAIL)–mediated apoptosis.[164] Lenalidomide-induced upregulation of CD40L is of particular interest, because the CLL cells also upregulate expression of CD40, CD80, and CD86, in a similar manner to CD40L-transfected CLL cells. The increased expression of these costimulatory ligands has been found to correlate with a unique aspect of the clinical activity of lenalidomide in CLL, the tumor flare reaction. This reaction is manifested by acute swelling of involved LNs, hepatosplenomegaly, rash, and fever, and is thought to be caused by lenalidomide-induced CLL-cell and T-cell activation.[178–180] There has been some suggestion that the presence of a tumor flare reaction correlates with clinical outcome, highlighting that the mechanisms underlying this phenomenon may also account for lenalidomide's antitumor effect.[181] The existence of this reaction, as well as the unexpected finding of increased hematologic toxicity, has meant that patients with CLL are generally unable to tolerate the same doses of lenalidomide that have been used in other hematological malignancies such as myeloma. Lenalidomide also has effects on other nonmalignant lymphocyte subsets. It has been shown to significantly inhibit the suppressor function and generation of T_{regs} in vitro, and was found to reduce numbers of T_{regs} in PB of patients with CLL.[182,183] Lenalidomide has also been shown to downregulate the expression of inhibitory receptors on NK cells, and to enhance antigen-specific expansion of NK T cells.[184,185] It seems to be particularly effective when used in combination with rituximab, because of its ability to augment NK cell–mediated cytotoxicity, potentially as a result of improved immunologic synapse formation.[106,186]

A recent article identified cereblon (CRBN) as a primary target of thalidomide teratogenicity. Thalidomide binds to CRBN, inhibiting the activity of a E3 ubiquitin ligase complex composed of CRBN, DNA damage–binding protein-1 (DDB1), cullin 4A, and ring-box protein-1 (RBX1, also known as Roc1). This binding was shown to lead to the downregulation of fibroblast growth factor genes and teratogenic effects in zebra fish and chick models.[187] CRBN is also implicated in other pathways, because it binds to a calcium-activated potassium channel in the brain, a chloride channel in the retina, and to adenosine monophosphate kinase, a master sensor of energy balance in eukaryotic cells.[188–190] In addition, a nonsense R419X mutation of CRBN is associated with autosomal recessive nonsyndromic mental retardation.[191] Further work has shown that CRBN binding is also a critical component of the activity of lenalidomide and pomalidomide, because its expression was required for the antimyeloma effect of these agents.[192] Furthermore, CRBN depletion is associated with the resistance of myeloma cell lines to both of these drugs, and to lack of clinical responses in patients on lenalidomide treatment. It is not clear what the implications of these findings are for CLL because, in contrast with myeloma, lenalidomide is not directly cytotoxic to CLL cells.[193] However, evidence is emerging that CRBN is also critical for the effect of lenalidomide and pomalidomide on T-cell activation, because siRNA knockdown of T-cell CRBN blocked the increase in production of IL-2 and TNF-α induced by these agents.[194]

Lenalidomide has been shown to have significant clinical activity in CLL, with an overall response rate as a single agent in treatment-naive patients of 56%. This finding compares well with responses seen with commonly used therapies such as fludarabine, alemtuzumab, bendamustine, and chlorambucil.[173] Furthermore, lenalidomide has been shown to have efficacy in patients with poor-risk cytogenetics with overall response rates of 38% in patients with del11q or del17p.[195] A recent phase II trial has shown similar activity in elderly ($\geq$65 years) patients, with lenalidomide being well tolerated.[196] Trials are underway to examine the efficacy of combining lenalidomide with other agents, but the presence of the tumor flare reaction and other toxicities has meant that the concurrent administration of fludarabine, rituximab, and lenalidomide was not well tolerated.[197] Given that T-cell activation seems to be a crucial component of this drug's effect in this disease, it can be postulated that combinations with T-cell–depleting agents such as fludarabine or alemtuzumab may be counterproductive. However, the situation may be more complex, because there is some evidence that lenalidomide can still be effective after T-cell depletion by alemtuzumab and high-dose glucocorticoids.[198] In contrast, the addition of rituximab to lenalidomide seems particularly attractive, with rituximab improving responses relative to single-agent lenalidomide, despite the patients having received this monoclonal antibody as part of previous therapy.[199,200] Trials to evaluate the efficacy of this combination as first-line treatment, and also to investigate the combination of lenalidomide and ofatumumab, are ongoing.[201,202] Furthermore, there is evidence that lenalidomide consolidation may prolong progression-free survival after induction treatment with pentostatin, cyclophosphamide, and rituximab.[203]

Adoptive T-Cell Therapies

Allogeneic hemopoietic stem cell transplantation remains the only curative option for CLL. Critical to its activity is the graft-versus-leukemia (GVL) effect, in which the transplanted hemopoietic stem cells differentiate into effector cells that mount an antitumor immune response. This effect is known to be primarily T-cell mediated, and is probably caused by a combination of improved T-cell function and the presence of allogeneic MHC molecules.[204] The major drawback of myeloablative allogeneic transplantation is that it is associated with unacceptably high rates of nonrelapse mortality, which can approach 50% even in younger patients[205] because of a combination of toxicity from the conditioning regimens, the prolonged period of immunosuppression during engraftment, and graft-versus-host disease (GVHD). One way of attempting to reduce nonrelapse mortality is to use reduced-intensity conditioning (RIC) to exploit the GVL effect while avoiding the significant morbidity and mortality associated with myeloablative conditioning. RIC regimens are associated with decreased mortality, but GVHD remains a significant problem.[206–208] Therefore, for most patients who are more than 65 years of age, allogeneic hemopoietic stem cell transplantation is not a reasonable option.

One approach to circumventing the problem of GVHD is the adoptive transfer of T cells with specificity for tumor antigens. By choosing T cells with specificity only for tumor cells, it should be possible to produce immune-mediated antitumor responses without the corresponding GVHD. There are 2 main strategies for generating tumor-specific T cells. The first involves the gene transfer of TCRs with known specificity into autologous or allogeneic T cells that are then expanded in vitro and infused into patients. This approach has had some successes, most notably in melanoma and the use of Epstein-Barr virus–specific T cells to treat posttransplant lymphoproliferative disorders.[209–211] However, a potential risk of this approach is that the alpha or beta subunit of the transgenic TCR could misassociate with the alpha or beta subunit of the endogenous TCR, resulting in an autoreactive T cell. Furthermore, a particular drawback to widespread clinical use is that the recognition of the tumor antigens is MHC restricted, and therefore the use of these T cells needs to be individualized on a patient-by-patient basis according to their MHC type. A second strategy involves the use of the single-chain variable fragment from an antibody molecule fused with an internal signaling domain such as CD3ζ, to form a CAR.[212] There are 2 important advantages to this approach. First, it eliminates MHC restriction, enabling the same CAR to be used for several different patients. Second, the use of an antibody receptor means that potential targets can be increased to include a wide range of surface proteins, sugars, and lipids.[213]

Several phase I/II clinical trials are underway using anti-CD19 CAR T cells for the treatment of B-cell malignancies.[214] One group has treated 8 patients with CLL in 2 cohorts. The first cohort of 3 patients did not receive any conditioning, and did not show any objective responses. They went on to give the next patient lymphodepleting conditioning with cyclophosphamide as part of the trial design. However, this patient rapidly developed hypotension, respiratory distress, and renal failure, and died within 48 hours of infusion of the T cells, highlighting the risks associated with this therapy.[215] They have gone on to treat a further 4 patients with cyclophosphamide conditioning and a reduced dose of T cells, with 3 out of 4 of the patients showing disease stabilization or LN responses.[216] A second group has investigated the use of anti-CD19 CAR T cells in 8 patients with progressive B-cell malignancies, including 4 patients with CLL. These patients received conditioning with cyclophosphamide and fludarabine, followed by infusion of anti-CD19 CAR T cells. They also received a postinfusion course of IL-2 to enhance in vivo T-cell expansion. Six of the 8 patients obtained objective remissions: of the 4 patients with CLL, 1 had a complete response, 2 had partial responses, and 1 had stable disease. This trial also investigated some of the potential adverse effects associated with the use of CAR T cells. Four out of the 8 patients had increased serum levels of IFN-γ and TNF, which correlated with the severity of acute toxicities. It is likely that the CAR T cells were a source of these inflammatory cytokines because T cells isolated from the patients after treatment produced IFN-γ and TNF-α ex vivo in a CD19-specific manner. These trials underscored the importance of the conditioning regimen in promoting T-cell engraftment and activation. As discussed earlier, it may be vital to use conditioning regimens that deplete the microenvironment of protumoral cell types such as regulatory T cells or immature dendritic cells. One important aspect of forthcoming clinical trials in this area will be the determination of which agents to use in the conditioning regimen, analogous to the impact of conditioning in allogeneic transplantation.

A key finding in preclinical studies of CAR T cells was that their efficacy could be significantly improved by the addition of a costimulatory domain such as CD28.[217] It is becoming apparent that the choice of costimulation can have significant impact on the clinical success of CAR T cell–based therapies. Many of the CAR T cells currently under investigation in clinical trials have incorporated the use of the CD28 costimulatory domain, including the 2 trials discussed earlier.[214] However, in a murine model of primary human pre–B-cell acute lymphoblastic leukemia, human T cells expressing anti-CD19 CARs containing the costimulatory domain CD137 (4-1BB) were significantly more effective and showed longer survival than cells expressing CARs containing the CD28 domain.[218] Furthermore, preclinical data suggest that CD137 is less likely to trigger IL-2 and TNF-α secretion, and hence induction of a cytokine storm and differentiation of regulatory T cells. In light of this, other investigators have trialed the use of anti-CD19 CAR T cells incorporating a CD137 costimulatory domain. A recent report documented a case of a heavily pretreated patient with refractory CLL who entered a complete remission after the adoptive transfer of anti-CD19 CAR T cells. A significant feature of this case was that these cells were still detectable at 6 months after infusion, and had started to express molecules associated with a central memory phenotype, which is known to be important in maintaining robust and persistent antitumor immune responses.[219] A further 2 cases have been reported, 1 of which also achieved complete remission after being heavily pretreated. Although this is encouraging, there remain many unresolved questions. One-hundred and sixty-nine days after infusion, the CAR T cells had high expression of CD45RA, PD-1, and CD57, which may reflect the extensive replication history of these cells leading to T-cell exhaustion and incipient loss of function.[220,221] This situation could lead to treatment failure in the long term and necessitate further infusions of these T cells to maintain clinical responses. Furthermore, the risk associated with profound long-term B-cell lymphopenia and hypogammaglobulinemia is still unknown, and could result in increased susceptibility to infections analogous to Bruton X-linked agammaglobulinemia. As discussed earlier, other issues remain, such as the best time to use these cells, the type of conditioning and costimulatory domain, and which antigen is best to target. The malignant cells may develop the ability to downregulate CD19, necessitating the use of CAR T cells targeting alternative tumor antigens such as CD23 and ROR1, or the use of combinations of CAR T cells specific for a range of antigens.[162,222] However, the potential of CAR T cells, and the possibility of engineering other cell types with CARs such as NK and NK T cells, means that this remains an exciting area of research.[223]

SUMMARY

Improvement in the understanding of the pathogenesis of CLL has resulted in a rapid increase in novel agents in the last decade. A key aspect of CLL is the immunodeficiency associated with this disease, which is a major contributor to patient morbidity and is often exacerbated by current treatments. In light of this, attempts to modulate immune responses are an attractive treatment strategy, because they have the potential to be useful in vulnerable patient subgroups such as the elderly. Furthermore, immune-mediated approaches do not necessarily have to target the tumor cells directly to be effective in the clinic, because reprogramming the microenvironment to remove protective niches, and reducing susceptibility to infections, would all be of potential benefit. There is an ever-expanding range of immune-based therapies that are been developed as a consequence of what is an active and fruitful area of research.

REFERENCES

1. National Cancer Institute. Surveillance epidemiology and end results, SEER stat fact sheets: chronic lymphocytic leukemia; 2012.
2. Hallek M, Fischer K, Fingerle-Rowson G, et al. Addition of rituximab to fludarabine and cyclophosphamide in patients with chronic lymphocytic leukaemia: a randomised, open-label, phase 3 trial. Lancet 2010;376:1164–74.

3. Catovsky D, Miliani E, Okos A, et al. Clinical significance of T-cells in chronic lymphocytic leukaemia. Lancet 1974;2:751–2.
4. Herrmann F, Lochner A, Philippen H, et al. Imbalance of T cell subpopulations in patients with chronic lymphocytic leukaemia of the B cell type. Clin Exp Immunol 1982;49:157–62.
5. Mills KH, Worman CP, Cawley JC. T-cell subsets in B-chronic lymphocytic leukaemia (CLL). Br J Haematol 1982;50:710–2.
6. Platsoucas CD, Galinski M, Kempin S, et al. Abnormal T lymphocyte subpopulations in patients with B cell chronic lymphocytic leukemia: an analysis by monoclonal antibodies. J Immunol 1982;129:2305–12.
7. Lauria F, Foa R, Catovsky D. Increase in T gamma lymphocytes in B-cell chronic lymphocytic leukaemia. Scand J Haematol 1980;24:187–90.
8. Pizzolo G, Chilosi M, Ambrosetti A, et al. Immunohistologic study of bone marrow involvement in B-chronic lymphocytic leukemia. Blood 1983;62:1289–96.
9. Tinhofer I, Marschitz I, Kos M, et al. Differential sensitivity of CD4+ and CD8+ T lymphocytes to the killing efficacy of Fas (Apo-1/CD95) ligand+ tumor cells in B chronic lymphocytic leukemia. Blood 1998;91:4273–81.
10. Nunes C, Wong R, Mason M, et al. Expansion of a CD8(+)PD-1(+) replicative senescence phenotype in early stage CLL patients is associated with inverted CD4:CD8 ratios and disease progression. Clin Cancer Res 2012;18:678–87.
11. te Raa GD, Tonino SH, Remmerswaal EB, et al. Chronic lymphocytic leukemia specific T-cell subset alterations are clone-size dependent and not present in monoclonal B lymphocytosis. Leuk Lymphoma 2012;53:2321–5.
12. Gonzalez-Rodriguez AP, Contesti J, Huergo-Zapico L, et al. Prognostic significance of CD8 and CD4 T cells in chronic lymphocytic leukemia. Leuk Lymphoma 2010;51:1829–36.
13. Chiorazzi N, Fu SM, Montazeri G, et al. T cell helper defect in patients with chronic lymphocytic leukemia. J Immunol 1979;122:1087–90.
14. Lauria F, Foa R, Mantovani V, et al. T-cell functional abnormality in B-chronic lymphocytic leukaemia: evidence of a defect of the T-helper subset. Br J Haematol 1983;54:277–83.
15. Prieto A, Garcia-Suarez J, Reyes E, et al. Diminished DNA synthesis in T cells from B chronic lymphocytic leukemia after phytohemagglutinin, anti-CD3, and phorbol myristate acetate mitogenic signals. Exp Hematol 1993;21:1563–9.
16. Mu X, Kay NE, Gosland MP, et al. Analysis of blood T-cell cytokine expression in B-chronic lymphocytic leukaemia: evidence for increased levels of cytoplasmic IL-4 in resting and activated CD8 T cells. Br J Haematol 1997;96:733–5.
17. Mainou-Fowler T, Proctor SJ, Miller S, et al. Expression and production of interleukin 4 in B-cell chronic lymphocytic leukaemia. Leuk Lymphoma 2001;42:689–98.
18. de Totero D, Reato G, Mauro F, et al. IL4 production and increased CD30 expression by a unique CD8+ T-cell subset in B-cell chronic lymphocytic leukaemia. Br J Haematol 1999;104:589–99.
19. Cerutti A, Kim EC, Shah S, et al. Dysregulation of CD30+ T cells by leukemia impairs isotype switching in normal B cells. Nat Immunol 2001;2:150–6.
20. Dancescu M, Rubio-Trujillo M, Biron G, et al. Interleukin 4 protects chronic lymphocytic leukemic B cells from death by apoptosis and upregulates Bcl-2 expression. J Exp Med 1992;176:1319–26.
21. Panayiotidis P, Ganeshaguru K, Jabbar SA, et al. Interleukin-4 inhibits apoptotic cell death and loss of the bcl-2 protein in B-chronic lymphocytic leukaemia cells in vitro. Br J Haematol 1993;85:439–45.

22. Buggins AG, Patten PE, Richards J, et al. Tumor-derived IL-6 may contribute to the immunological defect in CLL. Leukemia 2008;22:1084–7.
23. Fayad L, Keating MJ, Reuben JM, et al. Interleukin-6 and interleukin-10 levels in chronic lymphocytic leukemia: correlation with phenotypic characteristics and outcome. Blood 2001;97:256–63.
24. Kurzrock R, Redman J, Cabanillas F, et al. Serum interleukin 6 levels are elevated in lymphoma patients and correlate with survival in advanced Hodgkin's disease and with B symptoms. Cancer Res 1993;53:2118–22.
25. Bojarska-Junak A, Rolinski J, Wasik-Szczepaneko E, et al. Intracellular tumor necrosis factor production by T- and B-cells in B-cell chronic lymphocytic leukemia. Haematologica 2002;87:490–9.
26. Gallego A, Vargas JA, Castejon R, et al. Production of intracellular IL-2, TNF-alpha, and IFN-gamma by T cells in B-CLL. Cytometry B Clin Cytom 2003;56: 23–9.
27. Kiaii S, Choudhury A, Mozaffari F, et al. Signaling molecules and cytokine production in T cells of patients with B-cell chronic lymphocytic leukemia (B-CLL): comparison of indolent and progressive disease. Med Oncol 2005; 22:291–302.
28. Podhorecka M, Dmoszynska A, Rolinski J. Intracellular IFN-gamma expression by CD3+/CD8+ cell subset in B-CLL patients correlates with stage of the disease. Eur J Haematol 2004;73:29–35.
29. Zaki M, Douglas R, Patten N, et al. Disruption of the IFN-gamma cytokine network in chronic lymphocytic leukemia contributes to resistance of leukemic B cells to apoptosis. Leuk Res 2000;24:611–21.
30. Buschle M, Campana D, Carding SR, et al. Interferon gamma inhibits apoptotic cell death in B cell chronic lymphocytic leukemia. J Exp Med 1993;177:213–8.
31. Digel W, Stefanic M, Schoniger W, et al. Tumor necrosis factor induces proliferation of neoplastic B cells from chronic lymphocytic leukemia. Blood 1989;73: 1242–6.
32. Lotz M, Ranheim E, Kipps TJ. Transforming growth factor beta as endogenous growth inhibitor of chronic lymphocytic leukemia B cells. J Exp Med 1994;179: 999–1004.
33. Yoshizaki K, Nakagawa T, Kaieda T, et al. Induction of proliferation and Ig production in human B leukemic cells by anti-immunoglobulins and T cell factors. J Immunol 1982;128:1296–301.
34. Mainou-Fowler T, Craig VA, Copplestone JA, et al. Interleukin-5 (IL-5) increases spontaneous apoptosis of B-cell chronic lymphocytic leukemia cells in vitro independently of bcl-2 expression and is inhibited by IL-4. Blood 1994;84: 2297–304.
35. Reittie JE, Yong KL, Panayiotidis P, et al. Interleukin-6 inhibits apoptosis and tumour necrosis factor induced proliferation of B-chronic lymphocytic leukaemia. Leuk Lymphoma 1996;22:83–90.
36. Aderka D, Maor Y, Novick D, et al. Interleukin-6 inhibits the proliferation of B-chronic lymphocytic leukemia cells that is induced by tumor necrosis factor-alpha or -beta. Blood 1993;81:2076–84.
37. Yoshioka R, Shimizu S, Tachibana J, et al. Interleukin-7 (IL-7)-induced proliferation of CD8+ T-chronic lymphocytic leukemia cells. J Clin Immunol 1992;12: 101–6.
38. Long BW, Witte PL, Abraham GN, et al. Apoptosis and interleukin 7 gene expression in chronic B-lymphocytic leukemia cells. Proc Natl Acad Sci U S A 1995;92:1416–20.

39. Tangye SG, Weston KM, Raison RL. Interleukin-10 inhibits the in vitro proliferation of human activated leukemic CD5+ B-cells. Leuk Lymphoma 1998;31: 121–30.

40. Fluckiger AC, Durand I, Banchereau J. Interleukin 10 induces apoptotic cell death of B-chronic lymphocytic leukemia cells. J Exp Med 1994;179:91–9.

41. di Carlo E, de Totero D, Piazza T, et al. Role of IL-21 in immune-regulation and tumor immunotherapy. Cancer Immunol Immunother 2007;56:1323–34.

42. Van den Hove LE, Van Gool SW, Vandenberghe P, et al. CD57+/CD28- T cells in untreated hemato-oncological patients are expanded and display a Th1-type cytokine secretion profile, ex vivo cytolytic activity and enhanced tendency to apoptosis. Leukemia 1998;12:1573–82.

43. Van den Hove LE, Vandenberghe P, Van Gool SW, et al. Peripheral blood lymphocyte subset shifts in patients with untreated hematological tumors: evidence for systemic activation of the T cell compartment. Leuk Res 1998;22: 175–84.

44. Velardi A, Prchal JT, Prasthofer EF, et al. Expression of NK-lineage markers on peripheral blood lymphocytes with T-helper (Leu3+/T4+) phenotype in B cell chronic lymphocytic leukemia. Blood 1985;65:149–55.

45. Rossi E, Matutes E, Morilla R, et al. Zeta chain and CD28 are poorly expressed on T lymphocytes from chronic lymphocytic leukemia. Leukemia 1996;10:494–7.

46. Farace F, Orlanducci F, Dietrich PY, et al. T cell repertoire in patients with B chronic lymphocytic leukemia. Evidence for multiple in vivo T cell clonal expansions. J Immunol 1994;153:4281–90.

47. Goolsby CL, Kuchnio M, Finn WG, et al. Expansions of clonal and oligoclonal T cells in B-cell chronic lymphocytic leukemia are primarily restricted to the CD3(+)CD8(+) T-cell population. Cytometry 2000;42:188–95.

48. Rezvany MR, Jeddi-Tehrani M, Osterborg A, et al. Oligoclonal TCRBV gene usage in B-cell chronic lymphocytic leukemia: major perturbations are preferentially seen within the CD4 T-cell subset. Blood 1999;94:1063–9.

49. Wen T, Mellstedt H, Jondal M. Presence of clonal T cell populations in chronic B lymphocytic leukemia and smoldering myeloma. J Exp Med 1990;171:659–66.

50. Serrano D, Monteiro J, Allen SL, et al. Clonal expansion within the CD4+CD57+ and CD8+CD57+ T cell subsets in chronic lymphocytic leukemia. J Immunol 1997;158:1482–9.

51. Chidrawar S, Khan N, Wei W, et al. Cytomegalovirus-seropositivity has a profound influence on the magnitude of major lymphoid subsets within healthy individuals. Clin Exp Immunol 2009;155:423–32.

52. Khan N, Shariff N, Cobbold M, et al. Cytomegalovirus seropositivity drives the CD8 T cell repertoire toward greater clonality in healthy elderly individuals. J Immunol 2002;169:1984–92.

53. Mackus WJ, Frakking FN, Grummels A, et al. Expansion of CMV-specific CD8+CD45RA+CD27- T cells in B-cell chronic lymphocytic leukemia. Blood 2003;102:1057–63.

54. Pourgheysari B, Bruton R, Parry H, et al. The number of cytomegalovirus-specific CD4+ T cells is markedly expanded in patients with B-cell chronic lymphocytic leukemia and determines the total CD4+ T-cell repertoire. Blood 2010;116:2968–74.

55. Walton JA, Lydyard PM, Nathwani A, et al. Patients with B cell chronic lymphocytic leukaemia have an expanded population of CD4 perforin expressing T cells enriched for human cytomegalovirus specificity and an effector-memory phenotype. Br J Haematol 2010;148:274–84.

56. Gorgun G, Holderried TA, Zahrieh D, et al. Chronic lymphocytic leukemia cells induce changes in gene expression of CD4 and CD8 T cells. J Clin Invest 2005; 115:1797–805.

57. Ramsay AG, Johnson AJ, Lee AM, et al. Chronic lymphocytic leukemia T cells show impaired immunological synapse formation that can be reversed with an immunomodulating drug. J Clin Invest 2008;118:2427–37.

58. Bichi R, Shinton SA, Martin ES, et al. Human chronic lymphocytic leukemia modeled in mouse by targeted TCL1 expression. Proc Natl Acad Sci U S A 2002;99:6955–60.

59. Gorgun G, Ramsay AG, Holderried TA, et al. E(mu)-TCL1 mice represent a model for immunotherapeutic reversal of chronic lymphocytic leukemia-induced T-cell dysfunction. Proc Natl Acad Sci U S A 2009;106:6250–5.

60. Hofbauer JP, Heyder C, Denk U, et al. Development of CLL in the TCL1 transgenic mouse model is associated with severe skewing of the T-cell compartment homologous to human CLL. Leukemia 2011;25:1452–8.

61. Ramsay AG, Clear AJ, Fatah R, et al. Multiple inhibitory ligands induce impaired T cell immunological synapse function in chronic lymphocytic leukemia that can be blocked with lenalidomide. Blood 2012;120:1412–21.

62. Freeman GJ, Long AJ, Iwai Y, et al. Engagement of the PD-1 immunoinhibitory receptor by a novel B7 family member leads to negative regulation of lymphocyte activation. J Exp Med 2000;192:1027–34.

63. Tonino SH, van de Berg PJ, Yong SL, et al. Expansion of effector T cells associated with decreased PD-1 expression in patients with indolent B cell lymphomas and chronic lymphocytic leukemia. Leuk Lymphoma 2012;53:1785–94.

64. Cai G, Anumanthan A, Brown JA, et al. CD160 inhibits activation of human CD4+ T cells through interaction with herpesvirus entry mediator. Nat Immunol 2008;9:176–85.

65. Anumanthan A, Bensussan A, Boumsell L, et al. Cloning of BY55, a novel Ig superfamily member expressed on NK cells, CTL, and intestinal intraepithelial lymphocytes. J Immunol 1998;161:2780–90.

66. Junevik K, Werlenius O, Hasselblom S, et al. The expression of NK cell inhibitory receptors on cytotoxic T cells in B-cell chronic lymphocytic leukaemia (B-CLL). Ann Hematol 2007;86:89–94.

67. Curiel TJ, Coukos G, Zou L, et al. Specific recruitment of regulatory T cells in ovarian carcinoma fosters immune privilege and predicts reduced survival. Nat Med 2004;10:942–9.

68. Baecher-Allan C, Viglietta V, Hafler DA. Human CD4+CD25+ regulatory T cells. Semin Immunol 2004;16:89–98.

69. Jak M, Mous R, Remmerswaal EB, et al. Enhanced formation and survival of CD4+ CD25hi Foxp3+ T-cells in chronic lymphocytic leukemia. Leuk Lymphoma 2009; 50:788–801.

70. Gorczynski RM, Lee L, Boudakov I. Augmented induction of CD4+CD25+ Treg using monoclonal antibodies to CD200R. Transplantation 2005;79:1180–3.

71. Pallasch CP, Ulbrich S, Brinker R, et al. Disruption of T cell suppression in chronic lymphocytic leukemia by CD200 blockade. Leuk Res 2009;33:460–4.

72. Beyer M, Kochanek M, Darabi K, et al. Reduced frequencies and suppressive function of CD4+CD25hi regulatory T cells in patients with chronic lymphocytic leukemia after therapy with fludarabine. Blood 2005;106:2018–25.

73. Giannopoulos K, Schmitt M, Kowal M, et al. Characterization of regulatory T cells in patients with B-cell chronic lymphocytic leukemia. Oncol Rep 2008;20: 677–82.

74. Piper KP, Karanth M, McLarnon A, et al. Chronic lymphocytic leukaemia cells drive the global CD4+ T cell repertoire towards a regulatory phenotype and leads to the accumulation of CD4+ forkhead box P3+ T cells. Clin Exp Immunol 2011;166:154–63.

75. D'Arena G, Laurenti L, Minervini MM, et al. Regulatory T-cell number is increased in chronic lymphocytic leukemia patients and correlates with progressive disease. Leuk Res 2011;35:363–8.

76. D'Arena G, Rossi G, Minervini MM, et al. Circulating regulatory T cells in "clinical" monoclonal B-cell lymphocytosis. Int J Immunopathol Pharmacol 2011; 24:915–23.

77. D'Arena G, D'Auria F, Simeon V, et al. A shorter time to the first treatment may be predicted by the absolute number of regulatory T-cells in patients with Rai stage 0 chronic lymphocytic leukemia. Am J Hematol 2012;87:628–31.

78. Weiss L, Melchardt T, Egle A, et al. Regulatory T cells predict the time to initial treatment in early stage chronic lymphocytic leukemia. Cancer 2011;117:2163–9.

79. Perry C, Hazan-Halevy I, Kay S, et al. Increased CD39 expression on CD4(+) T lymphocytes has clinical and prognostic significance in chronic lymphocytic leukemia. Ann Hematol 2012;91:1271–9.

80. Pulte D, Furman RR, Broekman MJ, et al. CD39 expression on T lymphocytes correlates with severity of disease in patients with chronic lymphocytic leukemia. Clin Lymphoma Myeloma Leuk 2011;11:367–72.

81. Lee KM, Chuang E, Griffin M, et al. Molecular basis of T cell inactivation by CTLA-4. Science 1998;282:2263–6.

82. van der Merwe PA, Bodian DL, Daenke S, et al. CD80 (B7-1) binds both CD28 and CTLA-4 with a low affinity and very fast kinetics. J Exp Med 1997;185: 393–403.

83. Motta M, Rassenti L, Shelvin BJ, et al. Increased expression of CD152 (CTLA-4) by normal T lymphocytes in untreated patients with B-cell chronic lymphocytic leukemia. Leukemia 2005;19:1788–93.

84. Frydecka I, Kosmaczewska A, Bocko D, et al. Alterations of the expression of T-cell-related costimulatory CD28 and downregulatory CD152 (CTLA-4) molecules in patients with B-cell chronic lymphocytic leukaemia. Br J Cancer 2004;90:2042–8.

85. Ghia P, Strola G, Granziero L, et al. Chronic lymphocytic leukemia B cells are endowed with the capacity to attract CD4+, CD40L+ T cells by producing CCL22. Eur J Immunol 2002;32:1403–13.

86. Bagnara D, Kaufman MS, Calissano C, et al. A novel adoptive transfer model of chronic lymphocytic leukemia suggests a key role for T lymphocytes in the disease. Blood 2011;117:5463–72.

87. Burger JA, Tsukada N, Burger M, et al. Blood-derived nurse-like cells protect chronic lymphocytic leukemia B cells from spontaneous apoptosis through stromal cell-derived factor-1. Blood 2000;96:2655–63.

88. Farinha P, Masoudi H, Skinnider BF, et al. Analysis of multiple biomarkers shows that lymphoma-associated macrophage (LAM) content is an independent predictor of survival in follicular lymphoma (FL). Blood 2005;106:2169–74.

89. Tsukada N, Burger JA, Zvaifler NJ, et al. Distinctive features of "nurselike" cells that differentiate in the context of chronic lymphocytic leukemia. Blood 2002;99: 1030–7.

90. Collins RJ, Verschuer LA, Harmon BV, et al. Spontaneous programmed death (apoptosis) of B-chronic lymphocytic leukaemia cells following their culture in vitro. Br J Haematol 1989;71:343–50.

91. Nishio M, Endo T, Tsukada N, et al. Nurselike cells express BAFF and APRIL, which can promote survival of chronic lymphocytic leukemia cells via a paracrine pathway distinct from that of SDF-1alpha. Blood 2005;106:1012–20.
92. Bhattacharya N, Diener S, Idler IS, et al. Nurse-like cells show deregulated expression of genes involved in immunocompetence. Br J Haematol 2011; 154:349–56.
93. Ghobrial IM, Bone ND, Stenson MJ, et al. Expression of the chemokine receptors CXCR4 and CCR7 and disease progression in B-cell chronic lymphocytic leukemia/small lymphocytic lymphoma. Mayo Clin Proc 2004;79:318–25.
94. Burger JA, Burger M, Kipps TJ. Chronic lymphocytic leukemia B cells express functional CXCR4 chemokine receptors that mediate spontaneous migration beneath bone marrow stromal cells. Blood 1999;94:3658–67.
95. Burger JA, Quiroga MP, Hartmann E, et al. High-level expression of the T-cell chemokines CCL3 and CCL4 by chronic lymphocytic leukemia B cells in nurse-like cell cocultures and after BCR stimulation. Blood 2009;113:3050–8.
96. Sivina M, Hartmann E, Kipps TJ, et al. CCL3 (MIP-1alpha) plasma levels and the risk for disease progression in chronic lymphocytic leukemia. Blood 2011;117:1662–9.
97. Borge M, Nannini PR, Morande PE, et al. CXCL12 is a costimulator for CD4(+) T cell activation and proliferation in chronic lymphocytic leukemia patients. Cancer Immunol Immunother 2013;62:113–24.
98. Burger JA. Chemokines and chemokine receptors in chronic lymphocytic leukemia (CLL): from understanding the basics towards therapeutic targeting. Semin Cancer Biol 2010;20:424–30.
99. Ziegler HW, Kay NE, Zarling JM. Deficiency of natural killer cell activity in patients with chronic lymphocytic leukemia. Int J Cancer 1981;27:321–7.
100. Kay NE, Zarling JM. Impaired natural killer activity in patients with chronic lymphocytic leukemia is associated with a deficiency of azurophilic cytoplasmic granules in putative NK cells. Blood 1984;63:305–9.
101. Kay NE, Zarling J. Restoration of impaired natural killer cell activity of B-chronic lymphocytic leukemia patients by recombinant interleukin-2. Am J Hematol 1987;24:161–7.
102. Burton JD, Weitz CH, Kay NE. Malignant chronic lymphocytic leukemia B cells elaborate soluble factors that down-regulate T cell and NK function. Am J Hematol 1989;30:61–7.
103. Katrinakis G, Kyriakou D, Papadaki H, et al. Defective natural killer cell activity in B-cell chronic lymphocytic leukaemia is associated with impaired release of natural killer cytotoxic factor(s) but not of tumour necrosis factor-alpha. Acta Haematol 1996;96:16–23.
104. Maki G, Hayes GM, Naji A, et al. NK resistance of tumor cells from multiple myeloma and chronic lymphocytic leukemia patients: implication of HLA-G. Leukemia 2008;22:998–1006.
105. Buechele C, Baessler T, Schmiedel BJ, et al. 4-1BB ligand modulates direct and rituximab-induced NK-cell reactivity in chronic lymphocytic leukemia. Eur J Immunol 2012;42:737–48.
106. Gaidarova S, Li J, Corral LG, et al. Lenalidomide alone and in combination with rituximab enhances NK cell immune synapse formation in chronic lymphocytic leukemia (CLL) cells in vitro through activation of Rho and Rac1 GTPases [abstract 3441]. Blood 2009;114.
107. Palmer S, Hanson CA, Zent CS, et al. Prognostic importance of T and NK-cells in a consecutive series of newly diagnosed patients with chronic lymphocytic leukaemia. Br J Haematol 2008;141:607–14.

108. Kimby E, Mellstedt H, Nilsson B, et al. Differences in blood T and NK cell populations between chronic lymphocytic leukemia of B cell type (B-CLL) and monoclonal B-lymphocytosis of undetermined significance (B-MLUS). Leukemia 1989;3:501–4.

109. Bojarska-Junak A, Hus I, Sieklucka M, et al. Natural killer-like T CD3+/CD16+CD56+ cells in chronic lymphocytic leukemia: intracellular cytokine expression and relationship with clinical outcome. Oncol Rep 2010;24:803–10.

110. Guven H, Gilljam M, Chambers BJ, et al. Expansion of natural killer (NK) and natural killer-like T (NKT)-cell populations derived from patients with B-chronic lymphocytic leukemia (B-CLL): a potential source for cellular immunotherapy. Leukemia 2003;17:1973–80.

111. Zeya HI, Keku E, Richards F 2nd, et al. Monocyte and granulocyte defect in chronic lymphocytic leukemia. Am J Pathol 1979;95:43–54.

112. Sawicka-Powierza J, Jablonska E, Kloczko J, et al. Evaluation of TNF super-family molecules release by neutrophils and B leukemic cells of patients with chronic B-cell lymphocytic leukemia. Neoplasma 2011;58:45–50.

113. Gassner FJ, Weiss L, Geisberger R, et al. Fludarabine modulates composition and function of the T cell pool in patients with chronic lymphocytic leukaemia. Cancer Immunol Immunother 2011;60:75–85.

114. Maloney DG. Mechanism of action of rituximab. Anticancer Drugs 2001; 12(Suppl 2):S1–4.

115. Smyth MJ, Hayakawa Y, Takeda K, et al. New aspects of natural-killer-cell surveillance and therapy of cancer. Nat Rev Cancer 2002;2:850–61.

116. Fischer L, Penack O, Gentilini C, et al. The anti-lymphoma effect of antibody-mediated immunotherapy is based on an increased degranulation of peripheral blood natural killer (NK) cells. Exp Hematol 2006;34:753–9.

117. Weng WK, Levy R. Two immunoglobulin G fragment C receptor polymorphisms independently predict response to rituximab in patients with follicular lymphoma. J Clin Oncol 2003;21:3940–7.

118. Bologna L, Gotti E, Manganini M, et al. Mechanism of action of type II, glycoengineered, anti-CD20 monoclonal antibody GA101 in B-chronic lymphocytic leukemia whole blood assays in comparison with rituximab and alemtuzumab. J Immunol 2011;186:3762–9.

119. Le Garff-Tavernier M, Decocq J, de Romeuf C, et al. Analysis of CD16+CD56dim NK cells from CLL patients: evidence supporting a therapeutic strategy with optimized anti-CD20 monoclonal antibodies. Leukemia 2011;25:101–9.

120. Eskelund CW, Nederby L, Thysen AH, et al. Interleukin-21 and rituximab enhance NK cell functionality in patients with B-cell chronic lymphocytic leukaemia. Leuk Res 2011;35:914–20.

121. Moga E, Canto E, Vidal S, et al. Interleukin-15 enhances rituximab-dependent cytotoxicity against chronic lymphocytic leukemia cells and overcomes transforming growth factor beta-mediated immunosuppression. Exp Hematol 2011; 39:1064–71.

122. Lefebvre ML, Krause SW, Salcedo M, et al. Ex vivo-activated human macrophages kill chronic lymphocytic leukemia cells in the presence of rituximab: mechanism of antibody-dependent cellular cytotoxicity and impact of human serum. J Immunother 2006;29:388–97.

123. Hamblin TJ, Davis Z, Gardiner A, et al. Unmutated Ig V(H) genes are associated with a more aggressive form of chronic lymphocytic leukemia. Blood 1999;94:1848–54.

124. Wiestner A, Rosenwald A, Barry TS, et al. ZAP-70 expression identifies a chronic lymphocytic leukemia subtype with unmutated immunoglobulin genes, inferior clinical outcome, and distinct gene expression profile. Blood 2003;101:4944–51.

125. Minden MD, Ubelhart R, Schneider D, et al. Chronic lymphocytic leukaemia is driven by antigen-independent cell-autonomous signalling. Nature 2012;489: 309–12.

126. Flinn IW, Schreeder MT, Wagner-Johnson ND, et al. A phase 1 study of CAL-101, an isoform-selective inhibitor of phosphatidylinositol 3-kinase P110d, in combination with rituximab and/or bendamustine in patients with relapsed or refractory B-cell malignancies [abstract 2832]. Blood 2010;116.

127. Zent CS, LaPlant BR, Johnston PB, et al. The treatment of recurrent/refractory chronic lymphocytic leukemia/small lymphocytic lymphoma (CLL) with everolimus results in clinical responses and mobilization of CLL cells into the circulation. Cancer 2010;116:2201–7.

128. Burger J, O'Brien S, Fowler N, et al. The Bruton's tyrosine kinase inhibitor, PCI-32765, is well tolerated and demonstrates promising clinical activity in chronic lymphocytic leukemia (CLL) and small lymphocytic lymphoma (SLL): an update on ongoing phase 1 studies [abstract 57]. Blood 2010;116.

129. Andritsos L, Byrd JC, Jones J, et al. Preliminary results from a phase I dose escalation study to determine the maximum tolerated dose of plerixafor in combination with rituximab in patients with relapsed chronic lymphocytic leukemia [abstract 2450]. Blood 2010;116.

130. Hoellenriegel J, Meadows SA, Wierda W, et al. Phosphoinositide 3'-kinase (PI3K) delta inhibition with CAL-101 blocks B-cell receptor (BCR) signaling and the prosurvival actions of nurselike cells (NLC), in chronic lymphocytic leukemia [abstract 48]. Blood 2010;116.

131. Ponader S, Chen SS, Buggy JJ, et al. The Bruton tyrosine kinase inhibitor PCI-32765 thwarts chronic lymphocytic leukemia cell survival and tissue homing in vitro and in vivo. Blood 2012;119:1182–9.

132. Dazzi F, D'Andrea E, Biasi G, et al. Failure of B cells of chronic lymphocytic leukemia in presenting soluble and alloantigens. Clin Immunol Immunopathol 1995;75:26–32.

133. Yellin MJ, Sinning J, Covey LR, et al. T lymphocyte T cell-B cell-activating molecule/CD40-L molecules induce normal B cells or chronic lymphocytic leukemia B cells to express CD80 (B7/BB-1) and enhance their costimulatory activity. J Immunol 1994;153:666–74.

134. Ranheim EA, Kipps TJ. Activated T cells induce expression of B7/BB1 on normal or leukemic B cells through a CD40-dependent signal. J Exp Med 1993;177: 925–35.

135. Van den Hove LE, Van Gool SW, Vandenberghe P, et al. CD40 triggering of chronic lymphocytic leukemia B cells results in efficient alloantigen presentation and cytotoxic T lymphocyte induction by up-regulation of CD80 and CD86 costimulatory molecules. Leukemia 1997;11:572–80.

136. Noelle RJ, Roy M, Shepherd DM, et al. 39-kDa protein on activated helper T cells binds CD40 and transduces the signal for cognate activation of B cells. Proc Natl Acad Sci U S A 1992;89:6550–4.

137. Cantwell M, Hua T, Pappas J, et al. Acquired CD40-ligand deficiency in chronic lymphocytic leukemia. Nat Med 1997;3:984–9.

138. Kato K, Cantwell MJ, Sharma S, et al. Gene transfer of CD40-ligand induces autologous immune recognition of chronic lymphocytic leukemia B cells. J Clin Invest 1998;101:1133–41.

139. Takahashi S, Rousseau RF, Yotnda P, et al. Autologous antileukemic immune response induced by chronic lymphocytic leukemia B cells expressing the CD40 ligand and interleukin 2 transgenes. Hum Gene Ther 2001;12:659–70.

140. Buhmann R, Nolte A, Westhaus D, et al. CD40-activated B-cell chronic lymphocytic leukemia cells for tumor immunotherapy: stimulation of allogeneic versus autologous T cells generates different types of effector cells. Blood 1999;93:1992–2002.

141. Biagi E, Dotti G, Yvon E, et al. Molecular transfer of CD40 and OX40 ligands to leukemic human B cells induces expansion of autologous tumor-reactive cytotoxic T lymphocytes. Blood 2005;105:2436–42.

142. Romano MF, Lamberti A, Tassone P, et al. Triggering of CD40 antigen inhibits fludarabine-induced apoptosis in B chronic lymphocytic leukemia cells. Blood 1998;92:990–5.

143. Gricks CS, Zahrieh D, Zauls AJ, et al. Differential regulation of gene expression following CD40 activation of leukemic compared to healthy B cells. Blood 2004; 104:4002–9.

144. Chu P, Wierda WG, Kipps TJ. CD40 activation does not protect chronic lymphocytic leukemia B cells from apoptosis induced by cytotoxic T lymphocytes. Blood 2000;95:3853–8.

145. Kater AP, Evers LM, Remmerswaal EB, et al. CD40 stimulation of B-cell chronic lymphocytic leukaemia cells enhances the anti-apoptotic profile, but also Bid expression and cells remain susceptible to autologous cytotoxic T-lymphocyte attack. Br J Haematol 2004;127:404–15.

146. Wierda WG, Cantwell MJ, Woods SJ, et al. CD40-ligand (CD154) gene therapy for chronic lymphocytic leukemia. Blood 2000;96:2917–24.

147. Wierda WG, Castro JE, Aguillon R, et al. A phase I study of immune gene therapy for patients with CLL using a membrane-stable, humanized CD154. Leukemia 2010;24:1893–900.

148. Jak M, van Bochove GG, van Lier RA, et al. CD40 stimulation sensitizes CLL cells to rituximab-induced cell death. Leukemia 2011;25:968–78.

149. Scielzo C, Apollonio B, Scarfo L, et al. The functional in vitro response to CD40 ligation reflects a different clinical outcome in patients with chronic lymphocytic leukemia. Leukemia 2011;25:1760–7.

150. Law CL, Gordon KA, Collier J, et al. Preclinical antilymphoma activity of a humanized anti-CD40 monoclonal antibody, SGN-40. Cancer Res 2005;65:8331–8.

151. Luqman M, Klabunde S, Lin K, et al. The antileukemia activity of a human anti-CD40 antagonist antibody, HCD122, on human chronic lymphocytic leukemia cells. Blood 2008;112:711–20.

152. Byrd JC, Kipps TJ, Flinn IW, et al. Phase I study of the anti-CD40 humanized monoclonal antibody lucatumumab (HCD122) in relapsed chronic lymphocytic leukemia. Leuk Lymphoma 2012;53:2136–42.

153. Furman RR, Forero-Torres A, Shustov A, et al. A phase I study of dacetuzumab (SGN-40, a humanized anti-CD40 monoclonal antibody) in patients with chronic lymphocytic leukemia. Leuk Lymphoma 2010;51:228–35.

154. Lapalombella R, Gowda A, Joshi T, et al. The humanized CD40 antibody SGN-40 demonstrates pre-clinical activity that is enhanced by lenalidomide in chronic lymphocytic leukaemia. Br J Haematol 2009;144:848–55.

155. Krackhardt AM, Witzens M, Harig S, et al. Identification of tumor-associated antigens in chronic lymphocytic leukemia by SEREX. Blood 2002;100:2123–31.

156. Schmidt SM, Schag K, Muller MR, et al. Survivin is a shared tumor-associated antigen expressed in a broad variety of malignancies and recognized by specific cytotoxic T cells. Blood 2003;102:571–6.

157. Giannopoulos K, Li L, Bojarska-Junak A, et al. Expression of RHAMM/CD168 and other tumor-associated antigens in patients with B-cell chronic lymphocytic leukemia. Int J Oncol 2006;29:95–103.

158. Mayr C, Bund D, Schlee M, et al. MDM2 is recognized as a tumor-associated antigen in chronic lymphocytic leukemia by CD8+ autologous T lymphocytes. Exp Hematol 2006;34:44–53.

159. Favaro PM, de Souza Medina S, Traina F, et al. Human leukocyte formin: a novel protein expressed in lymphoid malignancies and associated with Akt. Biochem Biophys Res Commun 2003;311:365–71.

160. Mayr C, Bund D, Schlee M, et al. Fibromodulin as a novel tumor-associated antigen (TAA) in chronic lymphocytic leukemia (CLL), which allows expansion of specific CD8+ autologous T lymphocytes. Blood 2005;105:1566–73.

161. Bund D, Mayr C, Kofler DM, et al. CD23 is recognized as tumor-associated antigen (TAA) in B-CLL by CD8+ autologous T lymphocytes. Exp Hematol 2007;35:920–30.

162. Hudecek M, Schmitt TM, Baskar S, et al. The B-cell tumor associated antigen ROR1 can be targeted with T-cells modified to express a ROR1-specific chimeric antigen receptor. Blood 2010;116:4532–41.

163. Fukuda T, Chen L, Endo T, et al. Antisera induced by infusions of autologous Ad-CD154-leukemia B cells identify ROR1 as an oncofetal antigen and receptor for Wnt5a. Proc Natl Acad Sci U S A 2008;105:3047–52.

164. Lapalombella R, Andritsos L, Liu Q, et al. Lenalidomide treatment promotes CD154 expression on CLL cells and enhances production of antibodies by normal B cells through a PI3-kinase dependent pathway. Blood 2009;115:2619–29.

165. Janeway CA Jr, Sakato N, Eisen HN. Recognition of immunoglobulin idiotypes by thymus-derived lymphocytes. Proc Natl Acad Sci U S A 1975;72:2357–60.

166. Trojan A, Schultze JL, Witzens M, et al. Immunoglobulin framework-derived peptides function as cytotoxic T-cell epitopes commonly expressed in B-cell malignancies. Nat Med 2000;6:667–72.

167. Kwak LW, Campbell MJ, Czerwinski DK, et al. Induction of immune responses in patients with B-cell lymphoma against the surface-immunoglobulin idiotype expressed by their tumors. N Engl J Med 1992;327:1209–15.

168. Hsu FJ, Caspar CB, Czerwinski D, et al. Tumor-specific idiotype vaccines in the treatment of patients with B-cell lymphoma–long-term results of a clinical trial. Blood 1997;89:3129–35.

169. Harig S, Witzens M, Krackhardt AM, et al. Induction of cytotoxic T-cell responses against immunoglobulin V region-derived peptides modified at human leukocyte antigen-A2 binding residues. Blood 2001;98:2999–3005.

170. Hus I, Rolinski J, Tabarkiewicz J, et al. Allogeneic dendritic cells pulsed with tumor lysates or apoptotic bodies as immunotherapy for patients with early-stage B-cell chronic lymphocytic leukemia. Leukemia 2005;19:1621–7.

171. Hus I, Schmitt M, Tabarkiewicz J, et al. Vaccination of B-CLL patients with autologous dendritic cells can change the frequency of leukemia antigen-specific CD8+ T cells as well as CD4+CD25+FoxP3+ regulatory T cells toward an anti-leukemia response. Leukemia 2008;22:1007–17.

172. Spaner DE, Hammond C, Mena J, et al. A phase I/II trial of oxidized autologous tumor vaccines during the "watch and wait" phase of chronic lymphocytic leukemia. Cancer Immunol Immunother 2005;54:635–46.

173. Chen CI, Bergsagel PL, Paul H, et al. Single-agent lenalidomide in the treatment of previously untreated chronic lymphocytic leukemia. J Clin Oncol 2010;29:1175–81.

174. Corral LG, Haslett PA, Muller GW, et al. Differential cytokine modulation and T cell activation by two distinct classes of thalidomide analogues that are potent inhibitors of TNF-alpha. J Immunol 1999;163:380–6.

175. LeBlanc R, Hideshima T, Catley LP, et al. Immunomodulatory drug costimulates T cells via the B7-CD28 pathway. Blood 2004;103:1787–90.
176. Haslett PA, Hanekom WA, Muller G, et al. Thalidomide and a thalidomide analogue drug costimulate virus-specific CD8+ T cells in vitro. J Infect Dis 2003;187:946–55.
177. Xu Y, Li J, Ferguson GD, et al. Immunomodulatory drugs reorganize cytoskeleton by modulating Rho GTPases. Blood 2009;114:338–45.
178. Chanan-Khan AA, Cheson BD. Lenalidomide for the treatment of B-cell malignancies. J Clin Oncol 2008;26:1544–52.
179. Andritsos LA, Johnson AJ, Lozanski G, et al. Higher doses of lenalidomide are associated with unacceptable toxicity including life-threatening tumor flare in patients with chronic lymphocytic leukemia. J Clin Oncol 2008;26:2519–25.
180. Aue G, Njuguna N, Tian X, et al. Lenalidomide-induced upregulation of CD80 on tumor cells correlates with T-cell activation, the rapid onset of a cytokine release syndrome and leukemic cell clearance in chronic lymphocytic leukemia. Haematologica 2009;94:1266–73.
181. Chanan-Khan A, Miller KC, Lawrence D, et al. Tumor flare reaction associated with lenalidomide treatment in patients with chronic lymphocytic leukemia predicts clinical response. Cancer 2010;117:2127–35.
182. Galustian C, Meyer B, Labarthe MC, et al. The anti-cancer agents lenalidomide and pomalidomide inhibit the proliferation and function of T regulatory cells. Cancer Immunol Immunother 2009;58:1033–45.
183. Idler I, Giannopoulos K, Zenz T, et al. Lenalidomide treatment of chronic lymphocytic leukaemia patients reduces regulatory T cells and induces Th17 T helper cells. Br J Haematol 2009;148:948–50.
184. Dauguet N, Fournie JJ, Poupot R, et al. Lenalidomide down regulates the production of interferon-gamma and the expression of inhibitory cytotoxic receptors of human natural killer cells. Cell Immunol 2010;264:163–70.
185. Chang DH, Liu N, Klimek V, et al. Enhancement of ligand-dependent activation of human natural killer T cells by lenalidomide: therapeutic implications. Blood 2006;108:618–21.
186. Wu L, Adams M, Carter T, et al. lenalidomide enhances natural killer cell and monocyte-mediated antibody-dependent cellular cytotoxicity of rituximab-treated CD20+ tumor cells. Clin Cancer Res 2008;14:4650–7.
187. Ito T, Ando H, Suzuki T, et al. Identification of a primary target of thalidomide teratogenicity. Science 2010;327:1345–50.
188. Hohberger B, Enz R. Cereblon is expressed in the retina and binds to voltage-gated chloride channels. FEBS Lett 2009;583:633–7.
189. Jo S, Lee KH, Song S, et al. Identification and functional characterization of cereblon as a binding protein for large-conductance calcium-activated potassium channel in rat brain. J Neurochem 2005;94:1212–24.
190. Lee KM, Jo S, Kim H, et al. Functional modulation of AMP-activated protein kinase by cereblon. Biochim Biophys Acta 2011;1813:448–55.
191. Higgins JJ, Hao J, Kosofsky BE, et al. Dysregulation of large-conductance Ca2+-activated K+ channel expression in nonsyndromal mental retardation due to a cereblon p.R419X mutation. Neurogenetics 2008;9:219–23.
192. Zhu YX, Braggio E, Shi CX, et al. Cereblon expression is required for the antimyeloma activity of lenalidomide and pomalidomide. Blood 2011;118:4771–9.
193. Chanan-Khan A, Porter CW. Immunomodulating drugs for chronic lymphocytic leukaemia. Lancet Oncol 2006;7:480–8.

194. Lopez-Girona A, Mendy D, Ito T, et al. Cereblon is a direct protein target for immunomodulatory and antiproliferative activities of lenalidomide and pomalidomide. Leukemia 2012;26:2326–35.
195. Sher T, Miller KC, Lawrence D, et al. Efficacy of lenalidomide in patients with chronic lymphocytic leukemia with high-risk cytogenetics. Leuk Lymphoma 2010;51:85–8.
196. Badoux XC, Keating MJ, Wen S, et al. Lenalidomide as initial therapy of elderly patients with chronic lymphocytic leukemia. Blood 2011;118:3489–98.
197. Brown JR, Abramson J, Hochberg E, et al. A phase I study of lenalidomide in combination with fludarabine and rituximab in previously untreated CLL/SLL. Leukemia 2010;24:1972–5.
198. Arumainathan A, Kalakonda N, Pettitt AR. Lenalidomide can be highly effective in chronic lymphocytic leukaemia despite T-cell depletion and deletion of chromosome 17p. Eur J Haematol 2011;87:372–5.
199. Ferrajoli A, Badoux XC, O'Brien S, et al. The combination of lenalidomide and rituximab induces complete and partial responses in patients with relapsed and refractory chronic lymphocytic leukemia [abstract 1395]. Blood 2010;116.
200. Badoux XC, Keating M, O'Brien S, et al. Final analysis if a phase 2 study of lenalidomide and rituximab in patients with relapsed or refractory chronic lymphocytic leukemia (CLL) [abstract 980]. Blood 2011;118.
201. Ferrajoli A, O'Brien S, Wierda W, et al. Combination therapy with ofatumumab and lenalidomide in patients with relapsed chronic lymphocytic leukemia (CLL): results of a phase II trial [abstract 1788]. Blood 2011;118.
202. James DF, Brown JR, Werner L, et al. Lenalidomide and rituximab for the initial treatment of patients with chronic lymphocytic leukemia (CLL): a multicenter study of the CLL Research Consortium [abstract 291]. Blood 2011;118.
203. Shanafelt TD, Tun H, Hanson CA, et al. Lenalidomide consolidation after first-line chemoimmunotherapy for patients with previously untreated CLL [abstract 1379]. Blood 2010;116.
204. Kolb HJ. Graft-versus-leukemia effects of transplantation and donor lymphocytes. Blood 2008;112:4371–83.
205. Michallet M, Archimbaud E, Bandini G, et al. HLA-identical sibling bone marrow transplantation in younger patients with chronic lymphocytic leukemia. European Group for Blood and Marrow Transplantation and the International Bone Marrow Transplant Registry. Ann Intern Med 1996;124:311–5.
206. Schetelig J, Thiede C, Bornhauser M, et al. Evidence of a graft-versus-leukemia effect in chronic lymphocytic leukemia after reduced-intensity conditioning and allogeneic stem-cell transplantation: the Cooperative German Transplant Study Group. J Clin Oncol 2003;21:2747–53.
207. Dreger P, Brand R, Hansz J, et al. Treatment-related mortality and graft-versus-leukemia activity after allogeneic stem cell transplantation for chronic lymphocytic leukemia using intensity-reduced conditioning. Leukemia 2003;17:841–8.
208. Sorror ML, Maris MB, Sandmaier BM, et al. Hematopoietic cell transplantation after nonmyeloablative conditioning for advanced chronic lymphocytic leukemia. J Clin Oncol 2005;23:3819–29.
209. Rosenberg SA, Yang JC, Sherry RM, et al. Durable complete responses in heavily pretreated patients with metastatic melanoma using T-cell transfer immunotherapy. Clin Cancer Res 2011;17:4550–7.
210. Rooney CM, Smith CA, Ng CY, et al. Infusion of cytotoxic T cells for the prevention and treatment of Epstein-Barr virus-induced lymphoma in allogeneic transplant recipients. Blood 1998;92:1549–55.

211. Morgan RA, Dudley ME, Wunderlich JR, et al. Cancer regression in patients after transfer of genetically engineered lymphocytes. Science 2006;314:126–9.
212. June CH, Blazar BR, Riley JL. Engineering lymphocyte subsets: tools, trials and tribulations. Nat Rev Immunol 2009;9:704–16.
213. Cartellieri M, Bachmann M, Feldmann A, et al. Chimeric antigen receptor-engineered T cells for immunotherapy of cancer. J Biomed Biotechnol 2010; 2010:956304.
214. Koehler P, Schmidt P, Hombach AA, et al. Engineered T cells for the adoptive therapy of B-cell chronic lymphocytic leukaemia. Adv Hematol 2012;2012: 595060.
215. Brentjens R, Yeh R, Bernal Y, et al. Treatment of chronic lymphocytic leukemia with genetically targeted autologous T cells: case report of an unforeseen adverse event in a phase I clinical trial. Mol Ther 2010;18:666–8.
216. Brentjens RJ, Riviere I, Park JH, et al. Safety and persistence of adoptively transferred autologous CD19-targeted T cells in patients with relapsed or chemotherapy refractory B-cell leukemias. Blood 2011;118:4817–28.
217. Maher J, Brentjens RJ, Gunset G, et al. Human T-lymphocyte cytotoxicity and proliferation directed by a single chimeric TCRzeta/CD28 receptor. Nat Biotechnol 2002;20:70–5.
218. Milone MC, Fish JD, Carpenito C, et al. Chimeric receptors containing CD137 signal transduction domains mediate enhanced survival of T cells and increased antileukemic efficacy in vivo. Mol Ther 2009;17:1453–64.
219. Porter DL, Levine BL, Kalos M, et al. Chimeric antigen receptor-modified T cells in chronic lymphoid leukemia. N Engl J Med 2011;365:725–33.
220. Kalos M, Levine BL, Porter DL, et al. T cells with chimeric antigen receptors have potent antitumor effects and can establish memory in patients with advanced leukemia. Sci Transl Med 2011;3:95ra73.
221. Wherry EJ. T cell exhaustion. Nat Immunol 2011;12:492–9.
222. Giordano Attianese GM, Marin V, Hoyos V, et al. In vitro and in vivo model of a novel immunotherapy approach for chronic lymphocytic leukemia by anti-CD23 chimeric antigen receptor. Blood 2011;117:4736–45.
223. Boissel L, Betancur M, Wels WS, et al. Transfection with mRNA for CD19 specific chimeric antigen receptor restores NK cell mediated killing of CLL cells. Leuk Res 2009;33:1255–9.

The Significance of Stereotyped B-Cell Receptors in Chronic Lymphocytic Leukemia

Nikos Darzentas, PhD[a,b], Kostas Stamatopoulos, MD, PhD[b,c,*]

KEYWORDS

- CLL • Immunoglobulin gene • CDR3 • Antigen • Somatic hypermutation
- Stereotype • Subset

KEY POINTS

- Roughly 30% of patients with chronic lymphocytic leukemia (CLL) carry immunoglobulin receptors with highly similar primary sequences.
- Highly similar, quasi-identical immunoglobulins are termed stereotyped.
- Patients with CLL can be assigned to different subsets expressing different types of stereotyped immunoglobulin receptors.
- Just a few subsets account for more than 10% of the entire cohort.
- Reliable identification of stereotypy may assist in the molecular classification of CLL and thus better-guided, compartmentalized research.
- In several major subsets, stereotypy extends from shared primary sequences to shared clinicobiological features and outcome, even beyond *IGHV* gene mutational status.
- Reliable identification of stereotypy in CLL may pave the way for tailored treatment strategies applicable to each major stereotyped subset.

INTRODUCTION: A PRIMER ON MECHANISMS OF IMMUNOGLOBULIN DIVERSITY

All B cells express identical copies of immunoglobulin (IG) on their cell surface. The IGs, together with accessory proteins, constitute the surface complexes known as B-cell receptors (BcRs), which are critical for specific antigen recognition.[1] Each IG

This work was supported in part by: the ENosAI project (code 09SYN-13-880) co-funded by the EU and the Hellenic General Secretariat for Research and Technology to ND and KS; and the Cariplo Foundation (Milan, Italy) to KS.

[a] Molecular Medicine Program, Central European Institute of Technology, Masaryk University, 9, Zerotinovo street, 60177, Brno, Czech Republic; [b] Institute of Applied Biosciences, Center for Research and Technology Hellas, 6th Km Charilaou-Thermis street, Thermi, Thessaloniki 57001, Greece; [c] HCT Unit, Hematology Department, G. Papanicolaou Hospital, 59, Papanicolaou street, Exokhi, Thessaloniki 57010, Greece
* Corresponding author. HCT Unit, Hematology Department, G. Papanicolaou Hospital, Exohi, Thessaloniki 57010, Greece.
E-mail address: kostas.stamatopoulos@gmail.com

Hematol Oncol Clin N Am 27 (2013) 237–250
http://dx.doi.org/10.1016/j.hoc.2012.12.001
0889-8588/13/$ – see front matter © 2013 Elsevier Inc. All rights reserved.

hemonc.theclinics.com

molecule is a tetramer composed of 2 identical heavy chains (HCs) and 2 identical light chains (LCs), either κ or λ, each subdivided into a variable (V) and constant (C) domain.[2] The V domain is the part of the molecule that binds antigen, whereas the C domain determines the isotype of the molecule and has effector function.[3] Each V domain comprises 4 areas of limited diversity, known as the framework regions (FRs), interspersed with 3 regions of high variability, known as the complementarity determining regions (CDRs), which confer the IG molecule its unique specificity.[3]

The V domain of the IG HC of each B cell is generated somatically by the recombinatorial process and joining of distinct variable (IGHV), diversity (IGHD) and joining (IGHJ) genes at the IGH locus.[4] The V domain of IG LCs is generated in a similar fashion; however, the joining involves only variable (IGKV or IGLV, for κ or λ light chains, respectively) and joining (IGKJ or IGLJ) genes at the IGK and IGL loci. This recombinatorial assembly of IG HC and LC variable domains is known as V(D)J recombination.[5]

V(D)J recombination rests at the basis of the BcR IG diversity. The random assembly of one each of multiple distinct V, D (for IG HCs), and J genes leads to a variety of combinations (combinatorial diversity).[6] IG diversity increases significantly during V(D)J recombination by the trimming of nucleotides from the ends of the recombining genes and the insertion of random (nontemplated) nucleotides at the V-D, D-J, or V-J junctions located within the CDR3, the most diverse part of the V domain (junctional diversity).[7] It has been estimated that the combinatorial events of the IGH, IGK, and IGL loci create greater than 1.6×10^6 possible combinations for BcR IGs.

When the B cell encounters antigen to which the BcR adequately binds, affinity maturation of the IG occurs in specialized structures of the secondary lymphoid organs.[8] During this antigen-dependent phase of B-cell differentiation, diversity is increased exponentially as a result of somatic hypermutation (SHM) and class-switch recombination (CSR). SHM is characterized by the introduction of mutations within recombined genes, which increases IG diversity and produces IGs with higher specificity.[9] CSR replaces the constant (*IGHC*) gene to be expressed from *IGHM* to *IGHG* or *IGHE* or *IGHA*, switching the IG HC isotype without, however, changing antigen specificity.[10] SHM and CSR have been estimated to increase the potential for diversity 10^3-fold to 10^6-fold. Hence, altogether, the B-cell repertoire comprises, in principle, 10^{12} different antigen specificities. The theoretic probability that two independent B-cell clones might carry exactly the same BcR IG by chance alone is virtually negligible (10^{-12}).

BCR STEREOTYPY IN CLL: HOW IT ALL STARTED

Studies from the early 1990s offered the first hints for restrictions in the IG heavy variable (*IGHV*) gene repertoire of CLL.[11,12] Unrelated CLL cases were reported to carry distinctive VH CDR3 characterized by shared amino acid motifs.[13,14] A milestone in the immunogenetic study of CLL came in 1998, when it was convincingly shown that the *IGHV* gene repertoire of CLL is restricted, with certain genes, such as *IGHV1-69*, *IGHV4-34*, and *IGHV3-7*, overrepresented in CLL compared with normal IgM+ B cells.[15] Specific associations were identified between certain *IGHV* genes with certain *IGHD* and *IGHJ* genes, as shown by rearrangements using the *IGHV1-69* gene, which were frequently recombined with the *IGHD3-3* and *IGHJ6* genes. SHM was not uniform among rearrangements of *IGHV* genes: for example, the *IGHV1-69* gene carried few or no mutations as opposed to other genes (eg, *IGHV3-7*, *IGHV3-23* and *IGHV4-34*), which bore a significant SHM load.[15] On these grounds, it was proposed that selection by antigen is implicated in CLL ontogeny.

Another milestone followed soon. Less than a year later, 2 groups independently reported that the mutational status of the rearranged *IGHV* genes strongly correlated with patient survival.[16,17] In particular, patients carrying mutated *IGHV* genes were reported to follow a more indolent course than those with unmutated *IGHV* genes, who tend to show adverse cytogenetic profiles and follow aggressive disease courses characterized by clonal evolution and resistance to therapy. All studies since have corroborated the general rule: IGHV-unmutated = bad prognosis, IGHV-mutated = good prognosis.[18]

So far, the rule has had a single exception. Since the initial report in 2002,[19] accumulating evidence has suggested that usage of the *IGHV3-21* gene in CLL BcR IGs may represent an adverse prognostic factor, regardless of the SHM status.[20–23] CLL using the IGHV3-21 gene is also notable because many cases express distinctive IGs with highly similar VH CDR3s and biased association with λ LCs using the *IGLV3-21* gene.[24] Because this situation could not happen by chance alone, it was justifiably considered as evidence for common antigenic drive, perhaps of pathogenic significance.[24]

STEREOTYPED BCRS IN CLL: CONCEPTS, DEFINITIONS, AND STRATEGIES FOR IDENTIFICATION

Soon thereafter, as large datasets of IG sequences became available, groups from both Europe and the United States reported subsets of CLL cases with highly similar BcR IGs.[21,24–28] Hence, rather than an interesting curiosity, it was established beyond doubt that distinct prototypic BcR IGs existed in CLL, repeated with limited or no variation in different subsets of patients with either mutated or unmutated *IGHV* genes. This remarkable restriction, at odds with the logistics of IG synthesis, strongly supports an antigen-driven pathway to CLL development.[29]

Quasi-identical BcR IGs in unrelated CLL cases are conforming to a fixed or general pattern, thus amply fulfilling the definition of stereotype.[25] After almost a decade of intensive research, it is now established that different subsets of cases with distinct stereotyped VH CDR3 sequences within their BcRs collectively account for almost one-third of the CLL repertoire.[30,31] Furthermore, just a few major stereotyped subsets represent a substantial proportion of the entire cohort (**Fig. 1**), showing CLL-biased and often highly distinctive clinicobiological features and, even, outcome[31] (see later discussion). Therefore, the detection of BcR IG stereotypy may assist in the molecular classification of CLL into different categories, potentially paving the way for tailored treatment strategies applicable to each major stereotyped subset.[31]

This brings us to a fundamental question. How can BcR IG stereotypes be identified? The first set of criteria for the identification of stereotypy required potentially stereotyped BcR IGs to use the same *IGHV, IGHD, IGHJ* germline genes, use the same *IGHD* gene reading frame, and show VH CDR3 amino acid identity equal to or greater than 60% (**Table 1**).[25] However, the first criterion could not be met in all instances, because cases with overall high BcR IG similarity (ie, stereotyped) were found to use different *IGHV* genes. Hence, revised criteria were proposed, putting emphasis on (1) functional conservation of amino acids in case of sequence differences; and (2) also allowing the usage of different *IGHV* genes (see **Table 1**).[21]

The validity of this approach was made evident by a set of cases now defined as subset 1 that are characterized by usage of the *IGHD6-19* and *IGHJ4* genes in association with different IGHV genes (namely *IGHV1-2, IGHV1-3, IGHV1-18, IGHV1-8, IGHV5-a, IGHV7-4-1*).[21,25,27,28,31,32] The IGHV genes used in rearrangements assigned to subset 1 are all members of phylogenetic clan I,[33,34] which means that their germline

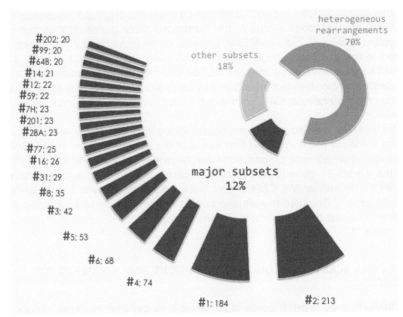

Fig. 1. Up to one-third of all CLL cases carry stereotyped BcRs. Patients can be allocated to different subsets based on shared VH CDR3 amino acid motifs and other criteria, with just a few major subsets accounting for more than 10% of the entire cohort.

sequences are closely and evolutionarily related, thus most probably producing overall similar VH domains when recombining with identical *IGHD* and *IGHJ* genes.

With the accumulation of IG sequence data for thousands of patients with CLL, these relatively straightforward approaches for identifying BcR IG stereotypy, essentially based on multiple sequence alignment, proved to have serious limitations with regards to efficiency, accuracy, and sensitivity. For this reason, purpose-built bioinformatics methods were developed based on de novo sequence pattern discovery and clustering, enabling sophisticated identification of VH CDR3 sequence similarities regardless of the IGHV/IGHD/IGHJ genes used (see **Table 1**).[30]

Table 1
Evolution of the criteria for the identification of BcR stereotypy in human B-cell malignancies

	Messmer et al,[25] 2004	Stamatopoulos et al,[21] 2007	Darzentas et al,[30] 2010	Agathangelidis et al,[31] 2012
VH CDR3 amino acid identity (%)	≥60	≥60	≥50	≥50
VH CDR3 amino acid similarity (%)	n/a[a]	n/a	≥70	≥70
IGHV genes	Same	Any	Any	Clan[b]
VH CDR3 length difference	?	≤3	≤2	=0
Offset of the pattern	n/a	n/a	≤2	=0
IGHD gene reading frame	Same	n/a	n/a	n/a

[a] n/a: nonapplicable.
[b] Clan: phylogenetic clan of IGHV genes.

A major advantage of this novel approach concerned the ability to document more distant relationships between sequences, thus forming a fuzzy treelike scheme, with first-level (ground-level) clusters merging, under certain conditions, into higher-level clusters with more relaxed membership criteria and more members (**Fig. 2**).[30] More recently, realizing that the phylogenetic relatedness of *IGHV* genes can be reflected in the gene composition of subsets, we refined our criteria for BcR IG stereotypy and now require that only sequences carrying *IGHV* genes of the same clan can be assigned to the same subset.[31] In addition, more stringent criteria were adopted related, indirectly, to the three-dimensional structure of the BcR, including the requirement for identical VH CDR3 lengths and identical locations of the shared patterns within the VH CDR3 of connected sequences (see **Table 1**).[31]

CLUES TO THE ONTOGENY OF CLL FROM THE ANALYSIS OF STEREOTYPED BCRS

CLL cells frequently express polyreactive and self-reactive antibodies with a reactivity profile similar to that of natural antibodies.[35–37] Natural antibodies, mainly produced from B1 and marginal zone (MZ) B cells, constitute a first line of defense against invading pathogens.[38–40] They are multireactive and tend to recognize nonprotein antigens widespread in diverse pathogenic and commensal organisms and, occasionally, by the host; therefore, many, if not all, natural antibodies may be both autoreactive (against self) and alloreactive (against antigens expressed by pathogens).[41–43] These attributes of natural antibodies may explain why B1 and MZ B cells show restricted IG gene usage and limited junctional diversity, thus ensuring the formation of archetypical BcR IGs, perhaps selected over evolutionary time for showing broad antigen reactivities.[44–46]

On these grounds, it is relevant that archetypical BcR IGs with widely shared sequence features are a feature of CLL with stereotyped BcRs. Within the stereotyped

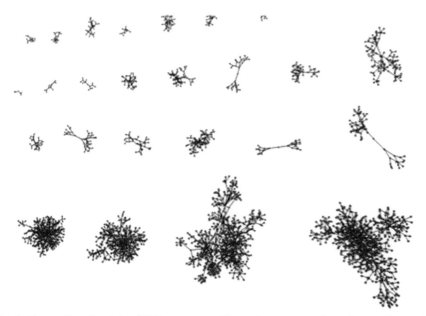

Fig. 2. Connecting the dots of BcR stereotypy. Network representation of more than 7400 CLL cases, linked at different levels according to the latest stereotypy identification criteria.

fraction of CLL, few genes (namely, *IGHV1-69, IGHV1-3, IGHV1-2, IGHV3-21, IGHV4-34, IGHV4-39*) account for more than 75% of cases.[30,31] This finding indicates that (1) the IG gene repertoire restrictions reported as typical for CLL are essentially a feature of cases expressing stereotyped BcRs IGs, whereas non-stereotyped CLL cases express a more diverse IGHV gene repertoire; and (2) that certain germline specificities may be selected for in the progenitors of at least subsets of CLL cases.[30]

A notable feature of several CLL subsets with stereotyped BcR IGs concerns the usage of different yet phylogenetically related *IGHV* genes, including subset 1 (*IGHV* genes belonging to clan I) as well as other examples (eg, subsets 12 [*IGHV1-2* and *IGHV1-46*], 59 [*IGHV1-58* and *IGHV1-69*] and 77 [*IGHV4-4* and *IGHV4-59*]), the latter including cases with mutated IGs.[31] This finding is similar to what has been described for recombinant monoclonal antibodies (mAbs) with similar reactivities using CDR shuffling approaches[47] and, recently, for potent broadly neutralizing CD4-binding site anti-human immunodeficiency virus antibodies that mimic binding to CD4.[48]

An animal model that reproducibly replicates abnormalities typical of CLL in the human is still lacking. However, CD5+ B-cell lymphoproliferative disorders similar to human CLL develop in mice manipulated in several different ways.[49–53] The leukemic BcR IGs in the mice show several molecular features reminiscent of the human disease, including BcR stereotypy. As recently shown by comparison of all available VH CDR3s of CD5+ lymphoproliferations from CLL mouse models,[53–55] 44% (29/66) of all cases could be assigned to 8 subsets of quasi-identical VH CDR3s.[53] In *TCL1* transgenic mice, one of the best characterized of CLL animal models,[49] antigen-binding studies have confirmed that selected TCL1 clones were polyreactive or autoreactive,[54] binding to a glycerophospholipid (PtC based on reactivity with Br-treated red blood cells), a lipoprotein (low-density lipoprotein), or polysaccharides (Fucα1-linkages). On these grounds, it has been suggested that the TCL1 clones likely derive from the B-1a subset,[54] consistent with finding the initial, preleukemic clonal expansions in the peritoneal cavity.[49]

Altogether, asymmetries in both the usage of IG genes and the molecular features of the antigen-binding site in CLL with stereotyped BcR IGs strongly recall B-1 cells, which show a distinct and considerably more biased IG repertoire than conventional B cells, with frequent occurrence of identical IG heavy and LC rearrangements.[44,45] The repertoire and reactivity pattern of B-1 cells is stable within each species and even across species, likely reflecting evolutionary pressure for maintaining broadly protective specificities against exogenous (ie, microbial pathogens) and endogenous (ie, apoptotic debris) risks.[56–58] Whether and how these observations are relevant for CLL ontogeny is unknown; however, the analogies to human disease are tantalizing and difficult to ignore.

STEREOTYPED BCRS, STEREOTYPED ANTIGEN REACTIVITY PROFILES?

The quest for the antigens recognized by CLL BcR IGs has been an intense activity for more than 2 decades. As already mentioned, earlier studies had shown that CLL-derived mAbs can be autoreactive and polyreactive[35,36]; however, substantial progress was made more recently with the advent of new methodologies for obtaining CLL mAbs, including recombinant DNA techniques,[37] cell lines derived from the neoplastic CLL clone by Epstein-Barr virus (EBV) transformation as well as primary ex vivo CLL cultures.[59]

As a result of these methodological advances, self-reactivity and polyreactivity were found to be more frequent in unmutated or low mutated rather than mutated CLL mAbs[37] and, furthermore CLL mAbs from the same subset could show similar antigen-binding profiles.[59–61] For instance, nonmuscle myosin HC IIA expressed on a subpopulation of apoptotic cells (called myosin-exposed apoptotic cells [MEACs]) was recognized by all tested CLL mAbs from subset 6 (*IGHV1-69/IGHD3-16/IGHJ3* stereotyped BcR IGs).[62] MEAC reactivity was not confined to subset 6 mAbs, but was rather shown by several other CLL mAbs, although variably.[63] However, CLL mAbs from the same subsets showed concordant patterns of MEAC reactivity,[63] strongly suggesting that the assignment of CLL cases into different subsets based on shared features of the primary IG gene sequences is functionally relevant.

Infections by common pathogens have also been linked to subgroups of CLL cases. First, a recent epidemiologic study[64] suggested that recurrent respiratory tract infections caused by *Streptococcus pneumoniae* and *Haemophilus influenzae* are associated with an increased risk of CLL. Furthermore, certain CLL Abs have been shown to react against various gram-positive and gram-negative bacterial strains (*Streptococcus pyogenes, Enterococcus faecium, Enterococcus faecalis, Enterobacter cloacae*), with unmutated *IGHV1-69* mAbs being the dominant binders.[60]

Persistent infections by EBV and cytomegalovirus have been correlated with the stereotyped *IGHV4-34* subset 4.[65] The BcR IGs of subset 4 show a series of distinctive immunogenetic features, including: (1) long and positively charged VH CDR3s, reminiscent of pathogenic anti-DNA antibodies in patients with lupus[66]; (2) shared (stereotyped) amino acid changes induced by SHM, of which particularly noteworthy are several changes leading to the introduction of negatively charged residues in both heavy and light variable domains,[32,67] similar to modifications editing anti-DNA reactivity in mouse models for human lupus[68,69]; (3) although heavily mutated, they all carry intact VH FR1 motifs for superantigenic-like recognition of the *N*-acetyllactosamine epitope present on both self-antigens and exogenous antigens.[32,70] On these grounds, it has been proposed that, in principle, progenitors of CLL subset 4 could be activated on infection by or reactivation of certain microbial pathogens or by material produced during apoptosis or inflammation, thus receiving signals that promote survival, expansion, malignant transformation, and, potentially, clonal evolution.[32,71,72]

The role of additional and concomitant ways of activating CLL cells through nonspecific immune receptors has remained largely overlooked, although, judging from normal B cells, highly relevant, given that these receptors collaborate with the BcR toward fine-tuning the outcome of interactions with the microenvironment.[73,74] CLL cases carrying mutated versus unmutated *IGHV* genes or assigned to different subsets with stereotyped BcR IGs were found to have significantly different expression profiles for toll-like receptors (TLRs) as well as other select genes in the TLR-signaling framework.[75] Furthermore, the functional outcomes of TLR and NOD-like receptor (NLR) stimulation were shown to be quantitatively and qualitatively different between (but similar within) subsets of CLL cases with different stereotyped BcR IGs, irrespective of the IGHV gene mutational status.[76] These results indicate distinct, subset-biased modalities of BcR collaboration with specific TLRs that may extend to the control of cell proliferation or apoptosis, B-cell anergy or TLR tolerance, thus affecting the biological behavior of the CLL clone and, likely, underlying the clinical phenotype.

Although the evidence is compelling that all CLL cells are antigen experienced, the jury is still out as to whether antigen involvement is restricted before the malignant transformation or whether it continues to trigger the CLL clone, thus promoting clonal evolution. The question is especially relevant in view of recent findings that CLL BcR IGs induce cell-autonomous signaling independently of extrinsic antigens through VH CDR3-mediated interactions with distinct epitopes on nearby BcR IGs.[77] These findings have prompted speculation that only certain VH CDR3s have this unique capacity, thus offering a potential explanation about the observed IG gene repertoire restrictions in CLL, which culminate in the existence of stereotyped BcR IGs.

In various lymphoma subtypes, intraclonal diversification (ID) within the clonotypic IG genes through ongoing SHM is a molecular imprint of continued interactions with antigen. In CLL, Sanger sequencing-based approaches have shown that ID is limited, with the outstanding exception of subset 4 cases, who show distinctive patterns of ID, leading to extensive subclone formation.[71,72] Therefore, (auto)antigenic stimulation after transformation is operating in at least subsets of CLL cases. It remains to be established whether this stimulation is also accompanied by a change in functional status and how it relates to clinical evolution and outcome. Concerning the issue of ID and ongoing SHM in CLL, revelations are expected from next-generation sequencing studies, once technical issues are fully resolved. Judging from the limited available data, clonal evolution at the IGH locus is complex in CLL, with subclones observed across IGHV-mutational categories and not simply restricted to patients with extensive SHM.[78]

CLINICAL IMPLICATIONS OF BCR STEREOTYPY IN CLL

The first evidence that immunogenetic features other than the SHM status of the clonotypic BcR IGs may have prognostic significance in CLL was provided by the case of the *IGHV3-21* gene,[19] spurring interest in other genes,[79,80] although with a poor yield. With hindsight, this finding is not unexpected for 2 related reasons: (1) BcR IGs using the same IGHV gene yet differing in VH CDR3 sequence and associated LC need not show similar antigen reactivity and, by extension, similar behavior; and (2) IGHV3-21-expressing CLL is remarkably homogeneous, with greater than 50% of cases assigned to a single subset with restricted VH CDR3s and restricted LC gene usage (see later discussion).

With hindsight, the turning point in searching for clinical implications of BcR IG features beyond *IGHV* gene mutational status was the realization that CLL expressing IGs encoded by the *IGHV3-21* gene can be subdivided into (1) cases carrying stereotyped BcRs with short and highly similar VH CDR3 and restricted usage of IGLV3-21 λ LCs; and (2) cases carrying heterogeneous BcR IGs.[81] The former, now known to belong to CLL subset 2, accounting for more than 50% of all IGHV3-21 CLL, were found to uniformly express CD38 and have progressive disease, whereas nonsubset 2 IGHV3-21 cases showed variable CD38 expression and followed variable clinical courses.[81] Since the original publication, several studies[21–23] have independently shown that expression of stereotyped subset 2 BcR IGs is associated with shorter time to progression and presence of other poor-prognostic markers.

Thus, a concept was established: prognostic information might be gleaned by defining not only the usage of specific genes (eg, *IGHV3-21*) and their mutational load but also the molecular features of the BcR IG among cases using similar *IGHV* genes. Although still a hypothesis rather than solid fact, mainly because numbers are not enough for robust statistical analysis (even major subsets account for no more than 2.5% of the cohort, thus hindering conclusive association studies), yet tantalizing hints have emerged by treading along the conceptual path of "stereotyped BcR IGs, stereotyped clinical behavior?".

One of the first studies to report associations between BcR IG stereotypy and clinical features concerned a subset of 5 cases expressing stereotyped *IGHV4-39/IGHD6-13/IGHJ5* BcR IGs (now known as subset 8).[82] Although these 5 CLL clones expressed IgG, the clonotypic IGHV and IGKV genes showed limited, if any, SHM, reminiscent of B-cell clonal expansion in response to T-independent antigens. Cases in subset 8 were reported to follow aggressive clinical courses complicated by severe recurrent infections, Richter transformation, or the occurrence of second solid tumors.[82] More recently, a large collaborative study reported that subset 8 shows the highest risk for Richter transformation among all CLL subgroups analyzed,[83] making it a paradigmatic subset for research into clonal evolution in CLL.

However, not all CLL stereotyped subsets are bad. A case in point is subset 4, defined by the expression of stereotyped mutated IGHV4-34/IGKV2-30 BcRs of the G isotype.[21,84] Cases assigned to subset 4 are significantly younger at diagnosis and have been reported to follow an indolent disease course even when compared with cases expressing mutated *IGHV4-34* BcR IGs but with nonsubset 4 molecular configuration.[21]

Altogether, the available evidence suggests possible links between certain stereotyped BcR IGs and clinical features at presentation or outcome, strongly implying that shared functional antigen reactivity profiles may underlie shared clonal behavior, eventually reflected in common prognosis.

A GLIMPSE INTO THE (NEAR) FUTURE: SYSTEMS BIOLOGY OF CLL SUBSETS WITH STEREOTYPED BCRS

The picture of B-cell biology in CLL is contrasting and complex, but decades of research and recent developments, many outlined earlier, have in part shattered an illusion of diversity and revealed a gradient of uniformity, unique among lymphoid malignancies.

From a mainly immunogenetic perspective, an apparently heterogeneous two-thirds of CLL cases have left the other third to fall into varyingly homogeneous subsets with stereotyped BcRs, around 20 of them now confirmed as major and the topic of intense scientific interest. Results from genomic aberrations, DNA methylation, and microRNA profiles, antigen reactivity studies, overtime ID occurrence, BcR/TLR/NLR signaling, clinical data, have provided a glimpse into the commonalities of CLL cases with stereotyped BcRs.

This enrichment of the knowledge around the subsets of patients with CLL with such diverse data allows for a systems-biology statistical recategorization of patients into more relevant and robust archetypes. These archetypes are readily amenable to further research and development toward tailored therapy protocols, probably targeting different cellular and molecular systems in different archetypes.

The relatively simplistic immunogenetic subsets, which have nevertheless been an already fruitful starting point, could eventually be upheld, split, or merged based on the integration of additional data, leading to a robust categorization of patients with unprecedented potential for targeted therapeutic interventions.

ACKNOWLEDGMENTS

We thank present and past members of our groups for their commitment and enthusiasm. A special thanks is due to our friends and fellow members of the IgCLL Group (www.igcll.org), Drs Belessi, Davi, Ghia, and Rosenquist for many years of stimulating and fruitful collaboration. Finally, we wish to sincerely thank Prof. Marie-Paule Lefranc and Dr Veronique Giudicelli, Laboratoire d'Immunogénétique Moléculaire, LIGM, Université Montpellier II, Montpellier, France, and IMGT, the international ImMunoGeneTics information system http://www.imgt.org, for their enormous support and help with IG sequence analysis.

REFERENCES

1. Kuby J. Immunobiology. 4th edition. San Francisco, CA: WH Freeman; 2001.

2. Janeway C, Travers P, Walport M, et al. The immune system in health and disease. 6th edition. New York, NY: Garland; 2004.
3. Lefranc MP, Lefranc G. The immunoglobulin FactsBook. London, San Diego, CA: Academic Press; 2001.
4. Schatz DG, Spanopoulou E. Biochemistry of V(D)J recombination. Curr Top Microbiol Immunol 2005;290:49–85.
5. Schatz DG, Swanson PC. V(D)J recombination: mechanisms of initiation. Annu Rev Genet 2011;45:167–202.
6. Schlissel MS. Regulating antigen-receptor gene assembly. Nat Rev Immunol 2003;3:890–9.
7. Maizels N. Immunoglobulin gene diversification. Annu Rev Genet 2005;39:23–46.
8. Victora GD, Nussenzweig MC. Germinal centers. Annu Rev Immunol 2012;30: 429–57.
9. Shlomchik MJ, Weisel F. Germinal center selection and the development of memory B and plasma cells. Immunol Rev 2012;247:52–63.
10. Xu Z, Zan H, Pone EJ, et al. Immunoglobulin class-switch DNA recombination: induction, targeting and beyond. Nat Rev Immunol 2012;12:517–31.
11. Schroeder HW Jr, Dighiero G. The pathogenesis of chronic lymphocytic leukemia: analysis of the antibody repertoire. Immunol Today 1994;15:288–94.
12. Efremov DG, Ivanovski M, Siljanovski N, et al. Restricted immunoglobulin VH region repertoire in chronic lymphocytic leukemia patients with autoimmune hemolytic anemia. Blood 1996;87:3869–76.
13. Hashimoto S, Dono M, Wakai M, et al. Somatic diversification and selection of immunoglobulin heavy and light chain variable region genes in IgG+ CD5+ chronic lymphocytic leukemia B cells. J Exp Med 1995;181:1507–17.
14. Johnson TA, Rassenti LZ, Kipps TJ. Ig VH1 genes expressed in B cell chronic lymphocytic leukemia exhibit distinctive molecular features. J Immunol 1997; 158:235–46.
15. Fais F, Ghiotto F, Hashimoto S, et al. Chronic lymphocytic leukemia B cells express restricted sets of mutated and unmutated antigen receptors. J Clin Invest 1998;102:1515–25.
16. Hamblin TJ, Davis Z, Gardiner A, et al. Unmutated Ig V(H) genes are associated with a more aggressive form of chronic lymphocytic leukemia. Blood 1999;94: 1848–54.
17. Damle RN, Ghiotto F, Valetto A, et al. B-cell chronic lymphocytic leukemia cells express a surface membrane phenotype of activated, antigen-experienced B lymphocytes. Blood 2002;99:4087–93.
18. Hillmen P. Using the biology of chronic lymphocytic leukemia to choose treatment. Hematology Am Soc Hematol Educ Program 2011;2011:104–9.
19. Tobin G, Thunberg U, Johnson A, et al. Somatically mutated Ig V(H)3-21 genes characterize a new subset of chronic lymphocytic leukemia. Blood 2002;99:2262–4.
20. Thorselius M, Krober A, Murray F, et al. Strikingly homologous immunoglobulin gene rearrangements and poor outcome in VH3-21-utilizing chronic lymphocytic leukemia independent of geographical origin and mutational status. Blood 2006; 107:2889–94.
21. Stamatopoulos K, Belessi C, Moreno C, et al. Over 20% of patients with chronic lymphocytic leukemia carry stereotyped receptors: pathogenetic implications and clinical correlations. Blood 2007;109:259–70.
22. Bomben R, Dal Bo M, Capello D, et al. Molecular and clinical features of chronic lymphocytic leukaemia with stereotyped B cell receptors: results from an Italian multicentre study. Br J Haematol 2009;144:492–506.

23. Oscier D, Wade R, Davis Z, et al. Prognostic factors identified three risk groups in the LRF CLL4 trial, independent of treatment allocation. Haematologica 2010;95: 1705–12.
24. Tobin G, Thunberg U, Johnson A, et al. Chronic lymphocytic leukemias utilizing the VH3-21 gene display highly restricted Vlambda2-14 gene use and homologous CDR3s: implicating recognition of a common antigen epitope. Blood 2003;101:4952–7.
25. Messmer BT, Albesiano E, Efremov DG, et al. Multiple distinct sets of stereotyped antigen receptors indicate a role for antigen in promoting chronic lymphocytic leukemia. J Exp Med 2004;200:519–25.
26. Widhopf GF 2nd, Rassenti LZ, Toy TL, et al. Chronic lymphocytic leukemia B cells of more than 1% of patients express virtually identical immunoglobulins. Blood 2004;104:2499–504.
27. Tobin G, Thunberg U, Karlsson K, et al. Subsets with restricted immunoglobulin gene rearrangement features indicate a role for antigen selection in the development of chronic lymphocytic leukemia. Blood 2004;104:2879–85.
28. Stamatopoulos K, Belessi C, Hadzidimitriou A, et al. Immunoglobulin light chain repertoire in chronic lymphocytic leukemia. Blood 2005;106:3575–83.
29. Chiorazzi N, Ferrarini M. Cellular origin(s) of chronic lymphocytic leukemia: cautionary notes and additional considerations and possibilities. Blood 2011; 117:1781–91.
30. Darzentas N, Hadzidimitriou A, Murray F, et al. A different ontogenesis for chronic lymphocytic leukemia cases carrying stereotyped antigen receptors: molecular and computational evidence. Leukemia 2010;24(1):125–32.
31. Agathangelidis A, Darzentas N, Hadzidimitriou A, et al. Stereotyped B-cell receptors in one-third of chronic lymphocytic leukemia: a molecular classification with implications for targeted therapies. Blood 2012;119:4467–75.
32. Murray F, Darzentas N, Hadzidimitriou A, et al. Stereotyped patterns of somatic hypermutation in subsets of patients with chronic lymphocytic leukemia: implications for the role of antigen selection in leukemogenesis. Blood 2008;111(3):1524–33.
33. Kirkham PM, Mortari F, Newton JA, et al. Immunoglobulin VH clan and family identity predicts variable domain structure and may influence antigen binding. EMBO J 1992;11:603–9.
34. Vargas-Madrazo E, Lara-Ochoa F, Ramirez-Benites MC, et al. Evolution of the structural repertoire of the human V(H) and Vkappa germline genes. Int Immunol 1997;9:1801–15.
35. Sthoeger ZM, Wakai M, Tse DB, et al. Production of autoantibodies by CD5-expressing B lymphocytes from patients with chronic lymphocytic leukemia. J Exp Med 1989;169:255–68.
36. Borche L, Lim A, Binet JL, et al. Evidence that chronic lymphocytic leukemia B lymphocytes are frequently committed to production of natural autoantibodies. Blood 1990;76:562–9.
37. Herve M, Xu K, Ng YS, et al. Unmutated and mutated chronic lymphocytic leukemias derive from self-reactive B cell precursors despite expressing different antibody reactivity. J Clin Invest 2005;115:1636–43.
38. Claflin JL, Berry J. Genetics of the phosphocholine-specific antibody response to *Streptococcus pneumoniae*. Germ-line but not mutated T15 antibodies are dominantly selected. J Immunol 1988;141:4012–9.
39. Shaw PX, Horkko S, Chang MK, et al. Natural antibodies with the T15 idiotype may act in atherosclerosis, apoptotic clearance, and protective immunity. J Clin Invest 2000;105:1731–40.

40. Baumgarth N, Tung JW, Herzenberg LA. Inherent specificities in natural antibodies: a key to immune defense against pathogen invasion. Springer Semin Immunopathol 2005;26:347–62.

41. Kasaian MT, Casali P. Autoimmunity-prone B-1 (CD5 B) cells, natural antibodies and self recognition. Autoimmunity 1993;15:315–29.

42. Mouthon L, Nobrega A, Nicolas N, et al. Invariance and restriction toward a limited set of self-antigens characterize neonatal IgM antibody repertoires and prevail in autoreactive repertoires of healthy adults. Proc Natl Acad Sci U S A 1995;92:3839–43.

43. Baumgarth N, Herman OC, Jager GC, et al. Innate and acquired humoral immunities to influenza virus are mediated by distinct arms of the immune system. Proc Natl Acad Sci U S A 1999;96:2250–5.

44. Seidl K, Wilshire J, MacKenzie J, et al. Predominant VH genes expressed in innate antibodies are associated with distinctive antigen-binding sites. Proc Natl Acad Sci U S A 1999;96:2262–7.

45. Seidl K, MacKenzie J, Wang D, et al. Frequent occurrence of identical heavy and light chain Ig rearrangements. Int Immunol 1997;9:689–702.

46. Milner EC, Anolik J, Cappione A, et al. Human innate B cells: a link between host defense and autoimmunity? Springer Semin Immunopathol 2005;26:433–52.

47. Jirholt P, Ohlin M, Borrebaeck CA, et al. Exploiting sequence space: shuffling in vivo formed complementarity determining regions into a master framework. Gene 1998;215:471–6.

48. Scheid JF, Mouquet H, Ueberheide B, et al. Sequence and structural convergence of broad and potent HIV antibodies that mimic CD4 binding. Science 2011;333:1633–7.

49. Bichi R, Shinton SA, Martin ES, et al. Human chronic lymphocytic leukemia modeled in mouse by targeted TCL1 expression. Proc Natl Acad Sci U S A 2002;99:6955–60.

50. ter Brugge PJ, Ta VB, de Bruijn MJ, et al. A mouse model for chronic lymphocytic leukemia based on expression of the SV40 large T antigen. Blood 2009;114:119–27.

51. Bertilaccio MT, Scielzo C, Simonetti G, et al. A novel Rag2-/-gammac-/- xenograft model of human CLL. Blood 2010;115:1605–9.

52. Salerno E, Yuan Y, Scaglione B, et al. The New Zealand black mouse as a model for the development and progression of chronic lymphocytic leukemia. Cytometry B Clin Cytom 2010;78(Suppl 1):S98–109.

53. Lia M, Carette A, Tang H, et al. Functional dissection of the chromosome 13q14 tumor-suppressor locus using transgenic mouse lines. Blood 2012;119:2981–90.

54. Yan XJ, Albesiano E, Zanesi N, et al. B cell receptors in TCL1 transgenic mice resemble those of aggressive, treatment-resistant human chronic lymphocytic leukemia. Proc Natl Acad Sci U S A 2006;103:11713–8.

55. Mercolino TJ, Locke AL, Afshari A, et al. Restricted immunoglobulin variable region gene usage by normal Ly-1 (CD5+) B cells that recognize phosphatidyl choline. J Exp Med 1989;169(6):1869–77.

56. Hardy RR. B-1 B cell development. J Immunol 2006;177(5):2749–54.

57. Wang H, Clarke S. Evidence for a ligand-mediated positive selection signal in differentiation to a mature B cell. J Immunol 2003;171:6381–8.

58. Wang H, Clarke SH. Positive selection focuses the VH12 B-cell repertoire towards a single B1 specificity with survival function. Immunol Rev 2004;197:51–9.

59. Lanemo Myhrinder A, Hellqvist E, Sidorova E, et al. A new perspective: molecular motifs on oxidized LDL, apoptotic cells, and bacteria are targets for chronic lymphocytic leukemia antibodies. Blood 2008;111:3838–48.

60. Hatzi K, Catera R, Ferrarini M, et al. B-cell chronic lymphocytic leukemia (B-CLL) cells express antibodies reactive with antigenic epitopes expressed on the surface of common bacteria. Blood 2006;108:12a.

61. Catera R, Silverman GJ, Hatzi K, et al. Chronic lymphocytic leukemia cells recognize conserved epitopes associated with apoptosis and oxidation. Mol Med 2008;14:665–74.

62. Chu CC, Catera R, Hatzi K, et al. Chronic lymphocytic leukemia antibodies with a common stereotypic rearrangement recognize nonmuscle myosin heavy chain IIA. Blood 2008;112:5122–9.

63. Chu CC, Catera R, Zhang L, et al. Many chronic lymphocytic leukemia antibodies recognize apoptotic cells with exposed non-muscle myosin heavy chain IIA: implications for patient outcome and cell of origin. Blood 2010;115:3907–15.

64. Landgren O, Rapkin J, Caporaso N, et al. Respiratory tract infections and subsequent risk of chronic lymphocytic leukemia. Blood 2007;109:2198–201.

65. Kostareli E, Hadzidimitriou A, Stavroyianni N, et al. Molecular evidence for EBV and CMV persistence in a subset of patients with chronic lymphocytic leukemia expressing stereotyped IGHV4-34 B-cell receptors. Leukemia 2009;23:919–24.

66. Jang YJ, Stollar BD. Anti-DNA antibodies: aspects of structure and pathogenicity. Cell Mol Life Sci 2003;60:309–20.

67. Hadzidimitriou A, Darzentas N, Murray F, et al. Evidence for the significant role of immunoglobulin light chains in antigen recognition and selection in chronic lymphocytic leukemia. Blood 2009;113:403–11.

68. Li H, Jiang Y, Prak EL, et al. Editors and editing of anti-DNA receptors. Immunity 2001;15:947–57.

69. Zhang J, Jacobi AM, Wang T, et al. Pathogenic autoantibodies in systemic lupus erythematosus are derived from both self-reactive and non-self-reactive B cells. Mol Med 2008;14:675–81.

70. Potter K, Hobby P, Klijn S, et al. Evidence for involvement of a hydrophobic patch in framework region 1 of human V4-34-encoded Igs in recognition of the red blood cell I antigen. J Immunol 2002;169:3777–82.

71. Sutton LA, Kostareli E, Hadzidimitriou A, et al. Extensive intraclonal diversification in a subgroup of chronic lymphocytic leukemia patients with stereotyped IGHV4-34 receptors: implications for ongoing interactions with antigen. Blood 2009;114:4460–8.

72. Kostareli E, Sutton L, Hadzidimitriou A, et al. Intraclonal diversification of immunoglobulin light chains in a subset of chronic lymphocytic leukemia alludes to antigen-driven clonal evolution. Leukemia 2010;24:1317–24.

73. Cerutti A, Puga I, Cols M. Innate control of B cell responses. Trends Immunol 2011;32:202–11.

74. Meyer-Bahlburg A, Khim S, Rawlings DJ. B cell intrinsic TLR signals amplify but are not required for humoral immunity. J Exp Med 2007;204:3095–101.

75. Arvaniti E, Ntoufa S, Papakonstantinou N, et al. Toll-like receptor signaling pathway in chronic lymphocytic leukemia: distinct gene expression profiles of potential pathogenetic significance in specific subsets of patients. Haematologica 2011;96:1644–52.

76. Ntoufa S, Vardi A, Papakonstantinou N, et al. Distinct innate immunity pathways to activation and tolerance in subgroups of chronic lymphocytic leukemia with distinct immunoglobulin receptors. Mol Med 2012;18:1281–91.

77. Minden MD, Ubelhart R, Schneider D, et al. Chronic lymphocytic leukaemia is driven by antigen-independent cell-autonomous signalling. Nature 2012;489:309–12.

78. Campbell P, Pleasance E, Stephens P, et al. Subclonal phylogenetic structures in cancer revealed by ultra-deep sequencing. Proc Natl Acad Sci U S A 2008;105: 13081–6.
79. Bomben R, Dal-Bo M, Benedetti D, et al. Expression of mutated IGHV3-23 genes in chronic lymphocytic leukemia identifies a disease subset with peculiar clinical and biological features. Clin Cancer Res 2010;16:620–8.
80. Matthews C, Catherwood M, Morris T, et al. V(H)3-48 and V(H)3-53, as well as V(H)3-21, gene rearrangements define unique subgroups in CLL and are associated with biased lambda light chain restriction, homologous LCDR3 sequences and poor prognosis. Leuk Res 2007;31:231–4.
81. Ghia P, Stamatopoulos K, Belessi C, et al. Geographic patterns and pathogenetic implications of IGHV gene usage in chronic lymphocytic leukemia: the lesson of the IGHV3-21 gene. Blood 2005;105:1678–85.
82. Ghiotto F, Fais F, Valetto A, et al. Remarkably similar antigen receptors among a subset of patients with chronic lymphocytic leukemia. J Clin Invest 2004;113: 1008–16.
83. Rossi D, Spina V, Cerri M, et al. Stereotyped B-cell receptor is an independent risk factor of chronic lymphocytic leukemia transformation to Richter syndrome. Clin Cancer Res 2009;15:4415–22.
84. Potter KN, Mockridge CI, Neville L, et al. Structural and functional features of the B-cell receptor in IgG-positive chronic lymphocytic leukemia. Clin Cancer Res 2006;12:1672–9.

MBL Versus CLL
How Important Is the Distinction?

Lydia Scarfò, MD[a,b], Claudia Fazi, PhD[a], Paolo Ghia, MD, PhD[a,b],*

KEYWORDS

- Monoclonal B-cell lymphocytosis • Chronic lymphocytic leukemia
- Immunoglobulin genes • Chromosomal aberrations • Progression • Prognosis
- Immunophenotype • Immune system

KEY POINTS

- The widespread availability of flow cytometric techniques showed that the detection of monoclonal B-cell populations with chronic lymphocytic leukemia (CLL) phenotype in the peripheral blood is not invariably linked to the diagnosis of a specific disease because this type of expansion can be detected frequently in otherwise healthy subjects.
- Monoclonal B-cell lymphocytosis (MBL) is defined as a clonal B-cell expansion where the B-cell count is less than 5×10^9/L and no symptoms or signs of lymphoproliferative disorders are detected.
- Based on the number of clonal B cells, MBL is further divided into low-count (median clone size, 1 cell/μL) and clinical MBL (median clone size, 2.9×10^9 cell/L).
- Low-count MBL appears to be rather distant from CLL based on both clinical and biologic characteristics and the reciprocal relationship between these 2 conditions seems to be more of interest for immunologists than hematologists, being more likely related to "immunosenescence."
- Clinical MBL is virtually indistinguishable from Rai stage 0 CLL regarding immunophenotypic, genetic, and molecular features and carries a risk of progression to CLL requiring treatment of 1% to 2% per year.
- CLL-like cells can be also found in lymph nodes without clinically relevant signs or symptoms of disease and a lymph node- equivalent of MBL, named "tissue involvement by CLL/SLL-like cells of uncertain significance" or "nodal (extranodal) MBL," has been recently proposed.
- As clinical MBL and CLL are overlapping entities, a deeper knowledge of the molecular pathways and of the microenvironmental influences critically involved in the disease evolution is needed and will likely help to differentiate nonprogressive and progressive cases that should be followed up intensively.

[a] Laboratory of B Cell Neoplasia, Division of Molecular Oncology, San Raffaele Scientific Institute, Università Vita-Salute San Raffaele, Via Olgettina 58, Milano 20132, Italy; [b] Clinical Unit of Lymphoid Malignancies, Department of Onco-Hematology, San Raffaele Scientific Institute and Università Vita-Salute San Raffaele, Via Olgettina 60, Milano 20132, Italy
* Corresponding author.
E-mail address: ghia.paolo@hsr.it

Hematol Oncol Clin N Am 27 (2013) 251–265
http://dx.doi.org/10.1016/j.hoc.2013.01.004
0889-8588/13/$ – see front matter © 2013 Elsevier Inc. All rights reserved.

hemonc.theclinics.com

INTRODUCTION

In the last 60 years, the improvement of laboratory techniques has radically changed the clinical presentation of chronic lymphocytic leukemia (CLL): the percentage of cases identified through a routine blood count has constantly increased from 10% (in the 1950s) to 80% (in the late 1990s).[1] Accordingly, they frequently present only with an asymptomatic lymphocytosis (Rai stage 0).[2]

At the same time, thanks to the widespread availability and use of flow cytometric analysis, the detection of monoclonal B-cell populations bearing the same immunophenotypic profile of CLL has become increasingly frequent, even in the absence of a detectable lymphocytosis.[3–7] This phenomenon, defined as CLL-like monoclonal B-cell lymphocytosis (MBL), has attracted great interest among CLL investigators.[8,9]

MBL, as a relatively new diagnostic entity, added a new piece in the complex puzzle of CLL biology. Although the alternative definition of "B-cell lymphocytosis of uncertain significance" has been long discarded because of the potential risk of creating anxiety in affected individuals, the "uncertain significance" is definitely characteristic of MBL. More than 7 years after the first consensus criteria publication,[8] a flurry of new information is animating the debate on the real essence of MBL and poses new and so far unanswered questions. On the one hand, it has been suggested that MBL might be a precursor state for CLL (like monoclonal gammopathy of undetermined significance for multiple myeloma).[10] On the other hand, it has been hypothesized that the presence of monoclonal B-cell expansions could be interpreted as part of the inevitable immune system modifications (ie, restriction) occurring with aging and should not be considered a truly preneoplastic condition per se.[11]

Several investigational studies in the last years shed some light on the biology of MBL as well as on the initial transforming events that occur in CLL.[12] All this new information can now be used to try to understand if and how these 2 conditions are related to each other and how important it might be to distinguish them.

HOW TO DEFINE MBL

Consensus guidelines,[8,9] World Health Organization classification,[13] and International Workshop on Chronic Lymphocytic Leukemia 2008 criteria[14] define MBL as a clonal B-cell expansion where the B-cell count is less than 5×10^9/L and no symptoms or signs of lymphoproliferative disorders (ie, B symptoms, hepatosplenomegaly, lymphadenopathies) are detected. In most (>75%) cases, the immunophenotypic profile of these clonal expansions is virtually indistinguishable from that of CLL cases (ie, CD5$^+$, CD23$^+$, CD20^{dim}, surface immunoglobulin expression at low levels [sIg^{dim}]). In the remaining 25% of affected subjects, B-cell clones exhibit a different immunophenotypic profile and are classified as the following:

- Atypical CLL MBL: CD5$^+$, CD20^{bright}, variable expression of CD23 (provided the lack of translocation involving the Cyclin-D1 locus);
- CD5-negative (or non-CLL) MBL: CD5$^-$, without evidence of other typical markers of lymphoproliferative disorders (eg, CD10 for follicular lymphomas).

Setting a numeric threshold (<5×10^9/L) made it clear that finding a monoclonal B-cell population in the peripheral blood should not necessarily lead to the diagnosis of a specific disease because this type of expansion can be detected frequently in otherwise healthy subjects.

How frequent is this finding? Although in the very beginning, this condition was detected at low incidence among healthy subjects (initial studies showed a prevalence of 0.60%),[15,16] more recent population studies demonstrated that CLL-like B-cell clones, in particular, are a rather common finding in the peripheral blood of otherwise healthy subjects regardless of their geographic origin or context (asymptomatic individuals performing routine blood tests for unrelated reasons as well as isolated communities involved in genetic studies).[3,4] The true frequency of this phenomenon varies between 3.5% and 12% and this variation mainly depends on the sensitivity of the flow cytometric technique used, which, in turn, is related to the number of fluorochromes used (2 vs 4 vs 5 vs 8 colors), the combination of monoclonal antibodies chosen, and the number of events acquired.[3–7] The more carefully one looks for it, the easier MBL can indeed be found. That notwithstanding, a plateau in MBL detection is now being approached despite the continuous technical improvement, as further gains in sensitivity apparently do not entail a proportional increase in ascertained cases.[11,17] In addition, all studies showed that the prevalence of this condition progressively increases with age, being detected in 45% to 75% of people aged 90 years or older, suggesting that, although not all individuals bear a CLL-like MBL clone at any given moment of life, virtually all have the possibility of carrying a B-cell expansion when aging.[17]

WHEN SIZE MATTERS: CLINICAL VERSUS LOW-COUNT MBL

After the definition, in 2005,[8] of the numerical cutoff of 5×10^9/L to distinguish MBL and CLL, several cases, falling below the threshold that in previous times would have been labeled *tout-court* as CLL, started being diagnosed as MBL. Given that they are mainly identified in a clinical context (ie, during blood tests performed in asymptomatic subjects showing mild lymphocytosis), they are now called "clinical" MBL and are characterized by the presence of clonal B cells in the range of ~ 0.5 to 5×10^9/L (median value, approximately 2.9×10^9/L with 95% of cases having more than 0.45×10^9/L clonal B cells), a concentration that can indeed be detected during routine flow cytometry testing.[18]

In contrast, when studies were performed in the general population using more sensitive techniques, it became clear that CLL-like B cells can be frequently observed also in healthy individuals although at definitely lower concentrations, the median number of clonal B-cells being 1 per microliter (95% of cases have less than 0.056×10^9/L clonal B cells). These CLL-like B cells are now defined as "low-count MBL" and are the cases that account for the high frequency of MBL in the general population (for this reason, also defined as "general population MBL").[18,19]

A cumulative meta-analysis of all MBL cases, regardless of the size of the clone, highlighted a bimodal distribution of the frequency confirming that MBL is a heterogeneous category comprising dramatically different entities at least in terms of size, although with identical phenotype.[18]

TO COUNT OR NOT TO COUNT: PROBLEMS AND PITFALLS IN DEFINING A B-CELL THRESHOLD

All these numerical thresholds and numerical differences may seem a bit arbitrary but it has been demonstrated that the absolute B-cell count at MBL presentation is indeed the most significant independent predictive factor for disease progression. Different studies performed in the clinical setting have shown that the B-cell count, as a continuous variable, correlates with the risk of progression, progression-free survival, and overall survival. In particular, the risk of progression to overt leukemia requiring treatment in clinical MBL has been reported as being 1% to 2%[5,20–23] and up to 4%[24] per year, making it comparable (although significantly different) to that of Rai stage 0 CLL (~ 5%). More importantly, in clinical MBL cases Kaplan-Meier curves for disease progression did not show a plateau over time, meaning that life-long periodic monitoring should be planned for these cases, similarly to what is the current practice for patients with Rai stage 0 CLL.[5]

In contrast, the few longitudinal studies investigating the course of low-count CLL-like MBL showed that these clonal expansions tend to remain stable over time, none apparently evolving into CLL or any other lymphoproliferative disorder.[25]

Based on this evidence, the discussion over MBL brought again to the attention of the scientific community the long-debated dilemma on the appropriate use of the term "leukemia" in CLL.[26] It is common knowledge that CLL pursues a heterogeneous clinical course with survival ranging from months to decades. In general, about one-third of patients will never require treatment during follow-up, showing a survival identical to age-matched unaffected individuals. The remaining patients will eventually need treatment at variable times after presentation and with different degrees of aggressiveness. Similarly, it is clear since the time of the original publication by Rai and colleagues[27] that Rai stage 0 CLL represents a melting pot, including cases bound to progress (in months or years) and patients who will never require treatment during the disease course. For this reason, in a relevant proportion of cases, mainly among those diagnosed with Rai stage 0 CLL, the "leukemia" definition carries an unnecessary psychological distress, given that some of these subjects bear an indolent nonprogressive condition that will never become clinically relevant.

Despite remarkable research efforts and a decade of studies on prognostic markers, it is not possible yet to predict at the time of diagnosis which individuals will require treatment and should therefore be intensively followed up and which will never suffer consequences from their disease and should be simply reassured and left unattended.

Based on these premises, several groups tested the possibility that by simply increasing the threshold of the B-cell count required for CLL diagnosis it would be possible to discriminate better the cases bound to progress versus the remaining ones.[28] A value of 10 to 11 $\times$ 10^9 B cells/L, proposed in different series,[21,29,30] is indeed able to enrich for individuals at risk of progression and would help to limit the CLL diagnosis to a greater number of individuals bound to progress. That notwithstanding, the potential tradeoff of this approach is that, using a higher cutoff value, the rate of progression of those not deserving a CLL diagnosis any longer would increase as well.[21]

Therefore the only solid conclusion that can be drawn with certainty from these studies is that no specific B-cell count cutoff alone will ever be able to segregate individuals with no risk of progression, given that these cases are strictly entangled with those with a worse prognosis.

It then becomes reasonable to postulate that dissecting specific molecular and biologic features associated with the risk of progression or with the stability of the condition might better hold the promise of identifying the subjects at risk who would deserve regular follow-ups.

LOW-COUNT MBL: THE UGLY DUCKLING STORY

Based on numerical as well as on clinical grounds, low-count MBL seems to be an entity clearly distinct from clinical MBL/Rai stage 0 CLL, although sharing with the latter the characteristic phenotype. This intrinsic difference is also supported by the few studies on its biologic features where it has been possible to isolate and analyze the tiny populations of CLL-like B cells in the peripheral blood.

Population-based studies clearly demonstrated that, in apparent contrast with MBL definition, CLL-like clones are not necessarily monoclonal, being sometimes polyclonal/oligoclonal.[6,31] This intriguing finding suggests that the acquisition of a CLL-like phenotype is not invariably linked to the occurrence of monoclonality but it might simply reflect a so far unknown functional state of activation.

Molecular studies of the immunoglobulin repertoire also supported the concept of a distinction between low-count MBL and CLL: it is well known that CLL is characterized by a preferential immunoglobulin heavy chain variable (IGHV) gene usage (including IGHV1-69, IGHV4-34, IGHV3-7, and IGHV3-23 genes),[32,33] highly restricted and biased as compared with the normal adult B-cell repertoire. This peculiar set of IGHV genes is underrepresented in small-size CLL-like clones and the genes most frequently used by low-count MBL are only rarely expressed by CLL, regardless of the mutational status of the expressed IGHV genes.[6] Moreover, in low-count MBL stereotyped receptors (ie, the presence of closely homologous, if not identical, complementarity determining region 3 sequences on immunoglobulin heavy and light chains) has been detected only in few cases, whereas they account for more than 30% of CLL cases.[34,35]

Interestingly, chromosomal analysis of low-count MBL provided unexpected results. It is common knowledge that 80% of CLL cases show a restricted number of fluorescence in situ hybridization (FISH)–detected genetic lesions that carry a prognostic value[36]: patients bearing 13q deletion have the most favorable prognosis, whereas subjects exhibiting a 17p deletion usually follow an aggressive clinical course.[36] Unexpectedly, several studies demonstrated that low-count MBL clones do carry the same cytogenetic abnormalities, with 13q deletion being detected at a frequency similar to CLL.[5,25] A few low-count MBL cases with 17p deletion have also been reported in the literature not showing sign of progression.[25,37] The detection of CLL-related abnormalities in low-count MBL strongly suggests that these lesions (and in particular 13q deletion) may occur early during MBL development (if not during B-cell development) resembling other lymphoma-related aberrations (ie, t14;18) that can be found frequently also in unaffected individuals.[38] In particular, this finding strongly supports the possibility that these aberrations are far from being causative of the disease, as corroborated by the murine model carrying a 13q14 deletion involving the DLEU2/mir15-a/16-1 cluster.[39] This alteration, known to reduce miR15a and miR16-1 expression, may give rise to a broad spectrum of lymphoproliferative disorders including MBL, CLL, and diffuse large B-cell lymphomas but only in a low percentage of animals and after several months of life, suggesting the necessity of additional, causative hits.[39]

Data reported from naturally occurring mouse models are in keeping with this scenario and confirm that oligoclonal and monoclonal CD5-positive B-cell expansions are a frequent phenomenon in different mouse strains with aging (eg, New Zealand Black[40] and New Zealand White[41] strains).[42]

LOW-COUNT MBL: SIMPLY A SIGN OF IMMUNOSENESCENCE?

The late appearance of low-count MBL, in both humans and mice, together with its stability over time, led to the hypothesis that this phenomenon might be related to "immunosenescence," the decreased immunocompetence status that occurs in elderly people.[43–45] This process is characterized by B-cell compartment changes that include a reduced antibody response associated with a limited heterogeneity in isotype, antigen-binding affinity, and immunoglobulin gene use, with the frequent detection of monoclonality.[46] T-cell alterations are also present and involve mainly the CD8$^+$ memory T-cell subgroup and the appearance of oligo-monoclonal CD4$^+$CD8$^+$ double-positive T lymphocytes.[47,48] T-cell expansions have been associated with persistent latent viral infections (eg, EBV and CMV) triggering a chronic immune stimulation.[49] Along this line of reasoning, an increased frequency of MBL clones has been demonstrated in HCV-infected patients, irrespective of age.[50] B-cell clonal expansions mainly with atypical CLL and CLL phenotype can be observed in about 30% of hepatitis C+ subjects and reach a peak of almost 40% in advanced hepatic disease.[50]

That CLL-like MBL clones might occur in the context of a diffuse modification of the immune system is a working hypothesis supported by different lines of evidence. Clonal T-cell expansions, especially within the double-positive CD4+CD8+ subgroup, have been detected with increased frequency in population screening CLL-like MBL cases.[25] These T-cell clones showed a preferential usage of specific T-cell receptors (TRBV2 and TRBV8), suggesting the fascinating (but still unproven) hypothesis that the occurrence of B-cell and T-cell proliferations may be triggered by common antigenic stimuli.[51] In particular, it has been recently reported that MBL detected in individuals with normal lymphocyte counts is associated with a decrease in immature and naive normal circulating B cells combined to T-cell subset dysregulation. These alterations, potentially leading to an impaired immunosurveillance, become more evident as the MBL cell count increases.[52]

IS THE DISTINCTION BETWEEN CLINICAL MBL AND RAI STAGE 0 CLL MEANINGFUL?

In contrast to low-count MBL, clinical MBL seems to be strictly connected to CLL in terms of risk of progression (and indeed all CLL are always preceded by an MBL stage).[10] One should also remember that before the publication of International Workshop on Chronic Lymphocytic Leukemia 2008 diagnostic criteria,[14] a great part of clinical MBL were indeed diagnosed until that moment as Rai stage 0 CLL. That notwithstanding, it is now known that both conditions are a mixture of real patients whose life expectancy will be affected by the disease but also of individuals who will never develop clinical signs and symptoms. Therefore, for a clinician it would be much more crucial to know how to identify subjects bound to progress regardless of the name label rather than to make a numerical distinction that does not exclude the need in either case of prolonged follow-ups.

Several studies have aimed at dissecting differences and/or similarities between these 2 conditions in addition to the numerical value and several factors deemed to be potentially involved have been actively investigated.

It is well known that genetic factors play a relevant role in CLL occurrence and evolution, as demonstrated by the fact that a family history of CLL or other lymphoproliferative disorder is a well-defined risk factor for developing CLL.[53] Interestingly, studies performed in relatives of familial CLL patients (ie, a family where at least 2 members are affected by CLL) demonstrated that MBL is detected at increased frequency in these subjects, regardless of their age.[54] The overall risk of detection of CLL-like MBL in CLL families is 17 times increased in individuals less than 40 years old, an age range where MBL is almost undetectable in the general population.[55] The higher incidence of MBL among relatives of CLL subjects is reported also in the sporadic setting whereby first-degree relatives have an MBL prevalence similar to that found in familial CLL relatives and definitely higher than that expected in the general population, again suggesting the MBL and CLL are tightly connected.[56,57] The specific genes involved in this process are yet to be defined, although some studies in CLL and MBL subjects showed a similar increased frequency of individual single nucleotide polymorphisms located in genes acting as regulators of B-cell development.[58,59]

Several other genetic and molecular features have been investigated in clinical MBL and Rai stage 0 CLL but none seem to be useful in differentiating these 2 conditions.

Studies comparing the distribution of IGHV gene mutation, CD38, and ZAP70 expression (all consolidated prognostic factors in CLL[60–62]) were not able to detect any significant difference between clinical MBL and Rai stage 0 CLL.[20,21] FISH—detected abnormalities were also comparable in most published studies (**Table 1**).[24] More recently, genome-wide sequencing studies identified relevant gene mutations, including NOTCH1,[63–66] SF3B1,[67–69] and BIRC3,[70] associated with advanced stages of CLL and risk of transformation. As these mutations appear in low frequency in CLL cases at diagnosis (NOTCH1 mutation as low as 4%,[63,65,66,71] SF3B1 mutation as low as 5%,[69] BIRC3 mutation as low as 4%[70]), it is not unexpected that the frequency of NOTCH1, SF3B1, and BIRC3 mutations in clinical MBL cohorts turned out to be particularly low (3.2%,[64] 1.5%,[68] and 0%,[70] respectively), therefore again not helping in narrowing down the patients at risk of progression.

Finally, clinical MBL and Rai stage 0 CLL seem to share the same immune system perturbation and in particular the increased risk of infections. Infectious complications usually represent one major cause of morbidity and mortality in CLL patients. Although mechanisms responsible for infectious complications are still not completely understood, they seem to be similarly present in clinical MBL. A recent multivariate analysis demonstrates that the MBL condition is independently associated with a shorter time to hospitalization for infection[72] and, in comparison to the control population, both MBL and CLL subjects have an increased rate of hospitalization for infections, again suggesting a similarity at a clinical level between the 2 conditions. Additional studies should address if this finding warrants preventive health recommendations in MBL subjects similar to that proposed to CLL patients.

MORE KNOWLEDGE, LESS CERTAINTY: WHAT ABOUT SLL AND MBL?

According to the World Health Organization classification of hematologic disorders,[13] a CLL diagnosis also includes the lymphoma form of the disease, still named, especially by pathologists, small lymphocytic lymphoma (SLL), when a count of $<5 \times 10^9/L$ B cells in the peripheral blood coexist with enlarged lymph nodes or spleens or infiltrated tissues.

CLL-like B cells can indeed be detected in lymph node biopsies performed for reasons other than the hematologic evaluation of a palpable lymphadenopathy as in the case of tissue biopsies for solid tumor staging or evaluation of lymphoadenopathies detected on radiologic studies.[73] These lymph nodes can show diffuse but also focal infiltration of CLL/SLL-like B cells not associated with a clinically relevant lymphocytosis. It has been recently proposed that such situations should be defined as "tissue involvement by CLL/SLL-like cells of uncertain significance"[73] or "nodal (extranodal) MBL."[74] Additional studies are warranted to define if this condition might be considered a tissue equivalent to clinical MBL rather than a full-fledged lymphoma (SLL), as currently diagnosed when detected in tissue specimens for histopathologic analysis.

This situation closely resembles the recently recognized entity of "in situ lymphomas,"[75] where tumor cells proliferate in the place usually occupied by their normal counterpart but without infiltrating surrounding structures. In situ follicular lymphoma and in situ mantle-cell lymphoma can represent isolated lesions not yet clinically relevant but maybe requiring a second hit to evolve and disseminate.[75]

The dissection of the SLL and MBL relationship is not only a semantic game but seems to be even more relevant considering that, in the case of CLL/SLL, the lymph node microenvironment is suspected to be the site where the disease might stem, likely in the context of the proliferative compartment located in the so-called

Table 1
Studies comparing clinical and biologic features of clinical MBL and Rai stage 0 CLL

Characteristics	Rossi et al,[24] 2009		Shanafelt et al,[20] 2009		Scarfò et al,[21] 2012	
	Clinical MBL	Rai Stage 0 CLL	Clinical MBL	Rai Stage 0 CLL	Clinical MBL	Rai Stage 0 CLL
Number of subjects	123	154	302	94[a]	184	430
Median ALC (range)	5.1×10^9/L (1.22–9.9×10^9/L)	12.9×10^9/L (9.2–17.8×10^9/L)[b]	5.4×10^9/L (0.3–9.6×10^9/L)	8.0×10^9/L (5.7–10.0×10^9/L)[b]	6.3×10^9/L (5.4–7.3×10^9/L)	12.4×10^9/L (9.8–17.5×10^9/L)[b]
Median B-cell count (range)	2.8×10^9/L (0.2–4.9×10^9/L)[c]	10.38×10^9/L (6.3–14.8×10^9/L)[b]	2.76×10^9/L (0.02–4.99×10^9/L)	6.06×10^9/L (5.0–9.29×10^9/L)[b]	3.4×10^9/L (2.5–4.2×10^9/L)	8.9×10^9/L (6.8–13.3×10^9/L)[b]
Age (y)[d]	68 (59–75)	68 (60–74)	69 (34–93)[e]	70 (45–92)[e]	64 (56–70)	63 (54–70)
Male sex (%)	60 (48.8%)	83 (53.9%)	175 (58%)	58 (62%)	98 (53.3%)	235 (54.7%)
IGHV identity ≥98%	21/105 (20.0%)	39/139 (28.1%)	25/109 (23%)	7/38 (18%)	26/100 (26%)	75/266 (28.2%)
IGHV4-34	17/105 (16.9%)	21/138 (15.2%)	n.e.	n.e.	11 (11.3%)	27 (10.1%)
IGHV3-23	12/105 (11.4%)	10/138 (7.2%)	n.e.	n.e.	9 (9.3%)	26 (9.7%)
IGHV1-69	9/105 (8.6%)	12/138 (8.7%)	n.e.	n.e.	8 (8.2%)	21 (7.9%)
IGHV3-30	5/105 (4.8%)	11/138 (8.0%)	n.e.	n.e.	7 (7.2%)	20 (7.5%)
Fluorescence in situ hybridization	105 pts	145 pts	126 pts	41 pts	118 pts	290 pts
Normal	45 (42.9%)	34 (23.4%)	39 (31%)	15 (37%)	40 (33.9%)	104 (35.9%)
del13q14	37 (35.2%)	68 (46.9%)	56 (44%)	19 (46%)	55 (46.6%)	126 (43.4%)

+12	19 (18.1%)	21 (14.5%)	23 (18%)	4 (10%)	11 (9.3%)	22 (7.6%)
del11q22-q23	0	9 (6.2%)[b]	2 (2%)	2 (5%)	7 (5.9%)	13 (4.5%)
del17p13	4 (3.8%)	13 (9.0%)[b]	4 (3%)	1 (2%)	5 (4.2%)	22 (7.6%)
Other (6q-)	n.e.	n.e.	2 (2%)	0	0	3 (1.0%)
TP53 mutation	2/66 (3.0%)	12/104 (11.5%)	n.e.	n.e.	n.e.	n.e.
CD38 ≥30%	27/119 (22.7%)	39/150 (26.0%)	60/274 (22%)	15/88 (17%)	25/146 (17.1%)	56/337 (16.6%)
ZAP70 ≥20%	39/97 (40.2%)	49/135 (36.3%)	23/120 (19%)	10/41 (24%)	n.e.	n.e.
Risk of progression to CLL requiring treatment	4% (≤6 y FU); 0% (>6 y FU)	n.a.	1.4% per y (5 y FU)	n.e.	1.5% per y (4 y FU)	5.2% per y (4 y FU)
Median TFS (mo)	Not reached	130.4[b]	n.e.	n.e.	Not reached	187[b]
Need for treatment	19/123 (15.4%)	47/154 (30.5%)	7/302 (2.3%)	9/94 (10%)[b]	23/180 (12.8%)	98/422 (23.2%)[b]
Median follow-up (mo)	42.7	48.2	18	18	45	45

Abbreviations: n.a., not applicable; n.e., not evaluated; pts, patients.

[a] Low count Rai 0 CLL defined by <10 × 10^9 B cells/L.

[b] P<.05.

[c] Median CLL-phenotype B-cell count.

[d] 25th to 75th percentiles.

[e] Range.

proliferation centers.[76] These pseudo-follicular areas, composed by focal aggregates of prolymphocytes, paraimmunoblasts admixed to small lymphocytes, are regarded as the hallmark of CLL in lymphoid tissues. Therefore, it is not unreasonable to postulate the existence of precursor (MBL?) cells also in the nodal compartment that can exist undetected (as less easily attainable) in a large fraction of healthy individuals as is happening in the peripheral blood.

SUMMARY

The distinction between a life-long asymptomatic laboratory alteration and a disease requiring treatment if not threatening life is an important one for the clinicians but especially for the patients.

The current distinction between MBL and CLL has somehow helped to create general awareness of the need of clarification for the sake of affected individuals, although it created inadvertently the wrong concept that an MBL diagnosis could be more reassuring than one of CLL.[77] It is now known that MBL is also a combination of nonprogressive and potentially progressive situations, as much as CLL includes ever-stable cases with mild lymphocytosis and cases needing to be treated sooner or later.

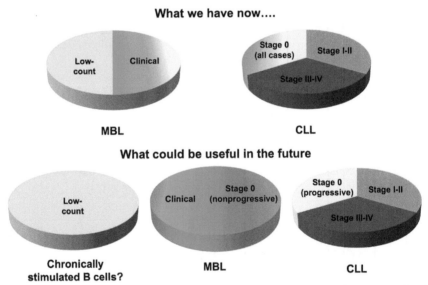

Fig. 1. The current and future paradigm of CLL-like clonal expansions. The current classification of CLL-like clonal expansions is shown on the top row: low-count and clinical MBL (on the left) are distinguished from CLL (on the right) based on the concentration of B lymphocytes in the peripheral blood (<5 × 10⁹/L for MBL cases) and on the absence of symptoms and signs of lymphoproliferative disorders. It is hoped that, in the future, low-count MBL (on the left), that is different from clinical MBL on both biologic and clinical grounds, will be defined as a separate biologic entity (maybe a not yet recognized category "immune-dysregulated"/activated B cells), whereas a better definition of biologic factors may help to segregate nonprogressive clinical MBL and Rai stage 0 cases (bound together under a new "MBL" definition) from progressive clinical MBL and Rai stage 0 CLL patients, who will appropriately receive a diagnosis of leukemia (CLL).

In this regard it has now become evident that a tiny population of CLL-like cells ("low-count MBL") has little to do with CLL as they seem to be a different condition from a clinical and a biologic point of view. Their reciprocal relationship should be deeply investigated but seems to be rather distant and these MBL cases should be more of interest for immunologists rather than hematologists, being potentially related to "immunosenescence" (**Fig. 1**).

In contrast, clinical MBL and CLL seem to be a continuum if not overlapping entities (in the case of Rai stage 0).[78] For all these cases, the main distinction should be between potentially progressive and nonprogressive cases rather than subjects below or above a numerical threshold. This distinction holds particularly true considering that life expectancy in European countries is constantly increasing. Given that both MBL and CLL frequency increases with age, in the next few years clinicians are likely going to deal with an epidemic of MBL cases, posing a relevant burden for national health care systems.

Efforts in the field of CLL diagnosis should aim in the future at finding a way to define as CLL only those cases that are or will be clinically relevant, needing to be intensively followed up because of the risk of progression to active disease (see **Fig. 1**). On the other hand, those cases now floating among clinical MBL/Rai stage 0 CLL should be clearly identified and labeled with the reassuring diagnosis of MBL and left unattended. This practice would help physicians to segregate the patients for whom they should refrain from unnecessary monitoring. It is reasonable to hypothesize that a deeper knowledge of the molecular pathways and of the microenvironmental influences critically involved in the disease evolution will help in reaching this ultimate goal in the near future.

ACKNOWLEDGMENTS

We thank Cristina Scielzo for helpful suggestions and support. This project was supported by: Associazione Italiana per la Ricerca sul Cancro AIRC (Investigator Grant and Special Program Molecular Clinical Oncology – 5 per mille #9965), PRIN – Ministero Istruzione, Università e Ricerca (MIUR), Roma, and Ricerca Finalizzata 2010 – Ministero della Salute, Roma.

REFERENCES

1. Rawstron AC. Monoclonal B-cell lymphocytosis. Hematology Am Soc Hematol Educ Program 2009;430–9.
2. Molica S, Levato D. What is changing in the natural history of chronic lymphocytic leukemia? Haematologica 2001;86:8–12.
3. Rawstron AC, Green MJ, Kuzmicki A, et al. Monoclonal B lymphocytes with the characteristics of "indolent" chronic lymphocytic leukemia are present in 3.5% of adults with normal blood counts. Blood 2002;100:635–9.
4. Ghia P, Prato G, Scielzo C, et al. Monoclonal CD5+ and CD5– B-lymphocyte expansions are frequent in the peripheral blood of the elderly. Blood 2004;103:2337–42.
5. Rawstron AC, Bennett FL, O'Connor SJ, et al. Monoclonal B-cell lymphocytosis and chronic lymphocytic leukemia. N Engl J Med 2008;359:575–83.
6. Dagklis A, Fazi C, Sala C, et al. The immunoglobulin gene repertoire of low-count chronic lymphocytic leukemia (CLL)-like monoclonal B lymphocytosis is different from CLL: diagnostic implications for clinical monitoring. Blood 2009;114:26–32.

7. Nieto WG, Almeida J, Romero A, et al. Increased frequency (12%) of circulating chronic lymphocytic leukemia-like B-cell clones in healthy subjects using a highly sensitive multicolor flow cytometry approach. Blood 2009;114:33–7.

8. Marti GE, Rawstron AC, Ghia P, et al. Diagnostic criteria for monoclonal B-cell lymphocytosis. Br J Haematol 2005;130:325–32.

9. Shanafelt TD, Ghia P, Lanasa MC, et al. Monoclonal B-cell lymphocytosis (MBL): biology, natural history and clinical management. Leukemia 2010;24:512–20.

10. Landgren O, Albitar M, Ma W, et al. B-cell clones as early markers for chronic lymphocytic leukemia. N Engl J Med 2009;360:659–67.

11. Scarfo L, Dagklis A, Scielzo C, et al. CLL-like monoclonal B-cell lymphocytosis: are we all bound to have it? Semin Cancer Biol 2010;20:384–90.

12. Caligaris-Cappio F, Ghia P. Novel insights in chronic lymphocytic leukemia: are we getting closer to understanding the pathogenesis of the disease? J Clin Oncol 2008;26:4497–503.

13. Müller-Hermelink HK, Montserrat E, Catovsky D, et al. In: Swerdlow SH, Campo E, Harris NL, et al, editors. WHO Classification of Tumours of Hematopoietic and Lymphoid Tissues. Lyon (France): International agency for Research on Cancer; 2008. p. 180–2.

14. Hallek M, Cheson BD, Catovsky D, et al. Guidelines for the diagnosis and treatment of chronic lymphocytic leukemia: a report from the International Workshop on Chronic Lymphocytic Leukemia updating the National Cancer Institute-Working Group 1996 guidelines. Blood 2008;111:5446–56.

15. Shim YK, Vogt RF, Middleton D, et al. Prevalence and natural history of monoclonal and polyclonal B-cell lymphocytosis in a residential adult population. Cytometry B Clin Cytom 2007;72:344–53.

16. Rachel JM, Zucker ML, Fox CM, et al. Monoclonal B-cell lymphocytosis in blood donors. Br J Haematol 2007;139:832–6.

17. Almeida J, Nieto WG, Teodosio C, et al. CLL-like B-lymphocytes are systematically present at very low numbers in peripheral blood of healthy adults. Leukemia 2011;25:718–22.

18. Rawstron AC, Shanafelt T, Lanasa MC, et al. Different biology and clinical outcome according to the absolute numbers of clonal B-cells in monoclonal B-cell lymphocytosis (MBL). Cytometry B Clin Cytom 2010;78(Suppl 1):S19–23.

19. Dagklis A, Fazi C, Scarfo L, et al. Monoclonal B lymphocytosis in the general population. Leuk Lymphoma 2009;50:490–2.

20. Shanafelt TD, Kay NE, Rabe KG, et al. Brief report: natural history of individuals with clinically recognized monoclonal B-cell lymphocytosis compared with patients with Rai 0 chronic lymphocytic leukemia. J Clin Oncol 2009;27:3959–63.

21. Scarfò L, Zibellini S, Tedeschi A, et al. Impact of B-cell count and imaging screening in cMBL: any need to revise the current guidelines? Leukemia 2012; 26:1703–7.

22. Fung SS, Hillier KL, Leger CS, et al. Clinical progression and outcome of patients with monoclonal B-cell lymphocytosis. Leuk Lymphoma 2007;48:1087–91.

23. Mulligan CS, Thomas ME, Mulligan SP. Monoclonal B-cell lymphocytosis and chronic lymphocytic leukemia. N Engl J Med 2008;359:2065–6 [author reply: 2066].

24. Rossi D, Sozzi E, Puma A, et al. The prognosis of clinical monoclonal B cell lymphocytosis differs from prognosis of Rai 0 chronic lymphocytic leukaemia and is recapitulated by biological risk factors. Br J Haematol 2009;146:64–75.

25. Fazi C, Scarfo L, Pecciarini L, et al. General population low-count CLL-like MBL persists over time without clinical progression, although carrying the same cytogenetic abnormalities of CLL. Blood 2011;118:6618–25.

26. Victor Hoffbrand A, Hamblin TJ. Is "leukemia" an appropriate label for all patients who meet the diagnostic criteria of chronic lymphocytic leukemia? Leuk Res 2007;31:273–5.

27. Rai KR, Sawitsky A, Cronkite EP, et al. Clinical staging of chronic lymphocytic leukemia. Blood 1975;46:219–34.

28. Shanafelt TD, Kay NE, Call TG, et al. MBL or CLL: which classification best categorizes the clinical course of patients with an absolute lymphocyte count >or= 5 x 10(9) L(-1) but a B-cell lymphocyte count <5 x 10(9) L(-1)? Leuk Res 2008;32: 1458–61.

29. Shanafelt TD, Kay NE, Jenkins G, et al. B-cell count and survival: differentiating chronic lymphocytic leukemia from monoclonal B-cell lymphocytosis based on clinical outcome. Blood 2009;113:4188–96.

30. Molica S, Mauro FR, Giannarelli D, et al. Differentiating chronic lymphocytic leukemia from monoclonal B-lymphocytosis according to clinical outcome: on behalf of the GIMEMA chronic lymphoproliferative diseases working group. Haematologica 2010;96:277–83.

31. Lanasa MC, Allgood SD, Volkheimer AD, et al. Single-cell analysis reveals oligoclonality among 'low-count' monoclonal B-cell lymphocytosis. Leukemia 2010;24: 133–40.

32. Ghiotto F, Fais F, Valetto A, et al. Remarkably similar antigen receptors among a subset of patients with chronic lymphocytic leukemia. J Clin Invest 2004;113: 1008–16.

33. Messmer BT, Albesiano E, Efremov DG, et al. Multiple distinct sets of stereotyped antigen receptors indicate a role for antigen in promoting chronic lymphocytic leukemia. J Exp Med 2004;200:519–25.

34. Stamatopoulos K, Belessi C, Moreno C, et al. Over 20% of patients with chronic lymphocytic leukemia carry stereotyped receptors: Pathogenetic implications and clinical correlations. Blood 2007;109:259–70.

35. Agathangelidis A, Darzentas N, Hadzidimitriou A, et al. Stereotyped B-cell receptors in one-third of chronic lymphocytic leukemia: a molecular classification with implications for targeted therapies. Blood 2012;119:4467–75.

36. Dohner H, Stilgenbauer S, Benner A, et al. Genomic aberrations and survival in chronic lymphocytic leukemia. N Engl J Med 2000;343:1910–6.

37. Lanasa MC, Allgood SD, Slager SL, et al. Immunophenotypic and gene expression analysis of monoclonal B-cell lymphocytosis shows biologic characteristics associated with good prognosis CLL. Leukemia 2011;25:1459–66.

38. Schuler F, Dolken L, Hirt C, et al. Prevalence and frequency of circulating t(14;18)-MBR translocation carrying cells in healthy individuals. Int J Cancer 2009;124: 958–63.

39. Klein U, Lia M, Crespo M, et al. The DLEU2/miR-15a/16-1 cluster controls B cell proliferation and its deletion leads to chronic lymphocytic leukemia. Cancer Cell 2010;17:28–40.

40. Phillips JA, Mehta K, Fernandez C, et al. The NZB mouse as a model for chronic lymphocytic leukemia. Cancer Res 1992;52:437–43.

41. Hamano Y, Hirose S, Ida A, et al. Susceptibility alleles for aberrant B-1 cell proliferation involved in spontaneously occurring B-cell chronic lymphocytic leukemia in a model of New Zealand white mice. Blood 1998;92:3772–9.

42. LeMaoult J, Manavalan JS, Dyall R, et al. Cellular basis of B cell clonal populations in old mice. J Immunol 1999;162:6384–91.

43. Wick G, Grubeck-Loebenstein B. The aging immune system: primary and secondary alterations of immune reactivity in the elderly. Exp Gerontol 1997;32:401–13.

44. Ghia P, Melchers F, Rolink AG. Age-dependent changes in B lymphocyte development in man and mouse. Exp Gerontol 2000;35:159–65.
45. Klinman NR, Kline GH. The B-cell biology of aging. Immunol Rev 1997;160: 103–14.
46. Nicoletti C. Antibody protection in aging: influence of idiotypic repertoire and antibody binding activity to a bacterial antigen. Exp Mol Pathol 1995;62:99–108.
47. Colombatti A, Doliana R, Schiappacassi M, et al. Age-related persistent clonal expansions of CD28(-) cells: phenotypic and molecular TCR analysis reveals both CD4(+) and CD4(+)CD8(+) cells with identical CDR3 sequences. Clin Immunol Immunopathol 1998;89:61–70.
48. Ghia P, Prato G, Stella S, et al. Age-dependent accumulation of monoclonal CD4+CD8+ double positive T lymphocytes in the peripheral blood of the elderly. Br J Haematol 2007;139:780–90.
49. Khan N, Shariff N, Cobbold M, et al. Cytomegalovirus seropositivity drives the CD8 T cell repertoire toward greater clonality in healthy elderly individuals. J Immunol 2002;169:1984–92.
50. Fazi C, Dagklis A, Cottini F, et al. Monoclonal B cell lymphocytosis in hepatitis C virus infected individuals. Cytometry B Clin Cytom 2010;78(Suppl 1):S61–8.
51. Marti GE. MBL: mostly benign lymphocytes, but…. Blood 2011;118:6480–1.
52. Hauswirth AW, Almeida J, Nieto WG, et al. Monoclonal B-cell lymphocytosis (MBL) with normal lymphocyte counts is associated with decreased numbers of normal circulating B-cell subsets. Am J Hematol 2012;87:721–4.
53. Goldin LR, Bjorkholm M, Kristinsson SY, et al. Elevated risk of chronic lymphocytic leukemia and other indolent non-Hodgkin's lymphomas among relatives of patients with chronic lymphocytic leukemia. Haematologica 2009;94:647–53.
54. Goldin LR, Lanasa MC, Slager SL, et al. Common occurrence of monoclonal B-cell lymphocytosis among members of high-risk CLL families. Br J Haematol 2010;151:152–8.
55. de Tute R, Yuille M, Catovsky D, et al. Monoclonal B-cell lymphocytosis (MBL) in CLL families: substantial increase in relative risk for young adults. Leukemia 2006;20:728–9.
56. Matos DM, Ismael SJ, Scrideli CA, et al. Monoclonal B-cell lymphocytosis in first-degree relatives of patients with sporadic (non-familial) chronic lymphocytic leukaemia. Br J Haematol 2009;147:339–46.
57. Del Giudice I, Mauro FR, De Propris MS, et al. Identification of monoclonal B-cell lymphocytosis among sibling transplant donors for chronic lymphocytic leukemia patients. Blood 2009;114:2848–9.
58. Di Bernardo MC, Crowther-Swanepoel D, Broderick P, et al. A genome-wide association study identifies six susceptibility loci for chronic lymphocytic leukemia. Nat Genet 2008;40:1204–10.
59. Crowther-Swanepoel D, Corre T, Lloyd A, et al. Inherited genetic susceptibility to monoclonal B-cell lymphocytosis. Blood 2010;116:5957–60.
60. Damle RN, Wasil T, Fais F, et al. Ig V gene mutation status and CD38 expression as novel prognostic indicators in chronic lymphocytic leukemia. Blood 1999;94: 1840–7.
61. Hamblin TJ, Davis Z, Gardiner A, et al. Unmutated Ig V(H) genes are associated with a more aggressive form of chronic lymphocytic leukemia. Blood 1999;94: 1848–54.
62. Crespo M, Bosch F, Villamor N, et al. ZAP-70 expression as a surrogate for immunoglobulin-variable-region mutations in chronic lymphocytic leukemia. N Engl J Med 2003;348:1764–75.

63. Puente XS, Pinyol M, Quesada V, et al. Whole-genome sequencing identifies recurrent mutations in chronic lymphocytic leukaemia. Nature 2011;475:101–5.
64. Rasi S, Monti S, Spina V, et al. Analysis of NOTCH1 mutations in monoclonal B-cell lymphocytosis. Haematologica 2012;97:153–4.
65. Fabbri G, Rasi S, Rossi D, et al. Analysis of the chronic lymphocytic leukemia coding genome: role of NOTCH1 mutational activation. J Exp Med 2011;208:1389–401.
66. Rossi D, Rasi S, Fabbri G, et al. Mutations of NOTCH1 are an independent predictor of survival in chronic lymphocytic leukemia. Blood 2012;119:521–9.
67. Wang L, Lawrence MS, Wan Y, et al. SF3B1 and other novel cancer genes in chronic lymphocytic leukemia. N Engl J Med 2011;365:2497–506.
68. Greco M, Capello D, Bruscaggin A, et al. Analysis of SF3B1 mutations in monoclonal B-cell lymphocytosis. Hematol Oncol 2012. [Epub ahead of print].
69. Quesada V, Conde L, Villamor N, et al. Exome sequencing identifies recurrent mutations of the splicing factor SF3B1 gene in chronic lymphocytic leukemia. Nat Genet 2011;44:47–52.
70. Rossi D, Fangazio M, Rasi S, et al. Disruption of BIRC3 associates with fludarabine chemorefractoriness in TP53 wild-type chronic lymphocytic leukemia. Blood 2012;119:2854–62.
71. Balatti V, Bottoni A, Palamarchuk A, et al. NOTCH1 mutations in CLL associated with trisomy 12. Blood 2012;119:329–31.
72. Moreira J, Rabe KG, Cerhan JR, et al. Infectious complications among individuals with clinical monoclonal B-cell lymphocytosis (MBL): a cohort study of newly diagnosed cases compared to controls. Leukemia 2013;27:136–41.
73. Gibson SE, Swerdlow SH, Ferry JA, et al. Reassessment of small lymphocytic lymphoma in the era of monoclonal B-cell lymphocytosis. Haematologica 2011;96:1144–52.
74. Ghia P. Another piece of the puzzle: is there a "nodal" monoclonal B-cell lymphocytosis? Haematologica 2011;96:1089–91.
75. Carbone A, Santoro A. How I treat: diagnosing and managing "in situ" lymphoma. Blood 2011;117:3954–60.
76. Bertilaccio MT, Scielzo C, Muzio M, et al. An overview of chronic lymphocytic leukaemia biology. Best Pract Res Clin Haematol 2010;23:21–32.
77. Ghia P, Caligaris-Cappio F. Monoclonal B-cell lymphocytosis: right track or red herring? Blood 2012;119:4358–62.
78. Kern W, Bacher U, Haferlach C, et al. Monoclonal B-cell lymphocytosis is closely related to chronic lymphocytic leukaemia and may be better classified as early-stage CLL. Br J Haematol 2012. http://dx.doi.org/10.1111/j.1365-2141.2011.09010.x.

The Role of Minimal Residual Disease Measurements in the Therapy for CLL
Is It Ready for Prime Time?

Sebastian Böttcher, MD[a],*, Michael Hallek, MD[b],
Matthias Ritgen, MD[a], Michael Kneba, MD, PhD[a]

KEYWORDS

- Chronic lymphocytic leukemia • Minimal residual disease • Prognostic factors
- MRD flow
- Allele-specific oligonucleotide *IGH* real-time quantitative polymerase chain reaction
- Progression-free survival

KEY POINTS

- The tumor load that remains after therapy in patients with chronic lymphocytic leukemia can be quantified by modern minimal residual disease (MRD) technology with a 1000-fold higher sensitivity compared with clinical staging.
- Quantitative multicolor flow cytometry or ASO primer real-time quantitative *IGH* PCR should be applied for standardized MRD monitoring with results evaluated with respect to thresholds at 10^{-4} and additionally at 10^{-2}.
- MRD is an independent predictor of progression-free and overall survival after conventional induction therapy adding significantly to the prognostic power of known pretreatment prognostic factors.
- MRD kinetics after allogeneic stem cell transplantation identifies patients who experience efficacious graft-versus-leukemia activity that leads to complete eradication of the malignant clone.
- MRD qualifies as a surrogate marker to identify the superior treatment arm in randomized clinical trials by a lower proportion of MRD-positive patients, but its general application for tailoring therapy in individual patients outside clinical trials is currently discouraged.

[a] Second Department of Medicine, University Hospital of Schleswig-Holstein, Campus Kiel, Chemnitzstrasse 33, Kiel 24116, Germany; [b] Department I of Internal Medicine, Centre of Integrated Oncology and CECAD, Cluster of Excellence Cellular Stress Responses in Aging-Associated Diseases, University of Cologne, Kerpener Strasse 62, Cologne 50924, Germany
* Corresponding author. Second Department of Medicine, University Hospital of Schleswig-Holstein, Campus Kiel, Chemnitzstrasse 33, Kiel 24116, Germany.
E-mail address: s.boettcher@med2.uni-kiel.de

Hematol Oncol Clin N Am 27 (2013) 267–288
http://dx.doi.org/10.1016/j.hoc.2013.01.005
0889-8588/13/$ – see front matter © 2013 Elsevier Inc. All rights reserved.

RATIONALE FOR MINIMAL RESIDUAL DISEASE ASSESSMENTS IN CHRONIC LYMPHOCYTIC LEUKEMIA

The number of leukemic cells in the body of patients with chronic lymphocytic leukemia (CLL) decreases when they respond to treatment. Considering residual leukemic cells as the source of relapse, one would intuitively hypothesize that a high tumor burden after therapy is associated with a short progression-free survival (PFS). Patients in whom regrowth of the leukemic clone starts from a larger number of malignant cells suffer an earlier clinical relapse, because a faster reoccurrence of clinical signs and symptoms of the leukemia is expected.

Minimal residual disease (MRD) is a very sensitive measurement of the tumor load that remains in the body of a patient after therapy. Therefore, the attainment of an MRD-negative status (ie, no detection of leukemia by sensitive methods) is expected to predict for long PFS. Because current MRD methods are approximately 1000-fold more sensitive than clinical staging, MRD status should much more exactly predict time to relapse. Moreover, modern MRD assessments are considered more accurate than clinical staging to quantitatively reflect the number of residual leukemia cells after treatment.

Current conventional therapy cannot cure CLL, as exemplified by a lack of a plateau in Kaplan-Meier plots for PFS.[1–9] It is expected, therefore, that all patients, even those from good risk subgroups treated with intensive therapy, eventually relapse. Consequently, the efficacy of therapies in CLL is primarily judged by median PFS (with overall survival used as a secondary end-point), thus resembling current concepts in many other peripheral B-cell malignancies (eg, multiple myeloma,[10–14] follicular[15–19] and mantle cell lymphomas[20–22]). Most current treatment strategies in CLL are characterized by an induction phase to reduce the tumor load followed by treatment-free observation. The general concept of MRD as a predictor of PFS after such a conventional induction therapy is depicted in **Fig. 1A**.

The predictive power of MRD in this situation depends on the assumption that regrowth kinetics are similar between different patients, do not relate to the MRD level achieved, and are constant over time. Logically, patients or patient cohorts who show faster regrowth kinetics are expected to present earlier with clinical signs or symptoms of relapse even if they have achieved low MRD levels directly after induction therapy (see **Fig. 1B**).

The absence of MRD is a prerequisite for but not identical to cure. Any MRD measurement has a finite sensitivity, so that the persistence of residual CLL cells below that limit of detection is possible. The minimum number of residual CLL cells necessary to eventually cause a relapse is unknown. However, patients who were MRD-negative at the lowest level measurable with the most sensitive available technology (1 CLL cell in more than 100,000 benign leukocytes) can show relapse.[23] That means that if there is a threshold for cure in CLL, it must be lower than 10^{-5}. The likelihood of relapse is therefore not only influenced by the treatment effects one can directly measure but also by treatment effects that occur in CLL cells below the limit of detection. It is assumed that treatment effects are similar below and above the detection threshold of MRD. To predict what will likely happen below the MRD limit of detection it is important to consider the duration and efficacy of treatment when interpreting MRD results.

Patients successfully treated with an allogeneic stem cell transplantation receive a very effective and long-lasting therapy mediated by graft-versus-leukemia effects, thus contrasting with the short-term efficacy in the induction therapy setting. After allogeneic transplantation the disappearance of CLL cells below the lowest measurable MRD level is likely a surrogate marker for effective graft-versus-leukemia activity.

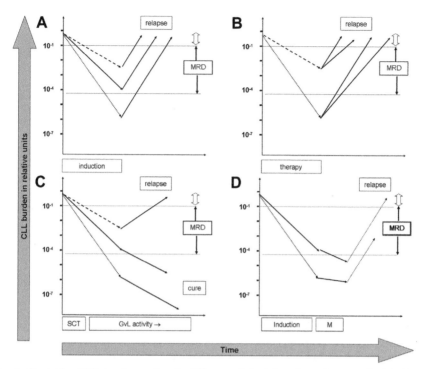

Fig. 1. Model for MRD load over time in different clinical situations. Compared with clinical assessments, CLL burden during and after therapy can be more accurately monitored using MRD. The *double-headed open arrow* symbolizes sensitivity of clinical staging. (*A*) Improved prediction of PFS using MRD quantification. (*B*) Regrowth kinetics impact on the predictive significance. (*C*) GvL activity can be monitored after allogeneic stem cell transplantation. (*D*) Effective maintenance therapy modulates regrowth kinetics. GvL, graft-versus-leukemia activity; M, maintenance; SCT, allogeneic stem cell transplantation.

Current data suggest that this activity not only reduces the malignant clone within the range of measurable MRD levels but is equally potent in suppressing or eradicating the disease at even lower levels, thus finally leading to cure in many patients (see **Fig. 1C**).

An intermediate situation between allogeneic stem cell transplantation and conventional therapy might be envisaged when patients receive an effective maintenance therapy that should lead to tumor suppression while given, thus modulating the kinetics of CLL regrowth (see **Fig. 1D**).

MRD assessments about 1000-fold extend the ability to directly measure treatment effects in CLL compared with clinical assessments, thus allowing better prediction of PFS after conventional therapy and better evaluation of graft-versus-leukemia activity after allogeneic stem cell transplantation.

TECHNIQUES TO DETECT MRD
Overview on Available Technology for MRD Detection

"Minimal residual disease" is not a registered trademark. The only feature common to all methods labeled "MRD" is the ability to detect CLL cells in patients without cytologic and histologic evidence of disease. However, clinicians have witnessed continuous technologic improvements over the last 30 years so that today's advanced methods are up to 100-fold more sensitive than the very early assays. In addition, state-of-the-art MRD technology is still not applied in all treatment protocols so that results with different sensitivity, quantitative accuracy, and reproducibility are reported. Differences in applied technology and data interpretation considerably contribute to different findings on the clinical significance of MRD. To allow clinicians a profound appraisal of the published data, general principles and performance features of MRD methods are reviewed next and summarized in **Table 1**. For reasons outlined in the following sections it is mandatory that sensitive, quantitatively accurate, standardized methods are used today.

Sensitive detection of MRD in CLL is currently possible using either the rearranged immunoglobulin genes of the CLL clone (polymerase chain reaction [PCR]-based MRD detection) or the unique immunophenotype of CLL cells (flow cytometric MRD detection). Both methods have advantages and drawbacks. Flow cytometry is generally more broadly available; faster (results available in 6 hours); less labor-intensive; and requires less specialized equipment. However, sensitive flow cytometry requires 20-fold more sample material than PCR. PCR-based MRD approaches target DNA, which is stable even at room temperature. PCR-based MRD assessments can therefore successfully be performed on older and even stored samples, whereas flow cytometry requires analysis within 48 hours from sample collection. Advanced PCR approaches can require several weeks before the results become available.

PCR-Based Methods for MRD Detection

PCR-based approaches in CLL are based on the detection of the clones' unique rearranged immunoglobulin gene. This so-called "genetic fingerprint" is inherited from the founder B-cell of the CLL clone in an individual patient.

The simplest technique to detect rearranged immunoglobulin genes uses primers matching conserved regions adjacent to the most diverse regions of the immunoglobulin gene (the complementary determining region 3 [CDR3]). PCR products of different lengths are obtained when such consensus primers are used in polyclonal samples. In contrast, CLL samples consisting of genetically uniform cells give rise to one single PCR product of defined length.[24] The sensitivity of this method, consensus-primer PCR, depends on the length of the monoclonal PCR product that represents the patient with CLL. The CLL clones with CDR3 lengths that are rarely represented in the benign B-cell repertoire can be more sensitively detected than PCR products of average size. Moreover, the abundance of residual benign B-cells impacts on sensitivity. Therefore, this method can be rather sensitive in certain clinical situations[25] but its sensitivity differs by sample and is often inferior to 10^{-4}.[26–29]

More sensitive are approaches that use primers directly matching the highly diverse CDR3. As opposed to the consensus PCR, which measures the length of the CDR3, this method identifies a part of the CDR3's sequence. However, the design of such an allele-specific oligonucleotide (ASO) primer requires sequencing of the CDR3 in diagnostic material of each patient before the design of a suitable, individual assay. Although the sensitivity (up to 10^{-5}) and specificity of ASO primer PCR is high and largely independent of the number of polyclonal B-cells in the sample, ASO primers differ in affinity to background cells. The sensitivity and specificity of individual ASO primer assays are consequently different from patient to patient. ASO primer PCR is not quantitative. The combination of a consensus PCR with a ASO primer–based PCR (nested ASO *IGH* PCR) can further improve specificities and sensitivities (reportedly up to 10^{-6})[23,30–32] but is a nonquantitative method.

Real-time quantitative (RQ) PCR measures the release of fluorochrome from a labeled probe during the PCR amplification process. The number of PCR cycles

Table 1
Overview on most commonly used methods for MRD detection

Method	Typical Sensitivity	Quantitative	Typical Quantitative Range	Sample Requirements	Assay Performance Influenced by	Standardization of Laboratory Procedures and Data Interpretation	Selected References on Methodologic Aspects
Consensus IGH PCR	10^{-3}	No	n/a	10^6 total leukocytes needed	Clone (PCR product size), number of benign B cells	Yes	24,26,27,29,69
Nested ASO IGH PCR	Up to 10^{-6}	No	n/a	10^6 total leukocytes needed	Clone (CDR3 region of patient)	None	30-32
ASO IGH RQ-PCR	10^{-5}	Yes	10^{-4}	10^6 total leukocytes needed	Clone (CDR3 region of patient)	Yes	27,34,35,44
Flow cytometry CD19/CD5	5×10^{-2}	No	n/a	Fresh (48 h)	Number of benign B cells Activation of benign B cells by previous therapy	None	40
Flow cytometry CD19/CD5/κ/λ	10^{-2}	No	n/a	Fresh (48 h)	Number of benign B cells Activation of benign B cells by previous therapy	None	40
Quantitative four-color MRD flow	10^{-4}	Yes	10^{-4}	Fresh (48 h), $\geq 10^7$ total leukocytes needed	Number of available leukocytes	Yes	29,43,44

Abbreviations: ASO, allele-specific oligonucleotide; RQ-PCR, real-time quantitative polymerase chain reaction.

required until this fluorescence signal becomes detectable can be converted into the tumor content of the sample. When RQ technology was combined with the ASO primer approach PCR-based quantification in lymphoid malignancies became possible.[33,34] Although ASO primer *IGH* RQ PCR is a very sensitive method for MRD quantification, it requires testing of the ASO assay for each individual patient. Two parameters, the quantitative range and the sensitivity, have to be determined experimentally for each individual ASO primer assay, making the method expensive and labor-intensive. However, definitions for quantitative range and sensitivity, and a standardized procedure for ASO RQ PCR-based MRD detection have been widely accepted, so that results are reproducible between laboratories.[35]

Flow Cytometric Methods to Detect MRD

Flow cytometric MRD analysis identifies CLL cells as a population of leukocytes that exhibit a combination of markers that are not observed in benign hematopoiesis. The following features are used for flow cytometric MRD detection in CLL:

- Expression of CD5 (otherwise seen on T cells and on a minor subpopulation of benign B cells)
- A predominance of either kappa or lambda immunoglobulin light chains (light chain restriction)
- Underexpression or overexpression of select antigens on CLL B cells when compared with benign CD5$^+$ B cells.

The simplest method to measure MRD by flow cytometry relies on the simultaneous detection of CD5 together with the B-cell markers CD19[36,37] or CD20.[38,39] Cases with more than 25% CD5$^+$ B cells of the total B cells were considered MRD positive. The approach lacks quantitative accuracy and specificity because the proportion of mature benign B cells that coexpress CD5 can reach at least 80% after intensive therapy.[40,41] The combination of light chain restriction with CD5/CD19 assessments can improve the specificity, but is still hampered by a low sensitivity.[40]

Current quantitative multicolor MRD flow is based on expression differences between benign CD19$^+$CD5$^+$ B cells and CLL cells. First systematic investigations in those expression differences revealed the use of CD20, CD79b, and CD38 for identification of CLL cells in samples that also contained normal B cells.[29] Later, the overexpression of CD43[26] and the combined underexpression of CD81 and CD22 were described as useful for MRD detection.[42] An international consortium under the auspices of the European Research Initiative on CLL tested 10 different four-color combinations and found the antibody-combinations CD20/CD38/CD19/CD5, CD22/CD81/CD19/CD5, and CD43/CD79b/CD19/CD5 to yield the most reproducible and specific results.[43] The international consortium also developed standard operating procedures for MRD cell identification and quantification to further improve reproducibility between laboratories.[43] The combined evaluation of expression levels (ie, number of molecules per cell) of the aforementioned antigens allows the distinction between benign B cells and minute CLL cell populations without overlap, so that the accurate flow cytometric quantification of residual leukemic cells at a level of 10^{-4} became possible. Because CLL cells and all benign cells can be reliably distinguished using the standardized antibody combinations, the sensitivity of MRD flow primarily depends on the availability of sufficient numbers of leukocytes in a sample.[43,44] Virtually all available data on the clinical significance of sensitive MRD quantification in CLL are based on the harmonized quantitative four-color MRD flow approach or, in case of studies that started before its publication,[45] on slight modifications of it (see **Table 2** for an overview).

Table 2
Clinical trials and series in CLL with analysis of MRD after current International Workshop on Chronic Lymphocytic Leukemia MRD definition of MRD thresholds

No.	Study (ref)	Number of Patients Assessed Using MRD	Therapy	Technique	MRD Threshold	PFS by MRD Group (MRD+ vs MRD−)	P Value
1	Moreno et al,[27] 2006	17	Auto SCT	ASO RQ-PCR	10^{-5}	19 mo vs NR	.02
		22		Quantitative three- or four-color MRD flow	10^{-4}	16 mo vs 75 mo	<.001
2	Bosch et al,[28] 2008	44	FCM	Quantitative four-color MRD flow	10^{-4}	MRD+ CR < MRD− CR (response duration)	.2
3	Kwok et al,[56] 2009	137	Various[a]	Quantitative four-color MRD flow	10^{-4}	24 mo vs 91 mo	<.001
4	Böttcher et al,[45] 2012	290[b]	FC/FCR	Quantitative four-color MRD flow	10^{-4} and 10^{-2}	$\geq 10^{-2}$ 15 mo NR; $\geq 10^{-4}$ to $<10^{-2}$ 41 mo; $<10^{-4}$ 69 mo	<.001
5	Fischer et al,[4] 2012	45	BR	Quantitative four-color MRD flow	10^{-4} and 10^{-2}	$\geq 10^{-2}$ 12 mo; $\geq 10^{-4}$ to $<10^{-2}$ 32 mo; $<10^{-4}$ NR	<.001
6	Pettitt et al,[60] 2012	29	alemtuzumab-HDMP	Quantitative four-color MRD flow	10^{-4}	10 mo vs 24 mo	.009

The most recent report only was cited in studies with published follow-up.

Abbreviations: BR, bendamustine rituximab; CR, complete remission; FC, fludarabine-cyclophosphamide; FCM, fludarabine-cyclophosphamide-mitoxantrone; FCR, fludarabine-cyclophosphamide-rituximab; HDMP, high dose methylprednisolone; NR, not reached; SCT, stem cell transplantation.

a For example, chlorambucil, fludarabine, FC (-R), alemtuzumab, auto SCT, or various others.

b Considering only 290 patients with MRD assessments in peripheral blood after induction therapy (final restaging).

A comparative analysis in 530 samples subsequently demonstrated that four-color MRD flow allows CLL quantification down to the 10^{-4} threshold with equal sensitivity as ASO primer RQ-PCR.[44] The PCR method was more effective in detecting CLL cells below that threshold. There was a high degree of quantitative correlation between PCR and MRD flow ($r = 0.95$), finally proving by cross-evaluation that both methods are quantitatively reliable.[44] MRD flow showed identical accuracy compared with ASO *IGH* RQ-PCR regardless of the therapeutic regimen (FCR, fludarabine-cyclophosphamide-rituximab, or FC, fludarabine-cyclophosphamide),[44] thus corroborating and extending earlier investigations.[27,43]

Quantitative four-color MRD flow and ASO RQ *IGH* PCR are the current reference methods for sensitive and quantitative MRD assessments in CLL.[46] Either of the two techniques should be applied for MRD monitoring. Novel technologies for MRD quantification (eg, next generation sequencing,[47] eight-color MRD flow) have to be thoroughly evaluated on clinical samples against these standards before clinical application.

MRD PREDICTS PFS

The prognostic significance of MRD is usually explained by an inverse correlation of tumor load after therapy and PFS (see **Fig. 1**A). That concept was inspired by data identifying clinical response or clinical complete remissions (CR) as predictors for longer time to progression.[1,9,28,48,49] For instance, in the German CLL study group (GCLLSG) CLL8 trial 75.9% of patients achieving a CR remained progression-free at 3 years postrandomization compared with 45.2% patients achieving only a partial response (PR) or nonresponse ($P<.0001$).[1] One can therefore conclude that residual tumor burden when assessed by the insensitive method, clinical staging, predicts PFS and hypothesize that this will be more accurately possible using MRD.

A survey of major investigations reporting a correlation between MRD and clinical outcome revealed data on 1328 patients with CLL included into 17 series or trials (see **Table 2**; **Table 3**). All those patients received induction therapy, but neither allogeneic transplants nor maintenance therapies.

Those investigations are heterogeneous with respect to the patient cohorts. MRD was often analyzed in CR patients only, whereas other researchers included partial and complete responders in their series. A comparison between studies is even more complicated because different technologies, different thresholds for the distinction between MRD-positive and -negative subgroups, and different sources of sampling material for MRD analysis (bone marrow or peripheral blood) were used. Finally, the treatment intensity differs between the investigations and in addition sampling time-points had not been fully standardized.

Despite the heterogeneity of investigations all of them reported an improved clinical outcome in MRD-negative patients (see **Tables 2** and **3**). Reported median PFS differed by more than 1 year between MRD-negative and -positive patients in all manuscripts so that the detected differences can be considered clinically relevant. The difference between MRD-negative and -positive patients was statistically significant for clinical outcome (usually PFS) in 14 out of 17 publications and not reported in one manuscript.

In a phase II trial investigating MRD after fludarabine-cyclophosphamide-mitoxantrone(FCM) treatment in 44 patients with CLL in clinical CR, MRD-negative patients enjoyed longer response duration compared with MRD-positive patients, but this difference did not reach statistical significance at 30 months follow-up.[28] In another investigation on 82 relapsed patients with CLL treated with FCR those with MRD-negative status had a longer time to progression than those with a positive result by qualitative PCR, but the difference was not significant with a median follow-up of 28 months.[50]

There is solid evidence from many investigations that patients who attain an MRD-negative status progress later than those who remain MRD positive. Of note, this could be demonstrated for different thresholds in different investigations ranging from 5×10^{-2} (marginally more sensitive than cytology) to 10^{-5}. The finding that MRD negativity is predictive of PFS independently from the threshold applied indirectly corroborates the assumption that there is a continuous inverse relationship between tumor burden and time to progression.

MRD LEVELS PREDICT PFS

For a long time results of MRD assessments were reported as positive versus negative, thus using the detection limits of the applied (often nonquantitative) technology as threshold. Logically, it would be much more reproducible to use predefined thresholds at certain MRD levels for reporting. Direct proof for the significance of MRD levels required the advent of quantitative MRD technology. One would predict that within the group of MRD-positive patients those with a higher MRD level would relapse earlier than MRD-positive patients presenting with a lower level. To date three reports could indeed demonstrate such a relationship.

The pivotal study by Moreno and colleagues[27] separated 12 MRD-positive patients after autologous stem cell transplantation into low- ($<10^{-3}$) and high-level ($\geq 10^{-3}$) subgroups. The five MRD-positive patients who belonged to the MRD low-level subgroup experienced a median PFS of 70 months, whereas PFS was 15 months only for seven MRD high-level patients.

Recent GCLLSG data extended and corroborated these early observations. Within the randomized CLL8 trial comparing FCR with FC treatment a significant inverse correlation between MRD levels and PFS was demonstrated at all time-points during and after therapy.[45] For instance, when MRD was analyzed 2 months after the completion of therapy an MRD level below 10^{-4} predicted a median PFS of 69 months, an intermediate level ($\geq 10^{-4}$ to $<10^{-2}$) predicted a median PFS of 41 months, and an even higher MRD level ($\geq 10^{-2}$) was associated with a PFS of 15 months ($P<.0001$). The hazard rates (HR) for the comparison within the range of MRD positivity ($\geq 10^{-4}$ to $<10^{-2}$ vs $\geq 10^{-2}$, HR 5.8) were higher than for the distinction between MRD negativity ($<10^{-4}$) and low-level MRD (HR, 2.5). Thus the prognostic significance of distinguishing MRD levels within the range of MRD positivity is at least as high as the distinction between MRD negative and MRD low positive. MRD levels were associated with almost identical median PFS in patients who were treated using FC compared with those who received FCR. This demonstrates that the attainment of low-level MRD but not the treatment regimen that induces the low-level state is important (**Fig. 2**).

The data could be reproduced in the recent GCLLSG CLL2M phase II study. When MRD was assessed in this cohort of patients receiving rituximab-bendamustine as first-line therapy, high-level MRD ($\geq 10^{-2}$) was associated with a median PFS of 12 months; intermediate MRD levels ($\geq 10^{-4}$ to $<10^{-2}$) were associated with a median PFS of 32 months; whereas median PFS has not been reached in the low-level MRD subgroup (median observation time 27 months; $P<.001$).[4]

The recent International Workshop on Chronic Lymphocytic Leukemia guidelines arbitrarily defined MRD negativity as an MRD level below 10^{-4} (ie, 1 CLL cell in 10,000 benign leukocytes).[46] This definition primarily reflects the current technologic standard of MRD detection, because quantitative four-color MRD flow and ASO *IGH* RQ-PCR can reliably quantify MRD at this level in most patients.[44]

Table 3
Clinical trials and series in CLL with analysis of MRD but with significant technical deviations from International Workshop on Chronic Lymphocytic Leukemia MRD definition

No.	Study (Ref)	Number of Patients with MRD Analysis	Therapy	Technique	MRD Threshold	Deviation from Current International Workshop on Chronic Lymphocytic Leukemia Standard	PFS by MRD Group (MRD+ vs MRD−)	P Value
1	Robertson et al,[38] 1992	66	Fludarabine + prednisone	Two-color flow	Not reported	Threshold not reported, qualitative	18 mo vs NR (TTF)[a]	<.001
2	Rawstron et al,[29] 2001	25	Auto SCT or alemtuzumab	Quantitative four-color MRD flow	5×10^{-4}	Higher threshold	19 mo vs NR (EFS)	.0001
3	Moreton et al,[53] 2005	91	Alemtuzumab ± auto/allo SCT	Quantitative four-color MRD flow	10^{-5}	Lower threshold	20 mo vs NR (TFS)	<.0001
4	Wierda et al,[50] 2005	82	FCR	Qualitative *IGHV* PCR	1×10^{-5}	Qualitative	27 mo vs 44 mo (TTP)[b]	Not significant
5	Hillmen et al,[48] 2007	36	Alemtuzumab vs chlorambucil	Qualitative CD19/CD5/κ/λ	Not reported (+ vs −)	Qualitative Threshold not reported	MRD+ CR < MRD− CR	Not reported

6	Kay et al,[49] 2007	52	PCR	Two-color flow	10^{-2}	Higher threshold, qualitative	18 mo vs 35 mo[c]	<.001
7	Tam et al,[9] 2008	266	FCR	Three-color flow	10^{-2}	Higher threshold, qualitative	49 mo vs 85 mo	<.001
8	Lamanna et al,[23] 2009	23	F→C→R	Nested ASO *IGH* PCR	10^{-5}	Qualitative	35 mo vs NR (CR)	.007
9	Maloum et al,[64] 2009	33	FC	Four-color flow	10^{-4}	Qualitative	28 mo vs NR	.0009
10	Ysebaert et al,[70] 2010	30	FCR	Quantitative four-color MRD flow	10^{-2}	Higher threshold, MRD assessed during FU	24 mo vs NR	<.01
11	Parikh et al,[63] 2011	57	CFAR	Three-color flow	5×10^{-2}	Higher threshold, qualitative	15 mo vs NR	<.001

The survey does not list reports on very small series, investigations using allogeneic stem cell transplantation or maintenance therapies, series without description of MRD methods, and series without centralized MRD assessments. The most recent report only was cited in studies with published follow-up.

Abbreviations: EFS, event free survival; FC, fludarabine-cyclophosphamide; FCR, fludarabine-cyclophosphamide-rituximab; FU, follow-up; NR, not reached; SCT, stem cell transplantation; TFS, treatment free survival; TTF, time to treatment failure; TTP, time to progression.

[a] Median TTF estimated from Fig. 4 of the manuscript.[38]
[b] Median TTP estimated from Fig. 3 of the manuscript.[50]
[c] Median PFS estimated from Fig. 3 of the manuscript.[49]

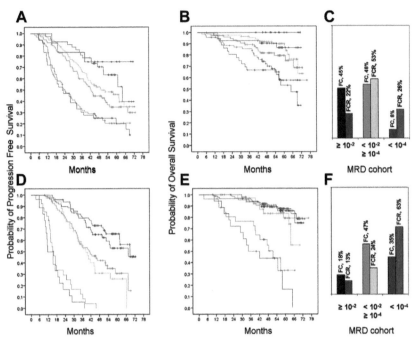

Fig. 2. Progression-free and overall survival can be predicted by MRD. Progression-free (*A, D*) and overall survival (*B, E*) grouped by MRD level and treatment regimen assessed after three (*A–C*) and after total six treatment cycles (*D, E*) in peripheral blood. Histograms *C* and *F* depict the frequency distributions of MRD groups at both analysis time-points. Percentages in the histograms denote frequency within a treatment arm. MRD $\geq 10^{-2}$: blue FC (fludarabine-cyclophosphamide), violet FCR (fludarabine-cyclophosphamide-rituximab). MRD $\geq 10^{-4}$ to $<10^{-2}$: green FC, yellow FCR. MRD $<10^{-4}$: brown FC, red FCR. (*From* Böttcher S, Ritgen M, Fischer K, et al. Minimal residual disease quantification is an independent predictor of progression free and overall survival in chronic lymphocytic leukemia. A multivariate analysis from the randomized GCLLSG CLL8 trial. J Clin Oncol 2012;30:980–8, with permission.)

However, there are residual leukemic cells below 10^{-4} in many if not all patients who receive chemotherapy, immunochemotherapy, or autologous stem cell transplantation. Those residual CLL cells below 10^{-4} can be directly measured using MRD flow or ASO *IGH* RQ-PCR.[40,44,51,52] Additional evidence for the existence of MRD below the current threshold comes from the observation that patients who had no measurable MRD at a level of 10^{-4} reconverted to MRD positivity over time. This observation could be made after such different treatment modalities as alemtuzumab,[53] FCM,[28] FC,[45] FCR,[45] and autologous stem cell transplantation.[52] In general, reconversion to MRD positivity preceded clinical relapse.[54]

A continuous relationship between tumor load as assessed by quantitative MRD and PFS is supported by available data. This relationship and evidence for residual CLL cells below any threshold that can be currently achieved strongly argue for the use of quantitative MRD technology and an international harmonization of thresholds. Thresholds should currently be set at 10^{-4}, according to International Workshop on Chronic Lymphocytic Leukemia guidelines[46] and in light of most recent data should subdivide MRD-positive patients using an additional threshold at 10^{-2}.[4,45]

FACTORS IMPACTING ON THE PROGNOSTIC SIGNIFICANCE OF MRD
The Prognostic Significance of MRD Is Independent from Pretherapeutic Risk Factors

The evidence accumulated over the last decades leaves little space for doubt on the prognostic significance of MRD. However, with the known heterogeneity of CLL and a myriad of pretherapeutic prognostic variables available, the added value of the correlation remained a matter of debate. It was hypothesized that MRD response would simply mirror biologic features of the disease in individual patients, implying that a good MRD response could be predicted by known pretherapeutic risk features.[55]

Data from the GCLLSG CLL8 trial have now convincingly proven the independent prognostic significance of MRD levels.[45] When MRD was tested in multivariate Cox models that initially included the additional risk factors clinical response, treatment (FCR vs FC), cytogenetics, pretherapeutic white blood cell count, thymidine kinase levels, β_2-microglobulin, and *IGHV* mutational status a significant association to PFS was retained. Notably, the treatment arm completely lost its prognostic significance in this model, because the higher efficacy of FCR over FC was fully reflected by a higher proportion of MRD-negative ($<10^{-4}$) patients in the combination therapy arm (FC, 35%; FCR, 63%; see **Fig. 2**). The same trial now also clarified the relationship between clinical staging and MRD response. Clinical staging was significantly correlated with MRD, because CR patients were more likely to present with low-level MRD ($<10^{-4}$) than PR patients (67% vs 39%; $P<.001$). PR patients who attain a low-level MRD status carry a similar risk for progression as complete responders of the same MRD level. A practical consequence of this observation is that MRD should be assessed in all responding patients.

Supporting evidence for the independent prognostic significance of MRD comes from a Leeds series that to date has been published only in abstract form[56] (and Rawstron, AC, personal communication, 2012). In this series MRD status was assessed in 137 first-line and relapsed patients treated with various regimens. The type of treatment, being predictive for PFS in univariate analysis, lost its significance in multivariate analysis. The only variables retaining their significance were treatment line (first-line vs relapse); clinical response; and as most significant factor, MRD status after therapy. Notably, this investigation lacked information on cytogenetic markers and *IGHV* mutational status.

It is likely that MRD levels as sensitive and quantitative representation of treatment response integrate an array of biologic features of the CLL clone (eg, apoptosis resistance to the applied therapy); pharmacogenetic and metabolic features of the patients (eg, polymorphisms within detoxifying enzymes, hepatic and renal function of the patient); and treatment-related causes of therapeutic efficacy (eg, number of treatment cycles, adherence to treatment schedule). As such MRD response cannot be predicted by known pretreatment factors or a combination thereof.

The data from the GCLLSG CLL8 trial and the series from Leeds strongly suggest that MRD levels after therapy are independent predictors of PFS after different induction treatment regimens.

MRD Regrowth Kinetics Relate to Biologic Features of the Clone

MRD levels achieved after therapy represent the nadir of the tumor burden in a patient, which might be independent from the speed of regrowth. It is tempting to speculate that factors correlated with the speed of regrowth are factors that modify median PFS predicted by a given MRD level (see **Fig. 1B**). Indeed, emerging evidence from the CLL8 trial demonstrates prognostic significance of MRD regrowth kinetics that is independent from the MRD level. Faster regrowth was significantly associated with unmutated *IGHV* status, 11q deletion, short time to treatment, and Binet C stage before therapy, whereas β_2 microglobulin and treatment arm had no impact on kinetics.[57]

Assuming identical regrowth kinetics within and below the range of measurable MRD one would hypothesize that the same features that are associated with fast regrowth kinetics also predict a short time of reconversion to MRD positivity from an MRD-negative status. Indeed, unmutated *IGHV* and deletion 11q were associated with a short MRD-negative period in an analysis after autologous stem cell transplantation.[58] An analysis from the Barcelona group in patients treated with FCM identified unmutated *IGHV* status and ZAP70 expression as predictors for early reconversion to MRD positivity.[28]

A scenario emerges that combines MRD levels at the end of therapy with select biologic factors that are associated with a fast CLL regrowth for most accurate prediction of PFS in patient cohorts.[59] Unmutated *IGHV* is the single feature with the most direct evidence for an association with fast regrowth from low MRD levels to clinical relapse.

What Median PFS Are Predicted by MRD Levels?

The ultimate goal of prediction is an estimate of median PFS for a group of patients, thus allowing one to counsel patients and to make educated decisions on possible maintenance and consolidation strategies after induction therapy. Considering the importance of MRD levels (as opposed to qualitatively reporting on positivity), attempts to compare median PFS with MRD results between trials should be restricted to investigations that used sensitive and quantitative methods and grouped patients according to the internationally accepted threshold of 10^{-4} (see **Table 2**). Six such investigations have been published with five of them reporting significant differences in PFS between MRD-negative and -positive patient groups.

Out of the five studies, Pettitt and coworkers[60] reported the by far shortest PFS for MRD-positive and -negative patients (10 vs 24 months). This trial tested the efficacy of alemtuzumab in combination with high-dose methylprednisolone exclusively in patients with a *TP53* deletion (ie, in a subgroup of patients known to experience the most aggressive clinical course). It is tempting to speculate that patients with 17p deletions not only often show resistance to conventional therapy but also fast regrowth kinetics, so that MRD-negative and -positive cohorts experience an early relapse.

Four trials and series included patients with active CLL but without selection according to risk features. Follow-up is mature enough in the Barcelona series, the Leeds series, and the GCLLSG CLL8 trial to estimate median PFS of the MRD-negative ($<10^{-4}$) groups at 75,[27] 91,[56] and 69 months,[45] respectively. The Leeds[56] and Barcelona[27] series found a median PFS of the total MRD-positive cohorts at 24 and 16 months, respectively. The groups of MRD-positive patients were subdivided in the prospective German CLL8[45] and CLL2M[4] trials, resulting in a median PFS of 15 and 12 months, respectively, for patients with an MRD level greater than or equal to 10^{-2} (MRD poor-risk group) and of 41 and 32 months for patients with an MRD level between 10^{-4} and 10^{-2} (MRD intermediate-risk group). Considering all patients with an MRD level of at least 10^{-4} (ie, intermediate plus poor risk) together, a median PFS of 28 months was estimated (Böttcher, S and Busch, R, unpublished data, 2011).

Current evidence suggests that in unselected patient cohorts an MRD level of at least 10^{-4} is associated with a median PFS of about 2 years, whereas median PFS is predicted at about 6 years for patients with an MRD level below 10^{-4}. Preliminary evidence is available to support a subdivision of the MRD-positive patient group using a threshold of 10^{-2}. This subdivision seems to delineate two patient cohorts with an estimated median PFS of approximately 1 and 3 years, respectively.

MEASURING MRD DURING THERAPY

MRD can be assessed only after therapy has been applied. Therefore, patients have to be subjected to side effects of therapy to measure MRD, even if the treatment turns out to be ineffective. The early prediction of treatment results (eg, after half of planned treatment cycles) by MRD would allow one to individualize the number of treatment cycles. That concept is supported by MRD monitoring in acute lymphoblastic leukemia, which convincingly demonstrated the prognostic significance of MRD when measured early in the course of treatment.[61]

First attempts to predict treatment efficacy early during the treatment were made in patients who received alemtuzumab for a planned 12 weeks. Patients who finally responded to the total length of therapy presented on average with lower levels of disease already after 2 and 4 weeks of therapy, but there was overlap in MRD levels between responders and nonresponders.[62] The prediction of nonresponders could be improved by additionally using the kinetics of B-cell depletion between weeks 2 and 4. Nonresponders were more likely than responders to show less than 10-fold reduction in tumor load during this period of time.

The GCLLSG CLL8 trial included MRD monitoring after three of the planned six cycles of FC or FCR therapy.[45] After three cycles of therapy more patients achieved MRD negativity below 10^{-4} in the FCR (26%) compared with the FC (8%) arm. After completion of therapy (ie, after additional three treatment cycles) the proportion of low-level MRD patients increased to 35% and 63% in the respective treatment arms (see **Fig. 2**). Although the proportion of MRD-negative patients more than doubled in both treatment arms, the prognostic significance of achieving low-level MRD after three cycles was similar to achieving low-level MRD after six cycles of therapy (median PFS, 64 vs 69 months). The data therefore show that the patient cohort as a whole profited from the last three cycles of therapy, because many patients converted to low-level MRD. However, the findings also suggest that the subgroup of patients who achieve a very good MRD response already after three cycles of therapy might be candidates for a clinical trial testing the de-escalation of treatment.

Similar trends on the prognostic significance of MRD assessments during therapy have been recently reported by a group from MD Anderson Cancer Center, even though a relatively insensitive three-color MRD flow assay was used. In patients planned to receive six cycles of fludarabine-cyclophosphamide-alemtuzumab-rituximab combination therapy, MRD assessments after three and six cycles of therapy were predictive of PFS.[63]

MRD assessments during induction therapy hold great promise for tailoring treatment according to response aiming at reducing side effects in good responders.

MRD PREDICTS OVERALL SURVIVAL

Many patients with CLL who suffer a relapse can be salvaged with a subsequent treatment line so that risk factors with impact on PFS often lack prognostic significance on overall survival. In general, a correlation to overall survival can be demonstrated if studies are performed with long follow-up, with large numbers of patients or in subgroups of poor-prognosis (eg, relapsed) patients. The correlation between MRD and overall survival is no exception to this rule.

First indication of the possibility to predict overall survival using MRD came with the pivotal study by Rawstron and colleagues[29] in mostly pretreated patients. They reported an improved overall survival when comparing 19 patients with MRD-negative CR with 6 compete responders who remained MRD positive ($P = .007$).

The same group later extended this series to 91 previously treated patients who received alemtuzumab until an MRD-negative status was achieved.[53] Patients in whom MRD negativity was not attainable had a median overall survival of 19 months only, whereas the median survival had not been reached in patients who became MRD negative. This series was the first to report an impact of MRD on overall survival in a larger cohort of patients. However, important pretherapeutic risk factors were not assessed, so that an independent prognostic significance of MRD response on survival remained a matter of debate.[55]

However, more recently the Leeds group reported a significant effect of MRD on overall survival when performing a multivariate analysis in 137 patients who received various treatment regimens.[56] In keeping with these results are data from the MD Anderson Cancer Center on 266 patients treated with FCR as first-line therapy. Using a relatively insensitive assay the investigators demonstrated a significant survival benefit for patients who became MRD negative compared with MRD-positive patients (6-year survival, 84% vs 65%; $P = .001$). Because MRD was not included in multivariate analyses the independent prognostic significance of the parameter on survival could not be proven.[9] A significantly longer overall survival in MRD responders has also been demonstrated in a small series from Barcelona after autologous stem cell transplantation.[27]

The most recent observations on the significance of MRD for overall survival were made in the CLL8 trial (see **Fig. 2**).[45] In this study the MRD status proved of independent prognostic significance for overall survival when tested in multivariate models that additionally included all major known risk factors. Of note, high-level MRD ($\geq 10^{-2}$) was the most significant risk factor for short survival (HR, 7.1; $P<.001$). The only additional risk features maintaining significance in the model were a poor performance status and the presence of a deletion 17p, whereas clinical response lost its impact on survival. With current follow-up (median, 52 months) the only difference in overall survival was detectable between MRD high-level ($\geq 10^{-2}$, median overall survival 48 months) and the other two MRD groups (intermediate- and low-level MRD, median survival not reached).

Given the aforementioned hurdles to demonstrate an impact of any risk factor on overall survival in CLL it is not surprising that there are also reports that did not detect a significant correlation to MRD status.[28,63,64]

There is evidence that MRD can not only predict PFS but also overall survival in CLL. The prediction is independent of other risk features but current data suggest that primarily patients with a very poor prognosis are identified. It is tempting to speculate that those patients have proven resistant to subsequent salvage therapies.

MRD AFTER ALLOGENEIC STEM CELL TRANSPLANTATION

Because of high treatment-related mortality and morbidity allogeneic stem cell transplantation is reserved for younger poor-risk patients with CLL (discussed elsewhere in this issue). Nevertheless, it is the only curative option for patients with CLL known to date. MRD assessments after this treatment modality therefore differ from all others in predicting cure, not time to relapse.

Quantitative MRD assessments were instrumental to delineate the mode of action of allogeneic stem cell transplantation in CLL.[52,65] They demonstrated that a decline in MRD levels occurred most often concomitantly with maneuvers that facilitated cellular immune attack on the malignant clone, such as the tapering of immunosuppression or the infusion of donor lymphocytes. After MRD negativity was achieved, this status proved durable with very few patients reconverting to MRD positivity even with prolonged follow-up.[32,66,67]

The delayed MRD response pattern is reflected by a high prognostic significance of attaining an MRD-negative status 12 months after allogeneic stem cell transplantation, when the tapering of immunosuppression is complete in most patients.[66] A clinical relapse occurred in between 0% and 11% of the MRD-negative patients with much higher relapse rates in MRD-positive patients (62% and 70%).[32,66] Typically, at least 85% of all MRD-negative patients could sustain their MRD-negative status with long-term follow-up.[27,66,68] A somewhat higher reoccurrence rate was detected in a study that mainly applied a very sensitive, but not quantitative method for MRD monitoring.[32]

Data from a total of four series on sensitive MRD monitoring after allogeneic stem cell transplantation are available, which in summary report only on 129 patients.[27,32,66,67] The general prognostic significance of MRD at 12 months after transplantation, the delayed MRD clearance patterns, and the durability of the MRD responses are recurring features in all those investigations and can therefore be considered as proven. Details as the exact clinical relapse rate in MRD-positive and -negative patients and the use of MRD-guided donor lymphocyte infusions to prevent clinical relapse merit prospective evaluation using quantitative MRD monitoring.

USE OF MRD FOR CLINICAL DECISION MAKING

Current evidence suggests that MRD assessments after completion of induction therapy are suited to identify the more efficacious arm in controlled randomized trials. Increased efficacy of one of the treatment arms will be detected by a higher rate of patients attaining low-level MRD. Because biologic risk features are balanced between the arms of a randomized trial, it is expected that average CLL regrowth speed will be comparable between the treatment arms. Therefore, significant differences in MRD negativity rates will very likely translate into different median PFS.

Patients who do not attain an MRD-negative response ($<10^{-4}$) to induction therapy are predicted to experience a median PFS of about 2 years. It is possible to further refine this subgroup using additional thresholds within the range of positivity or select biologic features that are related to regrowth kinetics. MRD poor responders are candidates for consolidation and maintenance strategies within the context of controlled clinical trials.

Judging from a limited number of observations a very good MRD response after half of the planned induction therapy cycles might identify patients who do not profit from additional therapy. Future clinical trials should investigate the noninferiority of a reduced treatment in this patient cohort.

Except for allogeneic stem cell transplantation, the use of MRD to tailor treatment in individual patients outside clinical trials is currently discouraged. Such application of the technology would require supportive evidence for the predictive power of MRD from multivariate analyses of high-quality MRD data generated in a few more randomized trials.

REFERENCES

1. Hallek M, Fischer K, Fingerle-Rowson G, et al. Addition of rituximab to fludarabine and cyclophosphamide in patients with chronic lymphocytic leukaemia: a randomised, open-label, phase 3 trial. Lancet 2010;376(9747):1164–74.
2. Eichhorst BF, Busch R, Hopfinger G, et al. Fludarabine plus cyclophosphamide versus fludarabine alone in first-line therapy of younger patients with chronic lymphocytic leukemia. Blood 2006;107(3):885–91.
3. Fischer K, Cramer P, Busch R, et al. Bendamustine combined with rituximab in patients with relapsed and/or refractory chronic lymphocytic leukemia: a multicenter phase II trial of the German Chronic Lymphocytic Leukemia Study Group. J Clin Oncol 2011;29(26):3559–66.

4. Fischer K, Cramer P, Busch R, et al. Bendamustine in combination with rituximab for previously untreated patients with chronic lymphocytic leukemia: a multicenter phase II trial of the German Chronic Lymphocytic Leukemia Study Group. J Clin Oncol 2012;30(26):3209–16.

5. Knauf WU, Lissichkov T, Aldaoud A, et al. Phase III randomized study of bendamustine compared with chlorambucil in previously untreated patients with chronic lymphocytic leukemia. J Clin Oncol 2009;27(26):4378–84.

6. Knauf WU, Lissitchkov T, Aldaoud A, et al. Bendamustine compared with chlorambucil in previously untreated patients with chronic lymphocytic leukaemia: updated results of a randomized phase III trial. Br J Haematol 2012;159(1):67–77.

7. Catovsky D, Richards S, Matutes E, et al. Assessment of fludarabine plus cyclophosphamide for patients with chronic lymphocytic leukaemia (the LRF CLL4 Trial): a randomised controlled trial. Lancet 2007;370(9583):230–9.

8. Flinn IW, Neuberg DS, Grever MR, et al. Phase III trial of fludarabine plus cyclophosphamide compared with fludarabine for patients with previously untreated chronic lymphocytic leukemia: US Intergroup Trial E2997. J Clin Oncol 2007; 25(7):793–8.

9. Tam CS, O'Brien S, Wierda W, et al. Long-term results of the fludarabine, cyclophosphamide, and rituximab regimen as initial therapy of chronic lymphocytic leukemia. Blood 2008;112(4):975–80.

10. Mateos MV, Oriol A, Martinez-Lopez J, et al. Maintenance therapy with bortezomib plus thalidomide or bortezomib plus prednisone in elderly multiple myeloma patients included in the GEM2005MAS65 trial. Blood 2012;120(13):2581–8.

11. Sonneveld P, Schmidt-Wolf IG, van der Holt B, et al. Bortezomib induction and maintenance treatment in patients with newly diagnosed multiple myeloma: results of the randomized phase III HOVON-65/GMMG-HD4 trial. J Clin Oncol 2012;30(24):2946–55.

12. Mateos MV, Richardson PG, Schlag R, et al. Bortezomib plus melphalan and prednisone compared with melphalan and prednisone in previously untreated multiple myeloma: updated follow-up and impact of subsequent therapy in the phase III VISTA trial. J Clin Oncol 2010;28(13):2259–66.

13. San Miguel JF, Schlag R, Khuageva NK, et al. Bortezomib plus melphalan and prednisone for initial treatment of multiple myeloma. N Engl J Med 2008;359(9): 906–17.

14. Palumbo A, Bringhen S, Rossi D, et al. Bortezomib-melphalan-prednisone-thalidomide followed by maintenance with bortezomib-thalidomide compared with bortezomib-melphalan-prednisone for initial treatment of multiple myeloma: a randomized controlled trial. J Clin Oncol 2010;28(34):5101–9.

15. Hiddemann W, Kneba M, Dreyling M, et al. Frontline therapy with rituximab added to the combination of cyclophosphamide, doxorubicin, vincristine, and prednisone (CHOP) significantly improves the outcome for patients with advanced-stage follicular lymphoma compared with therapy with CHOP alone: results of a prospective randomized study of the German Low-Grade Lymphoma Study Group. Blood 2005;106(12):3725–32.

16. Salles G, Seymour JF, Offner F, et al. Rituximab maintenance for 2 years in patients with high tumour burden follicular lymphoma responding to rituximab plus chemotherapy (PRIMA): a phase 3, randomised controlled trial. Lancet 2011;377(9759):42–51.

17. Martinelli G, Schmitz SF, Utiger U, et al. Long-term follow-up of patients with follicular lymphoma receiving single-agent rituximab at two different schedules in trial SAKK 35/98. J Clin Oncol 2010;28(29):4480–4.

18. van Oers MH, Van Glabbeke M, Giurgea L, et al. Rituximab maintenance treatment of relapsed/resistant follicular non-Hodgkin's lymphoma: long-term outcome of the EORTC 20981 phase III randomized intergroup study. J Clin Oncol 2010; 28(17):2853–8.

19. Marcus R, Imrie K, Solal-Celigny P, et al. Phase III study of R-CVP compared with cyclophosphamide, vincristine, and prednisone alone in patients with previously untreated advanced follicular lymphoma. J Clin Oncol 2008;26(28):4579–86.

20. Kluin-Nelemans HC, Hoster E, Hermine O, et al. Treatment of older patients with mantle-cell lymphoma. N Engl J Med 2012;367(6):520–31.

21. Forstpointner R, Unterhalt M, Dreyling M, et al. Maintenance therapy with rituximab leads to a significant prolongation of response duration after salvage therapy with a combination of rituximab, fludarabine, cyclophosphamide, and mitoxantrone (R-FCM) in patients with recurring and refractory follicular and mantle cell lymphomas: results of a prospective randomized study of the German Low Grade Lymphoma Study Group (GLSG). Blood 2006;108(13):4003–8.

22. Geisler CH, Kolstad A, Laurell A, et al. Long-term progression-free survival of mantle cell lymphoma after intensive front-line immunochemotherapy with in vivo-purged stem cell rescue: a nonrandomized phase 2 multicenter study by the Nordic Lymphoma Group. Blood 2008;112(7):2687–93.

23. Lamanna N, Jurcic JG, Noy A, et al. Sequential therapy with fludarabine, high-dose cyclophosphamide, and rituximab in previously untreated patients with chronic lymphocytic leukemia produces high-quality responses: molecular remissions predict for durable complete responses. J Clin Oncol 2009;27(4):491–7.

24. van Dongen JJ, Langerak AW, Bruggemann M, et al. Design and standardization of PCR primers and protocols for detection of clonal immunoglobulin and T-cell receptor gene recombinations in suspect lymphoproliferations: report of the BIOMED-2 Concerted Action BMH4-CT98-3936. Leukemia 2003;17(12):2257–317.

25. Bottcher S, Ritgen M, Buske S, et al. Minimal residual disease detection in mantle cell lymphoma: methods and significance of four-color flow cytometry compared to consensus IGH-polymerase chain reaction at initial staging and for follow-up examinations. Haematologica 2008;93(4):551–9.

26. Bottcher S, Ritgen M, Pott C, et al. Comparative analysis of minimal residual disease detection using four-color flow cytometry, consensus IgH-PCR, and quantitative IgH PCR in CLL after allogeneic and autologous stem cell transplantation. Leukemia 2004;18(10):1637–45.

27. Moreno C, Villamor N, Colomer D, et al. Clinical significance of minimal residual disease, as assessed by different techniques, after stem cell transplantation for chronic lymphocytic leukemia. Blood 2006;107(11):4563–9.

28. Bosch F, Ferrer A, Villamor N, et al. Fludarabine, cyclophosphamide, and mitoxantrone as initial therapy of chronic lymphocytic leukemia: high response rate and disease eradication. Clin Cancer Res 2008;14(1):155–61.

29. Rawstron AC, Kennedy B, Evans PA, et al. Quantitation of minimal residual disease levels in chronic lymphocytic leukemia using a sensitive flow cytometric assay improves the prediction of outcome and can be used to optimize therapy. Blood 2001;98:29–35.

30. Voena C, Ladetto M, Astolfi M, et al. A novel nested-PCR strategy for the detection of rearranged immunoglobulin heavy-chain genes in B cell tumors. Leukemia 1997;11(10):1793–8.

31. Noy A, Verma R, Glenn M, et al. Clonotypic polymerase chain reaction confirms minimal residual disease in CLL nodular PR: results from a sequential treatment CLL protocol. Blood 2001;97(7):1929–36.

32. Farina L, Carniti C, Dodero A, et al. Qualitative and quantitative polymerase chain reaction monitoring of minimal residual disease in relapsed chronic lymphocytic leukemia: early assessment can predict long-term outcome after reduced intensity allogeneic transplantation. Haematologica 2009;94(5):654–62.

33. Bruggemann M, van der Velden V, Raff T, et al. Rearranged T-cell receptor beta genes represent powerful targets for quantification of minimal residual disease in childhood and adult T-cell acute lymphoblastic leukemia. Leukemia 2004;18(4): 709–19.

34. van der Velden VH, Hochhaus A, Cazzaniga G, et al. Detection of minimal residual disease in hematologic malignancies by real-time quantitative PCR: principles, approaches, and laboratory aspects. Leukemia 2003;17(6):1013–34.

35. van der Velden VH, Cazzaniga G, Schrauder A, et al. Analysis of minimal residual disease by Ig/TCR gene rearrangements: guidelines for interpretation of real-time quantitative PCR data. Leukemia 2007;21(4):604–11.

36. Cabezudo E, Matutes E, Ramrattan M, et al. Analysis of residual disease in chronic lymphocytic leukemia by flow cytometry. Leukemia 1997;11(11):1909–14.

37. Vuillier F, Claisse JF, Vandenvelde C, et al. Evaluation of residual disease in B-cell chronic lymphocytic leukemia patients in clinical and bone-marrow remission using CD5-CD19 markers and PCR study of gene rearrangements. Leuk Lymphoma 1992;7(3):195–204.

38. Robertson LE, Huh YO, Butler JJ, et al. Response assessment in chronic lymphocytic leukemia after fludarabine plus prednisone: clinical, pathologic, immunophenotypic, and molecular analysis. Blood 1992;80(1):29–36.

39. Lenormand B, Bizet M, Fruchart C, et al. Residual disease in B-cell chronic lymphocytic leukemia patients and prognostic value. Leukemia 1994;8(6): 1019–26.

40. Rawstron AC, Bottcher S, Letestu R, et al. Improving efficiency and sensitivity: European Research Initiative in CLL (ERIC) update on the international harmonised approach for flow cytometric residual disease monitoring in CLL. Leukemia 2013;27:142–9.

41. Bomberger C, Singh-Jairam M, Rodey G, et al. Lymphoid reconstitution after autologous PBSC transplantation with FACS-sorted CD34+ hematopoietic progenitors. Blood 1998;91(7):2588–600.

42. Rawstron AC, de Tute R, Jack AS, et al. Flow cytometric protein expression profiling as a systematic approach for developing disease-specific assays: identification of a chronic lymphocytic leukaemia-specific assay for use in rituximab-containing regimens. Leukemia 2006;20(12):2102–10.

43. Rawstron AC, Villamor N, Ritgen M, et al. International standardized approach for flow cytometric residual disease monitoring in chronic lymphocytic leukaemia. Leukemia 2007;21(5):956–64.

44. Bottcher S, Stilgenbauer S, Busch R, et al. Standardized MRD flow and ASO IGH RQ-PCR for MRD quantification in CLL patients after rituximab-containing immunochemotherapy: a comparative analysis. Leukemia 2009;23(11):2007–17.

45. Böttcher S, Ritgen M, Fischer K, et al. Minimal residual disease quantification is an independent predictor of progression free and overall survival in chronic lymphocytic leukemia. A multivariate analysis from the randomized GCLLSG CLL8 trial. J Clin Oncol 2012;30:980–8.

46. Hallek M, Cheson BD, Catovsky D, et al. Guidelines for the diagnosis and treatment of chronic lymphocytic leukemia: a report from the International Workshop on Chronic Lymphocytic Leukemia updating the National Cancer Institute-Working Group 1996 guidelines. Blood 2008;111(12):5446–56.

47. Logan AC, Gao H, Wang C, et al. High-throughput VDJ sequencing for quantification of minimal residual disease in chronic lymphocytic leukemia and immune reconstitution assessment. Proc Natl Acad Sci U S A 2011;108(52):21194–9.
48. Hillmen P, Skotnicki AB, Robak T, et al. Alemtuzumab compared with chlorambucil as first-line therapy for chronic lymphocytic leukemia. J Clin Oncol 2007; 25(35):5616–23.
49. Kay NE, Geyer SM, Call TG, et al. Combination chemoimmunotherapy with pentostatin, cyclophosphamide, and rituximab shows significant clinical activity with low accompanying toxicity in previously untreated B chronic lymphocytic leukemia. Blood 2007;109(2):405–11.
50. Wierda W, O'Brien S, Wen S, et al. Chemoimmunotherapy with fludarabine, cyclophosphamide, and rituximab for relapsed and refractory chronic lymphocytic leukemia. J Clin Oncol 2005;23(18):4070–8.
51. Schweighofer CD, Ritgen M, Eichhorst BF, et al. Consolidation with alemtuzumab improves progression-free survival in patients with chronic lymphocytic leukaemia (CLL) in first remission: long-term follow-up of a randomized phase III trial of the German CLL Study Group (GCLLSG). Br J Haematol 2009;144(1):95–8.
52. Ritgen M, Stilgenbauer S, von Neuhoff N, et al. Graft versus leukemia effect may overcome therapeutic resistance of chronic lymphocytic leukemia with unmuted variable immunoglobulin heavy chain status: implications of minimal residual disease measurement with quantitative PCR. Blood 2004;104:2600–2.
53. Moreton P, Kennedy B, Lucas G, et al. Eradication of minimal residual disease in B-cell chronic lymphocytic leukemia after alemtuzumab therapy is associated with prolonged survival. J Clin Oncol 2005;23(13):2971–9.
54. Milligan DW, Fernandes S, Dasgupta R, et al. Results of the MRC pilot study show autografting for younger patients with chronic lymphocytic leukemia is safe and achieves a high percentage of molecular responses. Blood 2005;105(1):397–404.
55. Goodman M. Alemtuzumab until minimal residual disease for chronic lymphocytic leukemia: Is it a new standard? J Clin Oncol 2005;23(28):7240–1.
56. Kwok M, Rawstron AC, Varghese AM, et al. Minimal residual disease is a predictor for progression-free and overall survival in chronic lymphocytic leukemia (CLL) that is independent of the type or line of therapy [abstract]. Blood 2009;114:540.
57. Bottcher S, Ritgen M, Fischer K, et al. Minimal residual disease (MRD) re-growth kinetics are an independent predictor for progression free survival (PFS) in chronic lymphocytic leukemia (CLL) and are related to biologically defined CLL-subgroups- results from the CLL8 trial of the German CLL Study Group (GCLLSG) [abstract]. Blood 2011;118:1777.
58. Ritgen M, Lange A, Stilgenbauer S, et al. Unmutated immunoglobulin variable heavy-chain gene status remains an adverse prognostic factor after autologous stem cell transplantation for chronic lymphocytic leukemia. Blood 2003;101(5): 2049–53.
59. Fink A, Busch R, Pflug N, et al. Prediction of poor outcome in CLL patients treated with FCR (fludarabine, cyclophosphamide, rituximab) in the CLL8 Trial of the German CLL Study Group (GCLLSG) [abstract]. Blood 2011;118:977.
60. Pettitt AR, Jackson R, Carruthers S, et al. Alemtuzumab in combination with methylprednisolone is a highly effective induction regimen for patients with chronic lymphocytic leukemia and deletion of TP53: final results of the national cancer research institute CLL206 trial. J Clin Oncol 2012;30(14):1647–55.
61. Bruggemann M, Raff T, Flohr T, et al. Clinical significance of minimal residual disease quantification in adult patients with standard-risk acute lymphoblastic leukemia. Blood 2006;107(3):1116–23.

62. Rawstron AC, Kennedy B, Moreton P, et al. Early prediction of outcome and response to alemtuzumab therapy in chronic lymphocytic leukemia. Blood 2004; 103(6):2027–31.

63. Parikh SA, Keating MJ, O'Brien S, et al. Frontline chemoimmunotherapy with fludarabine, cyclophosphamide, alemtuzumab, and rituximab for high-risk chronic lymphocytic leukemia. Blood 2011;118(8):2062–8.

64. Maloum K, Settegrana C, Chapiro E, et al. IGHV gene mutational status and LPL/ADAM29 gene expression as clinical outcome predictors in CLL patients in remission following treatment with oral fludarabine plus cyclophosphamide. Ann Hematol 2009;88(12):1215–21.

65. Ritgen M, Bottcher S, Stilgenbauer S, et al. Quantitative MRD monitoring identifies distinct GVL response patterns after allogeneic stem cell transplantation for chronic lymphocytic leukemia: results from the GCLLSG CLL3X trial. Leukemia 2008;22(7):1377–86.

66. Dreger P, Dohner H, Ritgen M, et al. Allogeneic stem cell transplantation provides durable disease control in poor-risk chronic lymphocytic leukemia: long-term clinical and MRD results of the German CLL Study Group CLL3X trial. Blood 2010; 116(14):2438–47.

67. Caballero D, Garcia-Marco JA, Martino R, et al. Allogeneic transplant with reduced intensity conditioning regimens may overcome the poor prognosis of B-cell chronic lymphocytic leukemia with unmutated immunoglobulin variable heavy-chain gene and chromosomal abnormalities (11q- and 17p-). Clin Cancer Res 2005;11(21):7757–63.

68. Bottcher S, Ritgen M, Dreger P. Allogeneic stem cell transplantation for chronic lymphocytic leukemia: lessons to be learned from minimal residual disease studies. Blood Rev 2011;25(2):91–6.

69. Langerak AW, Groenen PJ, Bruggemann M, et al. EuroClonality/BIOMED-2 guidelines for interpretation and reporting of Ig/TCR clonality testing in suspected lymphoproliferations. Leukemia 2012;26(10):2159–71.

70. Ysebaert L, Gross E, Kuhlein E, et al. Immune recovery after fludarabine-cyclophosphamide-rituximab treatment in B-chronic lymphocytic leukemia: implication for maintenance immunotherapy. Leukemia 2010;24(7):1310–6.

17p Deletion in Chronic Lymphocytic Leukemia
Risk Stratification and Therapeutic Approach

Andrea Schnaiter, MD, Stephan Stilgenbauer, MD*

KEYWORDS

- CLL • 17p deletion • High-risk • Targeted therapy • BTK • PI3K • BH3 mimetic

KEY POINTS

- As there are also indolent clinical courses in the group of patients with 17p, criteria for treatment initiation should follow the recommendations of the International Workshop on Chronic Lymphocytic Leukemia.
- Physically fit patients with 17p-deleted CLL derive limited benefit from the current standard regimen for first-line therapy fludarabine/cyclophosphamide/rituximab.
- The most promising novel agents with a favorable risk profile, acting independently of the p53 signaling pathway are immunomodulatory drugs, PI3K inhibitors, BH3 mimetics and BTK inhibitors.

INTRODUCTION

The introduction of fluorescence in situ hybridization (FISH) of interphase nuclei in the routine diagnostics of chronic lymphocytic leukemia (CLL) has greatly advanced the evaluation of genetic abnormalities. Interphase FISH also allows the detection of genetic abnormalities in nondividing cells.[1] By FISH, genomic aberrations are detected in approximately 80% of CLL cases with a disease-specific probe set. If more than just 1 chromosomal aberration is detected, according to the hierarchical model of Döhner and colleagues,[2] the prognosis is determined by the most unfavorable alteration. Deletions of the short arm of chromosome 17 (17p deletion) are found in 3% to 10% of CLL cases at diagnosis and/or with first-line treatment indication[2–4] and in 30% to 50% of relapsed/refractory CLL.[5,6]

Breakpoints are distributed over the 17p10-p11.2 region.[7] TP53 is located in band 17p13.1, is always affected, and is the centerpiece of pathogenic importance of 17p deletions; 80% to 90% of cases with monoallelic 17p deletion harbor TP53 mutation

Supported by the CLL Global Research Foundation (Alliance), Else Kröner-Fresenius-Stiftung (2010_Kolleg24, Project 2012_A146), Virtual Helmholtz Institute (VH-VI-404, TP2), and DFG (SFB 1074 project B2).
Department of Internal Medicine III, Ulm University, Albert-Einstein-Allee 23, Ulm 89081, Germany
* Corresponding author.
E-mail address: stephan.stilgenbauer@uniklinik-ulm.de

Hematol Oncol Clin N Am 27 (2013) 289–301
http://dx.doi.org/10.1016/j.hoc.2013.01.008
0889-8588/13/$ – see front matter © 2013 Elsevier Inc. All rights reserved.

on the remaining allele. *TP53* mutation occurs in 8% to 15% of patients at first-line treatment and up to 35% to 50% of cases in refractory CLL.[5,8,9]

RISK STRATIFICATION

Genomic abnormalities identify subgroups of CLL patients with different time to progression and survival. It is widely acknowledged that patients with 17p deletion and/or *TP53* mutation belong to the ultra–high-risk group. In a multivariate analysis of 100 patients with B-cell CLL, B-prolymphocytic leukemia, or Waldenström macroglobulinemia, *TP53* mutation was the strongest prognostic factor for survival and predicted nonresponse to purine analogs, such as fludarabine and pentostatin.[4] Another study of 53 patients with B-cell CLL had reported an association of *TP53* gene mutations with poor clinical outcome and drug resistance.[10] In a prospective study of 560 untreated patients, samples were analyzed by conventional cytogenetics. Abnormalities of chromosome 17 were correlated to poor prognosis and observed as the only cytogenetic finding with independent prognostic value in multivariate analysis.[11] In a cohort of 325 patients with CLL analyzed by FISH, 17p deletions were found in 7%. In the multivariate analysis, 17p deletion was identified as a significant prognostic factor: patients with 17p deletion had the worst prognosis.[2]

Nevertheless, there seem to be prognostic differences in the 17p-deleted subgroup itself. There is evidence that acquired 17p deletion by clonal evolution harbors a poor prognosis.[12–15] A retrospective study of 99 CLL patients with 17p deletion at diagnosis showed clinical heterogeneity; some patients had an indolent clinical course. No progression within 18 months was a favorable sign for long-term stable disease. Risk factors for poor survival in this study were Rai stage 1 or higher, an unmutated immunoglobulin heavy chain variable (IGHV) status, and a 17p deletion in more than 25% of nuclei.[16] Another study described a small subset of patients with loss of *TP53* and stable disease at a median follow-up of 64 months. All patients with an indolent clinical course had mutated IGHV status.[17]

The cutoff values for determining 17p deletion by FISH vary (usually 3%–12%) and have to be established in every laboratory by hybridization of normal controls.[3,4,15,16,18] In one study, initially a level of 20% of 17p-deleted cells was defined as a critical threshold[3,19]; however, this 20% threshold seems to have resulted from technical artifact. Based on the same patient cohort, the cutoff was later revised and set to 10%.[18]

The clone with a 17p deletion might be suppressed by effective therapy: 15 patients with 17p deletion at diagnosis and response to therapy (nodular partial remission [PR] or complete remission [CR]) had no evidence for 17p deletion at the time of response. At the time of disease relapse or progression, however, the vast majority of patients again had 17p deletions.[16]

THERAPEUTIC APPROACH

17p deletion and *TP53* mutation are prognostic markers for nonresponse to conventional chemotherapy. Thus, alternative therapeutic approaches are needed, which act independently of the p53 signaling pathway (**Fig. 1**). As discussed previously, there are also indolent clinical courses in the group of patients with 17p deletion and, therefore, criteria for treatment initiation should be obeyed as set forth in the recommendations of the International Workshop on Chronic Lymphocytic Leukemia.[20] Outside clinical trials, treatment approaches for patients with 17p deletion and/or *TP53* mutation are chemoimmunotherapy, such as fludarabine, cyclophosphamide, and rituximab (FCR); alemtuzumab; and allogeneic stem cell transplantation. Novel treatment strategies, like targeted therapies, can be offered in clinical trials.

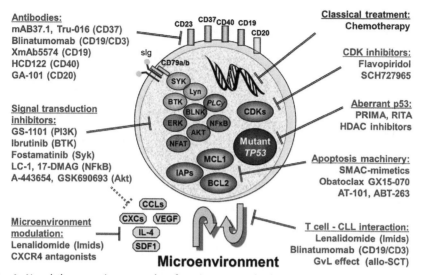

Antibodies:
mAB37.1, Tru-016 (CD37)
Blinatumomab (CD19/CD3)
XmAb5574 (CD19)
HCD122 (CD40)
GA-101 (CD20)

Signal transduction inhibitors:
GS-1101 (PI3K)
Ibrutinib (BTK)
Fostamatinib (Syk)
LC-1, 17-DMAG (NFkB)
A-443654, GSK690693 (Akt)

Microenvironment modulation:
Lenalidomide (Imids)
CXCR4 antagonists

Classical treatment:
Chemotherapy

CDK inhibitors:
Flavopiridol
SCH727965

Aberrant p53:
PRIMA, RITA
HDAC inhibitors

Apoptosis machinery:
SMAC-mimetics
Obatoclax GX15-070
AT-101, ABT-263

T cell - CLL interaction:
Lenalidomide (Imids)
Blinatumomab (CD19/CD3)
GvL effect (allo-SCT)

Microenvironment

Fig. 1. Novel therapeutic approaches focusing on CLL biology.

Fludarabine/Cyclophosphamide/Rituximab

Chemoimmunotherapy with FCR is today the standard of care in treatment-naive physically fit CLL patients.[21] In the CLL8 trial, 17p deletions were found in 10% (29/306) of patients in the fludarabine and cyclophosphamide (FC) arm versus 7% (22/315) of patients in the FCR arm. A significant improvement in overall response rate (ORR) and progression-free survival (PFS) was demonstrated for FCR versus FC treatment (**Fig. 2**). This was not the case for CR and 3-year overall survival (OS) (see **Fig. 2**, **Table 1**).

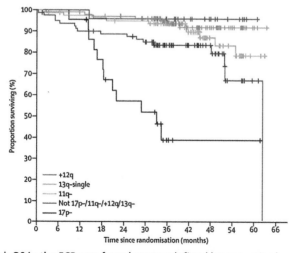

Fig. 2. CLL8 trial: OS in the FCR arm for subgroups defined by genomic aberrations. Patients with 17p deletion show the worst prognosis. (*From* Hallek M, Fischer K, Fingerle-Rowson G, et al. Addition of rituximab to fludarabine and cyclophosphamide in patients with chronic lymphocytic leukemia: a randomised, open-label, phase 3 trial. Lancet 2010;376:1164–74; with permission.)

Table 1
CLL8 trial: response and survival data for FC and FCR treatment of 17p deletion groups

	FC	FCR	P Value
17p Deletion	29/306 (10%)	22/315 (7%)	
CR	0/29 (0%)	1/22 (5%)	0.43
ORR	10/29 (34%)	15/22 (68%)	0.025
PFS at 3 y	0	18%	0.019
OS at 3 y	37%	38%	0.25

These experiences with the FCR combination show that physically fit patients with 17p-deleted CLL may derive some benefit from the current standard regimen for first-line therapy.

Alemtuzumab

The CD52 antibody, alemtuzumab, has been approved for the treatment of fludarabine-refractory CLL in the United States and European Union since 2001 and, since 2007/2008, for first-line treatment of CLL patients. In this context, it has generally been used primarily for those who are not expected to respond to fludarabine, primarily patients with 17p deletion and/or TP53 mutation. The producing company, however, has recently withdrawn the drug from the market.

Alemtuzumab has proved its efficacy, especially in high-risk CLL patients. One randomized trial investigated efficacy and safety of intravenous alemtuzumab compared with chlorambucil in CLL first-line treatment[22]; 297 patients were included. Alemtuzumab was significantly superior regarding the ORR (83% vs 55%, P<.0001) and rate of complete remissions (24% vs 2%, P<.0001). Alemtuzumab was able to eliminate minimal residual disease in 11 of 36 complete responders.

Another important trial on alemtuzumab evaluated efficacy, safety, and clinical benefit of alemtuzumab in 93 fludarabine-refractory CLL patients who had been exposed to alkylating agents.[23] The ORR was 33% with 2% CR and 31% PR; the median OS was 16 months. There was no information about cytogenetics. The CLL2H trial of the German CLL Study Group (GCLLSG) showed that subcutaneous administration of alemtuzumab in the refractory situation is equally effective as intravenous administration and harbors less adverse effects.[5] A comparatively high number of patients had a 17p deletion (31/103; 30%). Between the different cytogenetic subgroups there were no significant differences in ORR, OS (**Fig. 3**), PFS, or time to treatment failure. This finding confirms the efficacy of alemtuzumab independent of the p53 signaling pathway.

The combination of alemtuzumab with dexamethasone followed by alemtuzumab maintenance therapy or allogeneic stem cell transplantation in ultra–high-risk CLL (17p deletion or fludarabine refractoriness) was investigated in the CLL2O trial of the GCLLSG.[24] The results were updated at the American Society of Hematology annual meeting 2012; 70 of 131 eligible patients had a 17p deletion with either untreated (n = 42) or relapsed (n = 28) disease. The response rates were particularly high in untreated patients (ORR 98%) but also in the relapsed patients (ORR 79%). At a median follow-up time of 21 months, the median PFS was 38 months in first-line treatment and 10.3 months in relapsed patients. The median OS was not reached in the untreated and 21.3 months in the relapsed subgroup. Compared with the results of the FCR arm of the CLL8 trial (see **Table 1**; ORR 68%, PFS 11.3 months), response rates as well as PFS in the untreated subgroup were higher.[25] Another multicenter

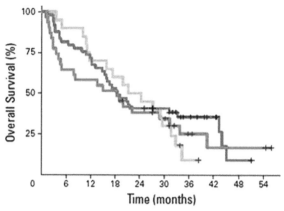

Fig. 3. CLL2H trial: no significant difference in OS between the genetic subgroups: 17p dele-tion (*blue*), 11q deletion (*yellow*), and other subgroups (*gray*) in fludarabine-refractory CLL treated with alemtuzumab. (*From* Stilgenbauer S, Zenz T, Winkler D, et al. Subcutaneous alemtuzumab in fludarabine-refractory chronic lymphocytic leukemia: clinical results and prognostic marker analyses from the CLL2H study of the German Chronic Lymphocytic Leukemia Study Group. J Clin Oncol 2009;27:3994–4001; with permission.)

study in 39 patients with *TP53* deletion tested the combination of alemtuzumab with methylprednisolone[26]; 39 patients (17 untreated, 22 previously treated) with 17p (*TP53*) deletion were included. The ORR was 85% and the CR rate was 36%. Con-cerning the previously untreated subgroup, the CR rate was even higher with 65% versus 14% in previously treated patients ($P = .003$). Also, PFS was longer in untreated compared with previously treated patients (18.3 vs 6.5 months, $P = .010$). Grades 3 to 4 infections occurred in 51% of the patients. In summary, the combination of Alemtuzumab with high-dose steroids led to high response rates, but survival was still inferior to the patients without *TP53* alterations in the CLL8 trial of the GCLLSG.

Allogeneic Stem Cell Transplantation

According to the European Group for Blood and Marrow Transplantation transplant consensus, indications for allogeneic hematopoietic stem cell transplantation in CLL include patients with p53 abnormalities requiring treatment.[27] In these patients, trans-plantation should be considered early during the course of the disease.

Several investigations have shown graft-versus-leukemia activity in CLL.[28–31] A retrospective review of European Group for Blood and Marrow Transplantation data was conducted to assess the curative potential of allogeneic hematopoietic stem cell transplantation in CLL patients with 17p deletion.[32] The course of 44 patients with a median age of 54 years was analyzed. The 3-year OS and PFS rates were 44% and 37%. CR after HCT was ongoing in 9 patients with a follow-up time between 4 and 8.5 years. The CLL3X trial of the GCLLSG investigated the long-term outcome of reduced-intensity conditioning allogeneic stem cell transplantation in CLL patients[33]; 13 of 72 (18%) patients who proceeded to transplantation harbored a 17p deletion. With a median follow-up of 43 months, 7 of these had still an ongoing complete remis-sion. The 4-year event-free survival and OS rates were 45% and 59%. Neither event-free survival nor OS was significantly different between the various cytogenetic subgroups, implicating that allogeneic stem cell transplantation may overcome the cytogenetic risk profile.

In summary, allogeneic stem cell transplantation should be recommended as a consolidation strategy for patients with 17p deletion requiring therapy with younger age, good performance status, and preferentially a remission after induction therapy as well as few prior therapies.

Flavopiridol

Flavopiridol (alvocidib) is a cyclin-dependent kinase inhibitor, which induces apoptosis in CLL cells, independently of p53, and decreases the expression of antiapoptotic molecules, such as Mcl-1 and XIAP. A prospective study in 64 relapsed CLL patients with 21 (33%) 17p-deleted cases showed no association of 17p deletion with response (P>.50), which was defined as CR, nodular PR, or PR. Furthermore, there was no significant difference in PFS between present and absent 17p deletion (12.1 vs 10.3 months; P = .94).[34] In a recently published follow-up of 112 patients, the ORRs did not differ between the cytogenetic subgroups (P = .17). CLL with 17p deletion showed an ORR of 48%. Also, PFS was not different between the subgroups with 10.4 months for 17p-deleted patients. Nevertheless, the risk for progression increased over time for patients with 17p deletion or 11q deletion: at 24 months, just 4% of 17p-deleted patients versus 24% in the group without 17p or 11q deletions were still progression-free. The median OS in 17p-deleted patients was 19.8 months and again not different from other cytogenetic subgroups.[35] The further commercial development of flavopiridol was stopped, however, based on results of a pivotal trial,[36] which showed satisfactory clinical activity in a high-risk subgroup but also considerable toxicity.

Lenalidomide

Lenalidomide is an orally bioavailable immunomodulatory drug derived from thalidomide. Its effects in CLL are mediated by stimulation of natural killer cells and cytotoxic T cells and by influencing the tumor microenvironment. Two adverse events are characteristic: tumor flare and tumor lysis. Two phase II trials showed the efficacy of lenalidomide in relapsed or refractory CLL with ORRs of 47% and 32%, respectively.[37,38] A separate analysis of cases with high-risk cytogenetics (17p or 11q deletion) was published for the first trial; 6 of 45 patients had a 17p deletion. In this small subgroup, no CR and just one PR were achieved.[39] In the second trial, 8 of 44 (18%) patients had a 17p deletion. Overall response in these patients was 13%.[37] A recent phase I trial identified 20 mg as the maximum tolerated dose in relapsed and refractory CLL.[40] Neutropenia and thrombocytopenia were the most common adverse events. Another phase II trial of lenalidomide combined with rituximab in 59 patients with relapsed and refractory CLL showed an ORR of 66%, with 12% CR and 12% nodular PR; 25% of the patients had a 17p deletion and the ORR in this subgroup was 53%. Moreover, patients with 17p deletion without refractoriness had a similar time to failure as patients with neither 17p deletion nor refractoriness (**Fig. 4**).[41] Currently, lenalidomide is being further investigated in first-line trials and as maintenance therapy after successful induction treatment (eg, CLLM1 trial of the GCLLSG).

Ofatumumab

Ofatumumab is a type I human anti-CD20 antibody (IgG1) with enhanced complement-dependent cytotoxicity. The drug has been approved since 2010 for the treatment of CLL refractory to fludarabine and alemtuzumab. In a phase 2 trial, ofatumumab was investigated in combination with FC in previously untreated patients. Ofatumumab was administered at doses of either 500 mg or 1000 mg and 8 of 61 (13%) patients had a 17p deletion. The OR rate in this subgroup was 63%; the CR

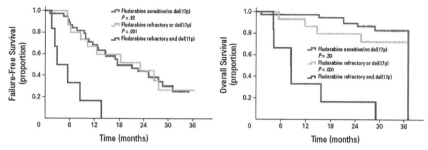

Fig. 4. Failure-free survival and OS in patients treated with lenalidomide and rituximab were significantly shorter for those with fludarabine-refractory disease and 17p deletion together, compared with those without or with just one of these characteristics. Patients with fludarabine-refractory disease or 17p deletion had a similar FFS and OS as patients without these characteristics. (*From* Badoux XC, Keating MJ, Wen S, et al. Phase II study of lenalidomide and rituximab as salvage therapy for patients with relapsed or refractory chronic lymphocytic leukemia. J Clin Oncol 2013;31:584–91; with permission.)

rate was 13%. Overall, the ORR was 75% and CR rate was 41%. Time-to-event analyses were limited by small patient numbers.[42]

As a single-agent, ofatumumab was investigated in fludarabine-refractory CLL; 138 patients were included in the interim analysis of the single-arm study, which led to the approval of ofatumumab by the FDA. The cohort was divided into 2 subgroups: fludarabine-refractory and alemtuzumab-refractory patients (FA-ref) and fludarabine-refractory patients with bulky disease (BF-ref). In 17p-deleted patients, ORR was 41% in the FA-ref subgroup and 14% in the BF-ref subgroup. Comparing subgroups based on pretreatment characteristics, 17p deletion was the only factor significantly associated with a lower response rate ($P = .0073$) just in the BF-ref patients.[43]

Ibrutinib

Ibrutinib (PCI-32765) is an orally bioavailable Bruton tyrosine kinase (BTK) inhibitor that modulates B-cell receptor signaling.[44] Loss-of-function mutations cause X-linked (Bruton) agammaglobulinemia with loss of B cells and lack of serum immunoglobulins. BTK inhibition in vitro leads to modest apoptosis induction, decreased proliferation, migration, and abrogation of downstream pathways, such as nuclear factor κB signaling.[44–46] Clinically, transient increase in lymphocytosis and rapid reduction of lymphadenopathy are typical findings in patients treated with ibrutinib, highlighting in vivo mechanisms of action in the tissue compartment.[45,46]

In a first-dose escalation study, 56 patients with relapsed or refractory B-cell malignancies (B-cell non-Hodgkin lymphoma, CLL, or Waldenström macroglobulinemia) were included. In this heavily pretreated phase I cohort, 11 of 16 CLL/small lymphocytic lymphoma patients achieved responses (2 of them CRs). Ibrutinib was well tolerated with self-limiting adverse events of grades 1 and 2. The median PFS over all cohorts was 13.6 months. Despite rapid absorption and elimination, BTK was occupied by ibrutinib for at least 24 hours, which is in accordance with irreversible inhibition.[47]

In a phase Ib/II study, 116 treatment-naive or relapsed/refractory CLL patients were treated with 2 fixed doses of ibrutinib (420 mg and 840 mg daily until disease progression). In the high-risk subgroup with either relapse within 2 years after combination chemoimmunotherapy or 17p deletion, the ORR was 50% with all of them

PRs. Response was independent of poor risk features with an ORR of 67% in relapsed/refractory patients with 17p deletion (3% CR, 64% PR, 20% PR with lymphocytosis). PFS seems somewhat inferior, however, in CLL with 17p deletion (**Fig. 5**).[48]

Another study evaluated the combination of ibrutinib plus rituximab in 40 high-risk patients (17p deletion/TP53 mutation or PFS less than 36 months after front-line chemoimmunotherapy or relapsed CLL with 11q deletion); 19 patients had either a 17p deletion or TP53 mutation. Median follow-up time was 4 months. At 3 months, 17 of 20 patients available for response assessment had a PR (ORR 85%).[49]

ABT-263 and ABT-199

ABT-263 (Navitoclax) is an orally bioavailable BH3-mimetic that induces apoptosis by binding to the antiapoptotic BCL-2 family members, BCL-2, BCL-XL, and BCL-W. Compared with ABT-263, the second-generation BH3-mimetic, ABT-199, is a potent selective BCL-2 inhibitor; thus, direct toxic effects on thrombocytes are reduced. An interim analysis of a phase I/IIa study of ABT-263 in 29 patients with relapsed or refractory CLL showed clinical activity in patients with refractory disease and in patients with bulky disease and 17p deletion.[50] A PR was achieved in 35% of 26 patients treated with doses of at least 110 mg daily. The median PFS was 25 months, which is astonishing in view of the high-risk nature of this population. Thrombocytopenia was the most common dose-limiting toxicity. Due to its higher specificity to BCL-2, the successor dru, ABT-199, is expected to exhibit similar efficacy paired with improved tolerability.

GS-1101

Activation of the B-cell receptor signaling pathway is essential for the survival of CLL cells (**Fig. 6**).[51] Phosphatidylinositol 3-kinase (PI3K) plays a major role in this signaling pathway and is involved in important cellular processes, such as proliferation,

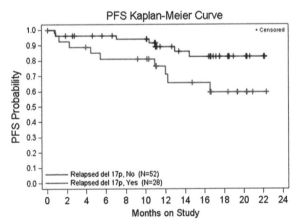

Fig. 5. PFS of relapsed CLL patients with (*red*) and without (*blue*) 17p deletion treated with ibrutinib. (*From* Byrd JC, Furman RR, Coutre S, et al. The Bruton's tyrosine kinase [BTK] inhibitor Ibrutinib [PCI-32765] promotes high response rate, durable remissions, and is tolerable in treatment naive [TN] and relapsed or refractory [RR] chronic lymphocytic leukemia [CLL] or small lymphocytic lymphoma [SLL] patients including patients with high-risk [HR] disease: new and updated results of 116 patients in a phase Ib/II study. Blood (ASH Annual Meeting Abstracts) 2012;120:189; with permission.)

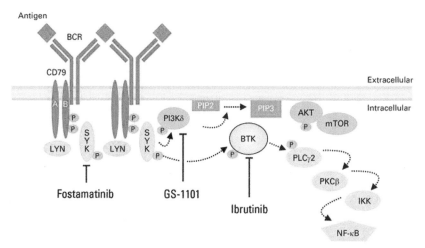

Fig. 6. The B-cell receptor signaling pathway as a target for novel therapeutic stategies (eg, fostamatinib, GS-1101, and ibrutinib). (*From* Wiestner A. Targeting B-Cell receptor signaling for anticancer therapy: the bruton's tyrosine kinase inhibitor ibrutinib induces impressive responses in B-Cell malignancies. J Clin Oncol 2013;31:128–30; with permission.)

differentiation, migration, and adhesion. In in vitro studies, the orally bioavailable specific PI3Kδ inhibitor, GS-1101 (idelalisib; formerly CAL-101), induced apoptosis in CLL cells by inhibition of B-cell receptor signaling.[52] Results of a phase I trial, combining GS-1101 with rituximab and/or bendamustine in 51 patients with relapsed or refractory CLL, have recently been presented at the the American Society of Hematology annual meeting.[53] Similar to ibrutinib treatment, a rapid reduction of lymphadenopathy is accompanied by transient lymphocytosis. The ORR was 78% (rituximab), 82% (bendamustine), and 87% (rituximab/bendamustine) in the 3 treatment groups, with 1-year PFS rates of 74%, 88%, and 87%, respectively. GS-1101 seemed to have activity in CLL with 17p deletion because responses were observed in this subgroup. Several phase III trials of GS-1101 in combination compared with the partner therapy alone are currently recruiting.

SUMMARY

CLL with 17p deletion and/or *TP53* mutation remains a major therapeutic challenge due to poor response to conventional approaches, rapid disease progression, and short survival. Although allogeneic hematopoietic stem cell transplantation offers promising long-term results, this approach is not suitable for elderly patients with comorbidities, who represent the largest portion of CLL patients. Alemtuzumab is not only effective but also of considerable toxicity and its approval in the United States and Europe has been withdrawn for economic reasons. Despite satisfactory clinical activity, the development of the cyclin-dependent kinase inhibitor, flavopiridol, has been stopped. Recently, many novel agents with a favorable risk profile, avoiding the p53 signaling pathway, have entered clinical trials: the immunomodulatory drug, lenalidomide; PI3K inhibitors, such as GS-1101; and BH3 mimetics, such as ABT-263 and ABT-199, as well as the BTK inhibitor, ibrutinib. These agents show promising results in phase I/II trials of refractory CLL, including in patients with 17p deletion/*TP53*, and are, therefore, specifically being investigated in this ultra–high-risk population at desperate unmet therapeutic need.

REFERENCES

1. Döhner H, Stilgenbauer S, Döhner K, et al. Chromosome aberrations in B-cell chronic lymphocytic leukemia: reassessment based on molecular cytogenetic analysis. J Mol Med 1999;77:266.
2. Dohner H, Stilgenbauer S, Benner A, et al. Genomic aberrations and survival in chronic lymphocytic leukemia. N Engl J Med 2000;343:1910–6.
3. Catovsky D, Richards S, Matutes E, et al. Assessment of fludarabine plus cyclophosphamide for patients with chronic lymphocytic leukaemia (the LRF CLL4 Trial): a randomised controlled trial. Lancet 2007;370:230–9.
4. Dohner H, Fischer K, Bentz M, et al. p53 gene deletion predicts for poor survival and non-response to therapy with purine analogs in chronic B-cell leukemias. Blood 1995;85:1580–9.
5. Stilgenbauer S, Zenz T, Winkler D, et al. Subcutaneous alemtuzumab in fludarabine-refractory chronic lymphocytic leukemia: clinical results and prognostic marker analyses from the CLL2H study of the German Chronic Lymphocytic Leukemia Study Group. J Clin Oncol 2009;27:3994–4001.
6. Lozanski G, Heerema NA, Flinn IW, et al. Alemtuzumab is an effective therapy for chronic lymphocytic leukemia with p53 mutations and deletions. Blood 2004;103:3278–81.
7. Fabris S, Mosca L, Todoerti K, et al. Molecular and transcriptional characterization of 17p loss in B-cell chronic lymphocytic leukemia. Genes Chromosomes Cancer 2008;47:781.
8. Zenz T, Häbe S, Denzel T, et al. Detailed analysis of p53 pathway defects in fludarabine-refractory chronic lymphocytic leukemia (CLL): dissecting the contribution of 17p deletion, TP53 mutation, p53-p21 dysfunction, and miR34a in a prospective clinical trial. Blood 2009;114:2589–97.
9. Zenz T, Kröber A, Scherer K, et al. Monoallelic TP53 inactivation is associated with poor prognosis in chronic lymphocytic leukemia: results from a detailed genetic characterization with long-term follow-up. Blood 2008;112:3322–9.
10. el Rouby S, Thomas A, Costin D, et al. p53 gene mutation in B-cell chronic lymphocytic leukemia is associated with drug resistance and is independent of MDR1/MDR3 gene expression. Blood 1993;82:3452–9.
11. Geisler CH, Philip P, Christensen BE, et al. In B-cell chronic lymphocytic leukaemia chromosome 17 abnormalities and not trisomy 12 are the single most important cytogenetic abnormalities for the prognosis: a cytogenetic and immunophenotypic study of 480 unselected newly diagnosed patients. Leuk Res 1997;21:1011.
12. Stilgenbauer S, Sander S, Bullinger L, et al. Clonal evolution in chronic lymphocytic leukemia: acquisition of high-risk genomic aberrations associated with unmutated VH, resistance to therapy, and short survival. Haematologica 2007;92:1242–5.
13. Shanafelt TD, Witzig TE, Fink SR, et al. Prospective evaluation of clonal evolution during long-term follow-up of patients with untreated early-stage chronic lymphocytic leukemia. J Clin Oncol 2006;24:4634–41.
14. Shanafelt TD, Hanson C, Dewald GW, et al. Karyotype Evolution on Fluorescent In Situ Hybridization Analysis Is Associated With Short Survival in Patients With Chronic Lymphocytic Leukemia and Is Related to CD49d Expression. J Clin Oncol 2008;26:e5–6.
15. Delgado J, Espinet B, Oliveira AC, et al. Chronic lymphocytic leukaemia with 17p deletion: a retrospective analysis of prognostic factors and therapy results. Br J Haematol 2012;157:67.

16. Tam CS, Shanafelt TD, Wierda WG, et al. De novo deletion 17p13.1 chronic lymphocytic leukemia shows significant clinical heterogeneity: the M. D. Anderson and Mayo Clinic experience. Blood 2009;114:957–64.
17. Best OG, Gardiner AC, Davis ZA, et al. A subset of Binet stage A CLL patients with TP53 abnormalities and mutated IGHV genes have stable disease. Leukemia 2008;23:212.
18. Oscier D, Wade R, Davis Z, et al. Prognostic factors identified three risk groups in the LRF CLL4 trial, independent of treatment allocation. Haematologica 2010;95:1705–12.
19. Catovsky D, Richards S, Matutes E, et al. Response to therapy and survival in CLL IS influenced by genetic markers. Preliminary analysis from the LRF CLL4 trial. ASH Annual Meeting Abstracts 2004;104:13.
20. Hallek M, Cheson BD, Catovsky D, et al. Guidelines for the diagnosis and treatment of chronic lymphocytic leukemia: a report from the International Workshop on Chronic Lymphocytic Leukemia updating the National Cancer Institute-Working Group 1996 guidelines. Blood 2008;111:5446–56.
21. Hallek M, Fischer K, Fingerle-Rowson G, et al. Addition of rituximab to fludarabine and cyclophosphamide in patients with chronic lymphocytic leukaemia: a randomised, open-label, phase 3 trial. Lancet 2010;376:1164–74.
22. Hillmen P, Skotnicki AB, Robak T, et al. Alemtuzumab compared with chlorambucil as first-line therapy for chronic lymphocytic leukemia. J Clin Oncol 2007;25:5616–23.
23. Keating MJ, Flinn I, Jain V, et al. Therapeutic role of alemtuzumab (Campath-1H) in patients who have failed fludarabine: results of a large international study. Blood 2002;99:3554–61.
24. Stilgenbauer S, Cymbalista F, Leblond V, et al. Alemtuzumab plus oral dexamethasone, followed by alemtuzumab maintenance or allogeneic transplantation in ultra high-risk CLL: interim analysis of a Phase II Study of the GCLLSG and fcgcll/MW. ASH Annual Meeting Abstracts 2011;118:2854.
25. Stilgenbauer S, Cymbalista F, Leblond V, et al. Alemtuzumab plus oral dexamethasone, followed by alemtuzumab maintenance or allogeneic transplantation in ultra high-risk CLL: updated results from a Phase II Study of the Gcllsg and fcgcll/MW. ASH Annual Meeting Abstracts 2012;120:716.
26. Pettitt AR, Jackson R, Carruthers S, et al. Alemtuzumab in combination with methylprednisolone is a highly effective induction regimen for patients with chronic lymphocytic leukemia and deletion of TP53: final results of the National Cancer Research Institute CLL206 Trial. J Clin Oncol 2012;30:1647–55.
27. Dreger P, Corradini P, Kimby E, et al. Indications for allogeneic stem cell transplantation in chronic lymphocytic leukemia: the EBMT transplant consensus. Leukemia 2006;21:12.
28. Mehta J, Powles R, Singhal S, et al. Clinical and hematological of chronic lymphocytic and prolymphocytic leukemia persisting after allogeneic bone marrow transplantation with the onset of acute graft-versus-host disease: possible role of graft-versus-leukemia. Bone Marrow Transplant 1996;17:371–5.
29. Esteve J, Villamor N, Colomer D, et al. Different clinical value of minimal residual disease after autologous and allogeneic stem cell transplantation for chronic lymphocytic leukemia. Blood 2002;99:1873–4.
30. Rondon G, Giralt S, Huh Y, et al. Graft-versus-leukemia effect after allogeneic bone marrow transplantation for chronic lymphocytic leukemia. Bone Marrow Transplant 1996;18:669–72.
31. Gribben JG, Zahrieh D, Stephans K, et al. Autologous and allogeneic stem cell transplantations for poor-risk chronic lymphocytic leukemia. Blood 2005;106:4389–96.

32. Schetelig J, van Biezen A, Brand R, et al. Allogeneic hematopoietic stem-cell transplantation for chronic lymphocytic leukemia with 17p deletion: a retrospective european group for blood and marrow transplantation analysis. J Clin Oncol 2008;26:5094–100.

33. Dreger P, Döhner H, Ritgen M, et al. Allogeneic stem cell transplantation provides durable disease control in poor-risk chronic lymphocytic leukemia: long-term clinical and MRD results of the German CLL Study Group CLL3X trial. Blood 2010; 116:2438–47.

34. Lin TS, Ruppert AS, Johnson AJ, et al. Phase II study of flavopiridol in relapsed chronic lymphocytic leukemia demonstrating high response rates in genetically high-risk disease. J Clin Oncol 2009;27:6012–8.

35. Woyach JA, Lozanski G, Ruppert AS, et al. Outcome of patients with relapsed or refractory chronic lymphocytic leukemia treated with flavopiridol: impact of genetic features. Leukemia 2012;26:1442.

36. Lanasa MC, Andritsos L, Brown JR, et al. Interim Analysis of EFC6663, a Multicenter Phase 2 Study of Alvocidib (flavopiridol), Demonstrates Clinical Responses Among Patients with Fludarabine Refractory CLL. ASH Annual Meeting Abstracts 2010;116:58.

37. Ferrajoli A, Lee BN, Schlette EJ, et al. Lenalidomide induces complete and partial remissions in patients with relapsed and refractory chronic lymphocytic leukemia. Blood 2008;111:5291–7.

38. Chanan-Khan A, Miller KC, Musial L, et al. Clinical efficacy of lenalidomide in patients with relapsed or refractory chronic lymphocytic leukemia: results of a phase II study. J Clin Oncol 2006;24:5343–9.

39. Sher T, Miller KC, Lawrence D, et al. Efficacy of lenalidomide in patients with chronic lymphocytic leukemia with high-risk cytogenetics. Leuk Lymphoma 2010;51:85–8.

40. Wendtner CM, Hillmen P, Mahadevan D, et al. Final results of a multicenter phase 1 study of lenalidomide in patients with relapsed or refractory chronic lymphocytic leukemia. Leuk Lymphoma 2012;53(3):417–23.

41. Badoux XC, Keating MJ, Wen S, et al. Phase II study of lenalidomide and rituximab as salvage therapy for patients with relapsed or refractory chronic lymphocytic leukemia. J Clin Oncol 2012. [Epub ahead of print].

42. Wierda WG, Kipps TJ, Dürig J, et al. Chemoimmunotherapy with O-FC in previously untreated patients with chronic lymphocytic leukemia. Blood 2011;117: 6450–8.

43. Wierda WG, Kipps TJ, Mayer J, et al. Ofatumumab as single-agent CD20 immunotherapy in fludarabine-refractory chronic lymphocytic leukemia. J Clin Oncol 2010;28:1749–55.

44. Herman SE, Gordon AL, Hertlein E, et al. Bruton tyrosine kinase represents a promising therapeutic target for treatment of chronic lymphocytic leukemia and is effectively targeted by PCI-32765. Blood 2012;117:6287–96.

45. Ponader S, Chen SS, Buggy JJ, et al. The Bruton tyrosine kinase inhibitor PCI-32765 thwarts chronic lymphocytic leukemia cell survival and tissue homing in vitro and in vivo. Blood 2012;119:1182–9.

46. de Rooij MF, Kuil A, Geest CR, et al. The clinically active BTK inhibitor PCI-32765 targets B-cell receptor and chemokine-controlled adhesion and migration in chronic lymphocytic leukemia. Blood 2012;119:2590–4.

47. Advani RH, Buggy JJ, Sharman JP, et al. Bruton Tyrosine Kinase Inhibitor Ibrutinib (PCI-32765) Has Significant Activity in Patients With Relapsed/Refractory B-Cell Malignancies. J Clin Oncol 2013;31(1):88–94.

48. Byrd JC, Furman RR, Coutre S, et al. The Bruton's Tyrosine Kinase (BTK) Inhibitor Ibrutinib (PCI-32765) Promotes High Response Rate, Durable Remissions, and Is Tolerable in Treatment Naive (TN) and Relapsed or Refractory (RR) Chronic Lymphocytic Leukemia (CLL) or Small Lymphocytic Lymphoma (SLL) Patients Including Patients with High-Risk (HR) Disease: New and Updated Results of 116 Patients in a Phase Ib/II Study. ASH Annual Meeting Abstracts 2012;120:189.
49. Burger JA, Keating MJ, Wierda WG, et al. The Btk Inhibitor Ibrutinib (PCI-32765) in Combination with Rituximab Is Well Tolerated and Displays Profound Activity in High-Risk Chronic Lymphocytic Leukemia (CLL) Patients. ASH Annual Meeting Abstracts 2012;120:187.
50. Roberts AW, Seymour JF, Brown JR, et al. Substantial susceptibility of chronic lymphocytic leukemia to BCL2 inhibition: results of a phase I study of navitoclax in patients with relapsed or refractory disease. J Clin Oncol 2012;30:488–96.
51. Wiestner A. Targeting B-Cell receptor signaling for anticancer therapy: the bruton's tyrosine kinase inhibitor ibrutinib induces impressive responses in B-Cell malignancies. J Clin Oncol 2013;31:128–30.
52. Hoellenriegel J, Meadows SA, Sivina M, et al. The phosphoinositide 3'-kinase delta inhibitor, CAL-101, inhibits B-cell receptor signaling and chemokine networks in chronic lymphocytic leukemia. Blood 2011;118:3603–12.
53. Coutre SE, Leonard JP, Furman RR, et al. Combinations of the Selective Phosphatidylinositol 3-Kinase-Delta (PI3Kdelta) Inhibitor GS-1101 (CAL-101) with Rituximab and/or Bendamustine Are Tolerable and Highly Active in Patients with Relapsed or Refractory Chronic Lymphocytic Leukemia (CLL): Results From a Phase I Study. ASH Annual Meeting Abstracts 2012;120:191.

Improving the Treatment Outcome of Patients with Chronic Lymphocytic Leukemia Through Targeted Antibody Therapy

Deborah M. Stephens, DO[a], John C. Byrd, MD[a,b],*

KEYWORDS

- Chronic lymphocytic leukemia • Monoclonal antibody • Immunotherapy
- Chemoimmunotherapy • Antibody

KEY POINTS

- Standard chemotherapeutic options for CLL cause significant immune suppression and myelosuppression, are not well-tolerated by the elderly population and have not consistently offered survival advantage and therefore, alternative immune therapies have been developed, including various monoclonal antibodies (mAbs).
- MAbs mechanisms of cytotoxicity include complement-dependent cytotoxicity, antibody-dependent cell-mediated cytotoxicity, antibody-dependent cell phagocytosis, and direct apoptosis.
- Rituximab was the first mAb approved by the FDA for marketing in the treatment of cancer, and over the last 10 years, rituximab and other mAbs including alemtuzumab and ofatumumab have become integral parts of the standard of care for CLL patients as single agents or in combination with chemotherapy or other immunotherapy.
- Following the introduction of rituximab, multiple subsequent novel mAbs have been designed to target CLL, are at various stages of development, and will continue to revolutionize therapy for CLL patients.

INTRODUCTION

Chronic lymphocytic leukemia (CLL) is the most common adult leukemia in the United States and Europe. CLL is predominantly a cancer of the elderly, with a median age at diagnosis of CLL of 72 years, and approximately 70% of patients are newly diagnosed

Funding sources: None.
Conflict of interest: None.
[a] Division of Hematology, Department of Internal Medicine, The Arthur G. James Comprehensive Cancer Center, The Ohio State University, 300 West 10th Avenue, Columbus, OH 43210, USA;
[b] Division of Medicinal Chemistry and Pharmacology, College of Pharmacy, The Ohio State University, 500 West 12th Avenue, Columbus, OH 43210, USA
* Corresponding author. 455 Wiseman Hall, 410 West 12th Avenue, Columbus, OH 43210.
E-mail address: john.byrd@osumc.edu

Hematol Oncol Clin N Am 27 (2013) 303–327
http://dx.doi.org/10.1016/j.hoc.2012.12.003   hemonc.theclinics.com
0889-8588/13/$ – see front matter Published by Elsevier Inc.

over the age of 65 years.[1] Despite recent advances in the field, CLL is a cancer that is considered incurable outside the setting of a stem cell transplant. The other approved, standard regimens available to treat symptomatic CLL patients are used with a goal of prolonging the time between treatment (treatment-free survival [TFS]). In recent years, many studies have identified select genomic and cellular features that help predict response to therapy and TFS, such as presence of del(17p13.1) and del(11q22.3) on interphase cytogenetics, complex karyotype by metaphase cytogenetics, immunoglobulin variable heavy chain (IgVH) mutational status, elevated β2-microglobulin, and presence of ZAP70 expression or methylation. Furthermore, at present there is no proven survival benefit with early therapy for CLL and, therefore, patients are observed until they become symptomatic from their leukemia.

Therapy for CLL has significantly changed over the years, from an emphasis on alkylator-based (chlorambucil and cyclophosphamide) therapies in the 1970s to fludarabine-based therapies in the early 1990s. These therapies can be toxic, with accompanying immunosuppression and myelosuppression in the majority of CLL patients who are generally elderly with multiple medical morbidities. In addition, these advances in treatment have modest effectiveness in patients with high-risk genomic features, such as del(17p13.1), p53 mutations, ZAP-70-unmethylated disease, and IgVH-unmutated disease[2] These factors prompted continued exploration of new therapeutic strategies for CLL.

For more than 3 decades the application of monoclonal antibodies (mAbs) as targeted therapy against cancer has been explored (as reviewed by Scott and colleagues[3]). mAbs have a fixed effector cell-binding region (Fc) and a variable region with affinity toward a specific antigen that can provide considerable selectivity. Tumor elimination can be mediated by mAbs through various mechanisms, including antibody-dependent cell-mediated cytotoxicity (ADCC), antibody-dependent cellular phagocytosis (ADCP), complement-dependent cytotoxicity (CDC), and direct cell toxicity through transmembrane signaling. ADCC is an immune reaction whereby the targeted tumor cell is coated with antibodies and subsequently destroyed by effector immune cells (ie, natural killer cells or macrophages) via cell lysis following cell membrane puncture by perforin and release of granzyme B or other cytotoxic cytokines. ADCP occurs when antibody-coated cells are engulfed by macrophages and related cells. CDC is an immune reaction whereby the formation of antibody-antigen complexes initiates the complement cascade wherein effector immune cells disrupt the target tumor cell surface membrane, causing water and solutes to exit the cell and thus mediating lysis of the tumor cell. These different mechanisms of cell killing are illustrated in **Fig. 1**.

In 1997, rituximab (Rituxan) became the first therapeutic antibody approved for marketing in CD20-positive low-grade B-cell non-Hodgkin lymphoma (NHL). Since then, significant advances have been made with both single-agent and combination therapies including rituximab in CLL and other B-cell malignancies. Because of the acclaimed success of this mAb, a significant amount of preclinical and clinical research has been produced with alternative CD20 mAbs and other target proteins found on the B-cell surface membrane (**Table 1**). The focus of this article is to review the laboratory concepts and clinical data available regarding mAb therapy for CLL (**Table 2**).

CD20 ANTIBODIES

CD20 is a protein expressed on the cell membrane of early pre–B cells and remains through B-cell development until postgerminal center cells differentiate into plasma cells.[4] CD20 is present on both resting and activated, and malignant and nonmalignant

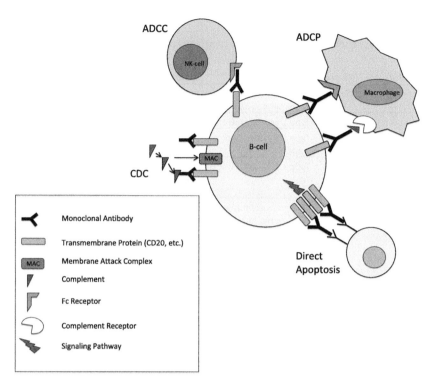

Fig. 1. Mechanisms of antibody cytotoxicity. Cells can be killed by at least 4 mechanisms. (1) Complement-dependent cytotoxicity (CDC). Antibody binds to transmembrane protein on B-cell surface. Complement cascade is activated. Membrane attack complex (MAC) is generated, which induces B-cell lysis. (2) Antibody-dependent cell-mediated cytotoxicity (ADCC). Antibody binds to transmembrane protein and stimulates interaction with Fc receptors on NK-cells, which leads to cell death. (3) Antibody-dependent cell phagocytosis (ADCP). Fc portion of antibody and complement fragments cause recognition by both Fc and complement receptors on macrophages, which stimulates phagocytosis and ADCC. (4) Direct apoptosis. Cross-linking of multiple (Type 1) antibodies and mobilization of the transmembrane protein into lipid rafts mediates interaction with Src kinase signaling pathway that leads to direct cell apoptosis. (Type II antibodies do not require cross-linking or lipid raft mobilization to induce apoptosis.)

Table 1
Location of cell-surface transmembrane proteins

Protein	Cell Types	Notably Not Present
CD20	Pre-B to mature B cells	Plasma cells
CD52	Most B and T cells, granulocytes, monocytes, macrophages, eosinophils, NK cells, and dendritic cells	Plasma cells
CD37	Pre–B cells to mature B cells, Minimally T cell, NK cells, monocytes	Plasma cells Platelets Red blood cells
CD40	B cells (including plasma), monocytes, dendritic cells, CD8 T cells, epithelial and endothelial cells, platelets	—
CD19	B cells, follicular dendritic cells	Plasma cells
HLA-DR	B cells, monocytes/macrophages, dendritic cells, thymic epithelial cells, and activated T cells and endothelial cells	—

Table 2
Monoclonal antibodies for the treatment of chronic lymphocytic leukemia

Antibody	Target	Antibody Characteristics	Comparison with Rituximab	Status
Rituximab	CD20	Type I, mouse/human chimeric IgG1	N/A	FDA approved
Ofatumumab	CD20	Type I, human IgG1	More effective CDC[55]	FDA approved
Obinutuzumab (GA-101)	CD20	Type II, humanized, IgG1	More potent ADCC and DCC, no CDC[69,71,72]	Phase I/II
Veltuzumab	CD20	Type I, humanized IgG1	Better off rate and CDC, enhanced binding avidity[80]	Phase I
Tru-016	CD37	SMIP, mouse/human chimeric, IgG1	Superior ADCC and DCC[104]	Phase I
37.1	CD37	SMIP, mouse/human chimeric, IgG1, engineered Fc portion	Superior DCD, clearance of CLL cells from whole blood samples[108]	Preclinical
37.2	CD37	SMIP, humanized, IgG1, engineered Fc portion	Superior DCD, clearance of CLL cells from whole blood samples[108]	Preclinical
Dacetuzumab (SGN-40)	CD40	Humanized, IgG1	Unknown	Phase I
Lucatumumab (HCD-122)	CD40	Humanized, IgG1	Superior ADCC	Phase I
XmAb5574	CD19	Human, IgG1, engineered Fc portion	Superior ADCC[123]	Phase I
MDX-1342	CD19	Human, nonfucosylated Fc portion	Unknown	Phase I
Apolizumab (Hu1D10)	HLA-DR	Humanized murine, IgG1	Unknown	Discontinued after phase I
IMMU-114	HLA-DR	Humanized murine, IgG4	Superior DCD[129]	Preclinical

Abbreviations: ADCC, antibody-dependent cell-mediated cytotoxicity; CDC, complement-dependent cytotoxicity; DCC, direct cell cytotoxicity; FDA, Food and Drug Administration; N/A, no data available; SMIP, small immunomodular pharmaceutical.

B cells,[5] making it an ideal target for B-cell malignancies. Of note, CLL cells express dim CD20 on their surface in comparison with normal B cells and most other B-cell malignancies.[6] The function of CD20 is still unknown, although studies derived from genetically engineered mice demonstrate that B-cell development and function is normal in the absence of this protein.[7]

Antibodies directed against CD20 have been classified into 2 major types, termed type I and type II. Type I antibodies show stronger C1q binding and potent induction of CDC, which may be related to inducing segregation of CD20 into plasma membrane lipid rafts.[8] A lipid raft is a microdomain on the plasma membrane consisting of glyco-phospholipids and protein receptors that are more organized and tightly packed than the surrounding bilayer membrane, but float freely in the membrane bilayer.[9] It is unclear as to why the translocation of CD20 into lipid rafts influences the antibody's ability to activate complement in such a significant manner. One theory is that the concentration of the antibodies into a comparatively small area of the plasma membrane provides an ideal density for the juxtaposed Fc regions to engage the C1q heads, thereby triggering the classic complement cascade. Another theory is that the raft provides a cholesterol-rich environment that is advantageous for complement activation through C3 deposition or by providing a region of the membrane that is more susceptible to penetration by the membrane attack complex (MAC).[8] In addition, type I antibodies cause low levels of direct signaling and cell death, with the requirement of a cross-linking antibody to mediate this process. By contrast, type II antibodies exhibit reduced binding to C1q, do not segregate CD20 into lipid rafts, and therefore cause lower levels of CDC. However, type II antibodies cause potent induction of direct cell death without requiring a cross-linking antibody. Rather, type II antibodies activate a caspase-independent, lysosomal-dependent mechanism of cell death that is dependent on homotypic adhesion.[10] For a direct comparison of type I and type II antibodies, see **Table 3**.

The contribution of different mechanisms of antibody killing in CLL by rituximab has been extensively explored and is still viewed as controversial. The authors' group was the first to demonstrate true in vivo caspase-dependent apoptosis and also downregulation of antiapoptotic proteins in CLL patients having a rapid blood response to rituximab.[11] Beum and colleagues[12] have demonstrated evidence of in vivo CDC activation and CD20 shaving (trogocytosis) in CLL, and have advocated for reduced dosing of antibody to avoid depleting complement. Although Fc receptor engagement by effector cells (ADCC and ADCP) has been shown to be important in many in vivo animal models,[13] surrogate evidence of the importance of these mechanisms is lacking in CLL, based on there being no correlation of response with FcγR-IIa and FcγR-IIIa polymorphisms associated with high-affinity binding and enhanced effector cell activation.[14] In addition, CLL has intrinsic immune defects as a consequence of both immunosuppressive cytokines and ligands that diminish natural killer (NK)-cell, monocyte, and macrophage dysfunction.[15]

Rituximab

Rituximab, the first approved antibody for cancer treatment, is a chimeric murine/human type I monoclonal immunoglobulin G1 (IgG1) directed against CD20. Rituximab mediates CDC, ADCC, and direct cell apoptosis in the treatment of B-cell malignancies.

Rituximab monotherapy

The initial landmark phase III trial, which earned approval for single-agent use of rituximab (375 mg/m^2 intravenously [IV] for 4 weekly doses) in NHL, included 33 patients with small lymphocytic lymphoma (SLL). Only 12% of these SLL patients achieved response (all partial response [PR]).[16] Several smaller studies (reviewed by Jaglowski

Table 3
Characteristics of CD20 monoclonal antibodies

Characteristic	Type I	Type II
Complement-dependent cytotoxicity	+++	+
Antibody-dependent cell-mediated cytotoxicity and phagocytosis	+++	+++
Direct cell cytotoxicity	+	+++
Localization of CD20 on lipid rafts	+	−

and Byrd[17]) showed similar modest clinical responses with single-agent rituximab in CLL patients, and it was unclear at that point whether rituximab would continue to be developed for CLL/SLL patients. Lower responses in CLL as opposed to NHL were thought to be secondary to diminished CD20 expression,[18] altered innate immune function,[19,20] or different pharmacokinetic features[21] of CLL in comparison with NHL. However, subsequent trials[22,23] using higher doses of rituximab administered either 3 times weekly or at higher weekly dosing (up to 2250 mg/m^2 per dose) showed improved responses in relapsed CLL patients with a response duration similar to those seen in NHL. These trials paved the way for further study of rituximab in CLL. Subsequently, a phase II trial using rituximab (375 mg/m^2) weekly for 4 doses in the front-line treatment of CLL showed a better response in the previously untreated patients (overall response rate [ORR] 51%) compared with the refractory/relapsed patients in previous trials (ORR 13%).[24] These trials prompted combinations of rituximab with chemotherapy (chemoimmunotherapy) in an attempt to further improve efficacy in CLL patients.

Rituximab chemoimmunotherapy

Multiple phase II studies have combined rituximab with various chemotherapeutic agents to show improved response. This section reviews the high-impact trials. Rituximab was combined with fludarabine (FR) in refractory (n = 11) and treatment-naïve (n = 20) CLL patients in a phase II trial that demonstrated an ORR of 87% with 32% complete response (CR).[25] Another phase II trial (CALGB-9712) evaluated the difference between the concurrent or sequential administration of fludarabine and rituximab in 104 treatment-naïve patients with CLL. The concurrent cohort experienced more severe hematologic and infusion-related toxicities, but demonstrated an ORR of 90% (CR 47%) compared with an ORR of 78% (CR 28%) in the sequential cohort.[26] Subsequent review of CALGB-9712 indicated that those patients with normal cytogenetics had a better 3-year overall survival (OS) (86%) than those patients with del(17p13.1) (33%) or del(11q22.3) (53%).[27] The retrospective comparison between patients on this trial and a similarly designed study (CALGB-9011), which used fludarabine alone, demonstrated that the patients who received FR had a significantly improved progression-free survival (PFS) and OS compared with those who received fludarabine alone.[28] Long-term follow-up of the patients on CALGB-9712 did not show an increased risk of therapy-related myeloid neoplasms.[29] Another phase II study using sequential fludarabine and rituximab in 60 treatment-naïve CLL patients demonstrated an ORR of 93% (CR 78%), providing further evidence of this regimen's activity in CLL.[30]

Rituximab in combination with fludarabine and cyclophosphamide (FCR) has been thoroughly investigated. In a large study, 300 treatment-naïve CLL patients who received FCR demonstrated an impressive ORR of 95% (CR 72%) and a 6-year PFS and OS of 51% and 77%, respectively. Most common adverse events were cytopenias and infections. There were 8 patients who developed therapy-related myelodysplasia.[31] In another large study, 177 relapsed/refractory CLL patients demonstrated an ORR of 73% (CR 25%). Median time to progression was 28 months. Common grade 3/4 toxicities were neutropenia (81%) and infection (16%).[32] Patients with del(11q22.3) appeared to benefit from the addition of cyclophosphamide to fludarabine and rituximab[33] as opposed to continued inferior outcomes in patients with del (17p13.1)[31] and IgVH-unmutated CLL.[34]

Pentostatin, a nucleoside analogue that is less myelotoxic than fludarabine, has been studied in combination with rituximab and cyclophosphamide (PCR). A study of PCR in 32 relapsed/refractory CLL patients demonstrated an ORR of 75% (CR 25%).

Common toxicities included myelosuppression and infection[35] A front-line study of PCR in 65 CLL patients demonstrated an ORR of 91% (CR 41%). The patients with del(11q22.3) again demonstrated that the addition of cyclophosphamide negates the poor prognosis associated with the marker. The most common adverse events were again myelosuppression and infection.[36]

The alkylator-like molecule bendamustine has recently been successfully combined with rituximab (BR) in CLL. In a newly published phase II study, 117 treatment-naïve CLL patients received BR and demonstrated an ORR of 88% (CR 23%). At a median observation time of 27 months, event-free survival was 34 months and 90.5% of the patients were still living at the time of publication. Patients with del(11q22.3), trisomy 12, del(17p13.1), and IgVH-unmutated disease demonstrated response to BR at rates of 90%, 95%, 38%, and 89%, respectively. Grade 3/4 adverse events observed were thrombocytopenia (22.2%), neutropenia (19.7%), anemia (19.7%), and infection (7.7%).[37] The same group reported the preliminary results of a phase II study of 81 relapsed/refractory patients who received BR and achieved an ORR of 77% (CR 15%; 62 patients were evaluable). Severe toxicities included myelosuppression and infection, with 3 patients dying of infections related to neutropenia caused by treatment.[38] Longer-term analysis of this study is pending. A randomized phase III study comparing BR with FCR in front-line CLL therapy is ongoing (CLL10 Trial).

For rituximab chemoimmunotherapy in phase III studies, 2 landmark trials confirmed improved response rates and OS with FCR in both front-line[39] and relapsed/refractory[40] CLL patients. In the CLL8 trial, 817 CLL patients were randomized to receive either FCR or FC. The ORR was significantly better in the FCR group, at 90% versus 80% in the FC group ($P<.0001$). The median PFS was significantly improved in the FCR group, at 51.8 months versus 32.8 months in the FC group ($P<.0001$; hazard ratio [HR] 0.56; 95% confidence interval [CI] 0.46–0.69). In addition, the 3-year estimated OS was significantly improved in the FCR group, at 87% in the FCR group versus 83% in the FC group ($P = .012$; HR 0.76; 95% CI 0.48–0.92). No increase in the number of infections was noted with the addition of rituximab, and more patients on the FC arm died during the trial.[39] In the relapsed/refractory setting, the REACH trial randomized 552 CLL patients who had received a median of one line of therapy (mostly single-agent alkylator therapy) to receive either FCR or FC. The ORR was significantly improved in the FCR group, at 69.9% versus 58.0% in the FC group ($P = .0034$). The median PFS was significantly improved in the FCR group, at 30.6 months versus 20.6 months in the FC group ($P<.001$; HR 0.65; 95% CI 0.51–0.82). Hematologic toxicity was the most significant adverse event.[40] These 2 studies have placed rituximab as a standard addition to front-line and subsequent lines of therapy for CLL.

Rituximab immunomodulation therapy

Lenalidomide is an immunomodulatory drug, which is active as a single agent in CLL. In vitro, the agent enhances NK-cell–mediated ADCC of rituximab against CLL cells,[41] making lenalidomide an attractive agent to use in combination with rituximab in clinical trials (LR). In a phase II trial, 59 relapsed/refractory CLL patients received LR and demonstrated an ORR of 66% (CR 10%). Of note, the patients with del(17p13.1) (n = 15) in the study demonstrated an ORR of 53%. Reported 2-year OS was 83%. There were 3 patient deaths while on therapy that were thought to be unrelated to the study drug. Two second malignancies were observed (1 colon cancer and 1 myelodysplastic syndrome). The most common grade 3/4 adverse events were neutropenia (47%), infection (31%), thrombocytopenia (22%), anemia (10%), and 1 tumor lysis syndrome. Tumor flare reactions (27%) were all grade 2 or less.[42] In the front-line setting, a phase-II trial, 2-arm study of 69 CLL patients (arm A = patients <65 years old, arm B = patients ≥65 years) who received LR has been reported. At the time of publication, 57 patients were available for analysis. Preliminary results of the study indicate an ORR of 94% (CR 20%) in arm A and 77% (CR 9%) in arm B. Neutropenia was the most common grade 3/4 adverse event. Infusion and tumor flare reactions were more frequent in the first cycle. A lower proportion of arm B patients were able to complete 7 full cycles of therapy (16 of 27) compared with those in arm A (35 of 39), mainly secondary to toxicity.[43] Pending final publication of the study, this regimen appears to be efficacious and tolerable in CLL.

Rituximab maintenance therapy

Rituximab has been studied as a maintenance regimen for patients who achieved response with standard chemoimmunotherapy regimens. In one phase II study, 75 patients received 4 weekly doses of rituximab (375 mg/m^2) as maintenance therapy following response to fludarabine. Those patients who continued to have minimal residual disease (MRD) then received 4 monthly doses of rituximab at 375 mg/m^2 followed by 12 monthly doses at 150 mg/m^2. The MRD patients receiving consolidation had a significantly longer 5-year PFS than the patients who did not receive consolidation (87% vs 32%, $P = .001$).[44] Several ongoing phase III trials are assessing the efficacy of maintenance rituximab in CLL (www.clinicaltrials.gov), and this approach should still be viewed as investigational.

Rituximab therapy for the autoimmune complications of CLL

Another proposed use of rituximab in CLL is for the autoimmune complications that commonly occur with CLL, including autoimmune hemolytic anemia (AIHA), immune thrombocytopenia (ITP), and pure red cell aplasia. Rituximab was initially described in the treatment of steroid-refractory pure red cell aplasia and AIHA.[45] Subsequently, successful treatment of 2 patients with pure red cell aplasia with rituximab (375 mg/m^2) weekly for 2 weeks was described.[46] Eight patients with steroid-refractory AIHA were treated with rituximab and dexamethasone, and all patients achieved remission of AIHA. Retreatment was also successful for relapses in this group.[47] In a case series of CLL patients with AIHA treated with rituximab, 12 of 14 patients had increased hemoglobin levels.[48] In the ITP setting, 3 CLL patients who developed ITP while on fludarabine therapy and who were refractory to both steroids and intravenous immunoglobulin were treated with rituximab for 4 weekly doses. These patients all had a rapid and durable response to rituximab therapy.[49] Although there are limited randomized data, these reports in conjunction with the experience at the authors' institution provide evidence for rituximab's effectiveness in the setting of autoimmune complications of CLL.

In general, rituximab is very well tolerated. The most common adverse event is infusion-related toxicity, and although more than 90% of patients experience some type of infusion-related reaction, it is generally mild to moderate in severity.[16,50] Patients with CLL and those with an increased number of circulating lymphocytes are at a higher risk of the more severe adverse events, such as respiratory insufficiency and tumor lysis syndrome.[51] Rare cases of hepatitis B[52] or JC polyomavirus[53] reactivation have been reported.

Ofatumumab (Arzerra, HuMax-CD20)

Because of the success of rituximab, many other CD20 antibodies have been developed to enhance select mechanisms of killing. Ofatumumab is the other currently approved type I humanized CD20 IgG1 antibody. In contrast to rituximab, it binds to a different epitope of CD20, which is composed of both the small and large extracellular loops of the CD20 molecule[54] that facilitates enhanced CDC, direct killing (with cross-linking), and ADCC against CLL cells in comparison with rituximab. **Fig. 2** depicts the binding sites of rituximab and ofatumumab on the CD20 protein. Ofatumumab has mediated CDC against rituximab-resistant Raji cell and CLL cells with low expression of CD20 in vitro. The agent appears to cause more potent CDC, has a slower off rate, and more stable CD20 binding than rituximab.[55] The improved CDC may be the result of the greater proximity of the small-loop binding site to the cell membrane, which could potentially lead to more effective deposition of complement on the cell surface.[54–56]

Ofatumumab has shown clinical efficacy in relapsed/refractory CLL patients. A phase I/II study of single-agent ofatumumab in 33 relapsed/refractory CLL patients demonstrated an ORR of 50%. Toxicity analysis indicated that infusion-related reactions were similar to those of rituximab, with decreased rate after the first infusion. Infections occurred in 51% of the patients, including 1 fatal infection.[57] The interim analysis of the landmark trial, which led to the approval of single-agent ofatumumab for relapsed/refractory CLL, included 138 patients with refractory CLL to fludarabine or alemtuzumab (FA-group) or bulky lymphadenopathy (>5 cm [BF-group]). Patients on this trial received ofatumumab for 8 weekly doses followed by 4 monthly doses for a total 24-week treatment period (dose 1 = 300 mg; doses 2–12 = 2000 mg). The ORR was 58% and 47%, the median PFS was 5.7 months and 5.9 months, and the OS was 13.7 months and 15.4 months in the FA-group and BF-group, respectively. The most common adverse events were infusion reactions and infections, which were primarily grade 1 and 2 events. Hematologic adverse events included neutropenia and anemia.[58] Subsequent ad hoc analysis of 117 CLL patients on this trial who were previously treated with rituximab (89 patients were rituximab-refractory) and

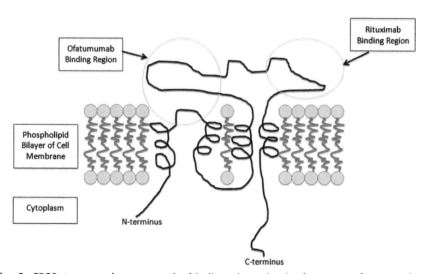

Fig. 2. CD20 transmembrane protein binding sites: rituximab versus ofatumumab. In contrast to rituximab, ofatumumab binds to a different epitope of CD20, composed of both the small and large extracellular loops of the CD20 molecule, which facilitates enhanced complement-dependent cytotoxicity, direct killing (with cross-linking), and antibody-dependent cell-mediated cytotoxicity against chronic lymphocytic leukemia cells in comparison with rituximab.

89 patients who were rituximab-naïve demonstrated no differences in ORR, median PFS, or OS between the 3 groups.[59] This analysis indicates that ofatumumab is an effective treatment for CLL regardless of prior rituximab therapy. Similarly, ofatumumab appeared to offer clinical benefit across all genomic groups except in patients with 17p deletion and bulky lymph node (>5 cm) disease.

Recently, Flinn and colleagues[60] from the Sarah Cannon Research Institute reported a phase II trial whereby 42 older CLL patients (median age 69 years; range 47–88 years) or patients who refused fludarabine-based regimens received weekly ofatumumab (300 mg, week 1; 2000 mg, weeks 2–8) as front-line therapy. Patients who achieved response or did not progress after 8 weeks of therapy (n = 24 at the time of publication) received maintenance ofatumumab (2000 mg) every 2 months for a total of 2 years (for a planned total of 12 doses). After the initial 8 weeks, the lymphocyte count normalized in 85% of patients. Of the 30 patients evaluable for response at time of publication, 44% (n = 13) achieved response (all PR) and 53% (n = 16) had stable disease, with only 1 patient (3%) with progressive disease. Ofatumumab therapy was well tolerated with infrequent adverse effects. Two patients were hospitalized with events possibly related to the antibody: grade 2 fever and grade 3 anemia and pneumonia. Only 1 patient experienced a significant infusion-related reaction. These preliminary data indicate that ofatumumab is highly active and well tolerated when used as front-line therapy in this patient population. Continued toxicity and efficacy assessment is ongoing.

Based on the success of ofatumumab as a single agent in CLL, multiple trials have been initiated combining ofatumumab with other chemoimmunotherapy agents. A phase II study combining ofatumumab with fludarabine and cyclophosphamide (O-FC) in previously untreated CLL was recently published. Sixty-one patients received standard doses of fludarabine (25 mg/m^2 IV on day 1) plus cyclophosphamide (250 mg/m^2 IV on days 1–3) in combination with ofatumumab, 300 mg for the first dose followed by either 500 mg (group A) or 1000 mg (group B) of ofatumumab every 4 weeks for 6 cycles. The ORR was 77% and 73% with a CR of 32% and 50% for groups A and B, respectively. Median follow-up was 8 months at the time of publication and did not allow for meaningful calculation of PFS or OS. The most common grade 3 and 4 adverse events were neutropenia (48%), thrombocytopenia (15%), anemia (13%), and infection (8%).[61] This study indicated that O-FC is an active and safe regimen in the first-line treatment of CLL. Multiple phase II studies with ofatumumab in combination are ongoing with standard agents such as lenalidomide,[62] pentostatin and cyclophosphamide,[63] high-dose methylprednisolone,[64] bendamustine,[65] and novel agents, which target the B-cell receptor pathway, such as ibrutinib[66] and GS-1101.[67] Ofatumumab is currently viewed as an acceptable salvage therapy for relapsed/refractory CLL. Multiple phase III studies in the front-line, relapsed/refractory, and maintenance settings are ongoing to assess the efficacy of ofatumumab, with the hope of expanding it to being fully approved as therapy by the Food and Drug Administration.

Obinutuzumab (GA-101)

Obinutuzumab is a novel humanized anti-CD20 type II IgG1 monoclonal antibody (mAb) currently under clinical development. Obinutuzumab was developed with a glycol-engineered Fc segment that binds with increased affinity to Fc receptor displayed by immune effector cells.[68] The antibody initiates nonapoptotic cell death via an actin-dependent lysosome-mediated mechanism that is dependent on cell-to-cell contact.[10,69] While CDC activity is low, as described previously with type II antibodies, owing to the lack of CD20 localization into lipid rafts, obinutuzumab binds with high affinity to the CD20 epitope, which causes potent induction of NK-cell ADCC. Induction of ADCC has been demonstrated to be 5 to 100 times greater than that of rituximab.[69–73] In whole blood samples, the antibody demonstrates depletion of CLL cells and may be more potent than rituximab at similar concentrations.[72,73] In contrast to rituximab and ofatumumab, obinutuzumab does not mediate as effective ADCP. The agent demonstrates increased antitumor activity compared with type I antibodies in human tumor xenograft models, both as a single agent[74,75] and in combination with chemotherapy,[75] and has shown excellent B-cell–depleting activity in the lymphoid tissue (lymph nodes and spleen) of nonhuman primates.[74]

Early clinical data are available for obinutuzumab. In a recently published phase I/II study, 21 patients with heavily pretreated relapsed/refractory CD20+ malignancies received doses from 50 mg to 2000 mg. Infusion-related reactions were the most common grade 3/4 adverse events, mostly during the first infusion. The ORR in this early study was 43%, demonstrating encouraging activity for this well-tolerated agent. There were no CLL patients on this trial, and 1 patient with SLL.[76] A phase I study of 13 heavily pretreated CLL patients, the majority expressing high-risk genetic features, received doses of obinutuzumab from 400 mg to 2000 mg IV on days 1, 8, and 22 for 9 total infusions. The most common adverse events were grade 1/2 infusion reactions, generally limited to the first infusion. Grade 3/4 hematologic toxicities were neutropenia (n = 9), febrile neutropenia (n = 1), and transient thrombocytopenia (n = 1). Although 17 episodes of infection were reported, only 3 were grade 3. The ORR was 62%, indicating promising efficacy in this group and tolerable adverse events.[77] In the phase II portion of this study, 20 patients received obinutuzumab (1000 mg) weekly for a total of 10 infusions. The antibody was well tolerated, with infusion-related reactions as the most common adverse event (n = 13; grade 3/4-n = 6), which occurred mainly during the first infusion. Following the last infusion, the ORR was 25% (4 PR, 5 stable disease). Those patients with greater than 2400 mm^2 of tumor burden (by lymph node measurement on computed tomography scan) did not respond as well as the patients with lower tumor burden, indicating that obinutuzumab will likely need to be used in combination in the setting of bulky adenopathy. This phase II trial further supported that obinutuzumab has promising clinical activity in the heavily pretreated CLL population.[78] Another recently published phase I study investigated the use of obinutuzumab induction followed by 2 years of maintenance in 22 patients with relapsed CD20+ lymphoid malignancies. Five patients had CLL, 4 with intermediate risk (Rai stage I/II) disease. In this study, cohorts of 3 to 6 patients received obinutuzumab (200–2000 mg) IV weekly for 4 weeks. Subsequently, patients who achieved CR or PR went on to receive obinutuzumab every 3 months for a maximum of 8 doses. Infusion-related reactions were the most common adverse events (all grades 73%, grades 3/4 18%), followed by infection (32%), pyrexia (23%), neutropenia (23%), headache (18%), and nausea (18%). At the end of induction, 5 (23%) patients had PR and 12 (54%) had stable disease. Eight patients received maintenance therapy, with ORR of 32% (n = 6) with 1 CR. The study demonstrated tolerability and promising efficacy in this population.[79] There are multiple ongoing trials using obinutuzumab in CLL, including a phase II trial in untreated CLL patients, and a large phase III trial in untreated comorbid CLL patients comparing monotherapy with chlorambucil, chlorambucil plus rituximab, and chlorambucil plus obinutuzumab (CLL11 Trial).

Other CD20 mAbs

Veltuzumab (IMMU-106, hA20) is a type I, humanized, IgG1 monoclonal antibody with complementary determining regions, similar to rituximab. In vitro, this antibody has a stronger effect on CDC and a reduced off rate in some lymphoma cell lines when compared with rituximab.[80] A phase I/II study of low dose subcutaneous veltuzumab contained 11 CLL patients (4 were treatment-naïve). These patients tolerated the agent well but demonstrated lower serum levels than their NHL counterparts, indicating that more frequent or prolonged dosing will be needed for CLL patients.[81] Two radiolabeled CD20 monoclonal antibodies are currently in use for the treatment of NHL. Ibritumomab tiuxetan (Zevalin) and tositumomab (Bexxar) are conjugated with ytrrium-90 and iodine-131, respectively. Studies of ibritumomab in CLL noted limited efficacy and significant hematologic toxicity[82] that stopped study in this area. Although tositumomab has been found to have less hematologic toxicity,[83] there is limited interest in pursuing this molecule for CLL therapy. Multiple other CD20 antibodies are currently in development for CLL in addition to NHL, as recently reviewed by Robak and Robak.[84] For additional CD20 antibody descriptions, see **Table 2**.

CD52 ANTIBODY

CD52 is a membrane-anchored glycoprotein, which is highly expressed on all B and T lymphocytes (with the exception of plasma cells), granulocytes, monocytes, macrophages, eosinophils, NK cells, and dendritic cells.[85] CD52 is an attractive therapeutic target for hematologic malignancies, as it is expressed on tumor cells of CLL, T-cell prolymphocytic leukemia, hairy cell leukemia, NHL, and acute lymphoblastic leukemia.[86]

Alemtuzumab (Campath-1H)

Alemtuzumab is a recombinant DNA-derived humanized IgG1 κ mAb that recognizes CD52. Although its precise mechanism of action is unknown, alemtuzumab has been shown to cause CDC[72] and/or ADCC through its IgG Fc region.[87,88] In vitro, the agent is capable of direct CLL cell death through a membrane raft–dependent mechanism, which is independent of p53 status and caspase activation.[89] This cell-death mechanism is important for patients with del(17p13.1) or otherwise dysfunctional p53 who are difficult to treat. Early in vivo studies demonstrated responses independent of del(17p13.1) status,[90,91] supporting a mechanism of action independent of p53 pathway.

Alemtuzumab was initially approved as a single agent for relapsed/refractory CLL following the landmark CAM 211 trial. In this study, 93 CLL patients received gradually increased doses of alemtuzumab, followed by 30 mg IV 3 times weekly for a total of 12 weeks. The ORR was 33%, with bulky lymphadenopathy (>5 cm) correlating with poor response. The median PFS was 4.7 months and median OS was 16 months.[92] As nearly all patients experienced infusion reactions, subcutaneous (SQ) dosing was trialed. In a phase II study, 103 relapsed/refractory CLL patients received alemtuzumab SQ 30 mg 3 times weekly for up to 12 weeks. The ORR, median PFS, and OS were 34%, 7.7 months, and 19.1 months, respectively.[93] Responses were achieved even in the del(17p13.1) population, further confirming the results from earlier trials.[90,91] The major adverse events noted in these trials were hematologic toxicity and infections related to profound immune suppression, most commonly reactivation of herpesviruses including cytomegalovirus (CMV). These findings led to a recommendation of prophylactic therapy for opportunistic infections in patients treated with alemtuzumab.

Because of the efficacy of alemtuzumab in relapsed/refractory CLL patients and initial efficacy in pilot studies, the agent was studied in the front-line setting as monotherapy. In a large phase III study, 297 untreated CLL patients were randomized to receive either IV alemtuzumab, 30 mg 3 times weekly for up to 12 weeks or oral chlorambucil, 40 mg/m^2 every 4 weeks for up to 12 cycles. The alemtuzumab group demonstrated a significantly higher ORR (83% vs 56%) and improved median PFS (14.6 vs 11.7 months) when compared with the chlorambucil group. Alemtuzumab again showed improved efficacy in the patients with del(17p13.1). Although hemato-logic toxicities were similar between the 2 groups, 52% of the patients in the alemtu-zumab group developed CMV reactivation, compared with 2% in the chlorambucil group.[94] Alemtuzumab was approved for front-line monotherapy following this trial; however, concerns about infections commonly limit its use.

Alemtuzumab has been studied in the setting of consolidation[95–99] and in combina-tion with various chemoimmunotherapy agents; however, severe infectious toxicities and limited improved efficacy have prohibited development of the agent in these settings. Alemtuzumab was recently removed from the commercial market for CLL therapy to allow more expansion into alternative applications such as multiple scle-rosis. Alemtuzumab will still be available compassionately to patients with CLL who meet indications for its use.

CD37 ANTIBODIES AND SMALL MODULAR IMMUNE PHARMACEUTICALS

CD37, a tetraspanin transmembrane protein, features 4 possible membrane-spanning regions.[100,101] CD37 is an intriguing target in the treatment of CLL, as it is found on the cell membranes of developing B cells, from pre–B cell to mature peripheral B cells, but not plasma cells. The protein is also expressed at very low levels on T cells, NK cells, and monocytes,[102] but is not found on the cell surface of platelets or red blood cells.[103]

TRU-016

TRU-016 is a small modular immunopharmaceutical (SMIP), which is a structurally modified IgG1 anti-CD37 mAb that lacks the constant heavy-chain region 1 (CH1) domain of the IgG antibody. In vitro, TRU-016 has been shown to have ADCC and direct cell death superior to rituximab and alemtuzumab when directed against CLL cells.[104] It has recently been shown that the ligation of CD37 causes tyrosine phos-phorylation of the protein, and can act as an immunoreceptor tyrosine-based inhibition motif (ITIM) and immunoreceptor tyrosine-based activation motif (ITAM), which leads to association with proximal signaling molecules (SHP1 and p110δ), initiating a cascade of events that leads to cell apoptosis[105] or survival signaling depending on the region of the protein activated.

TRU-016 is currently under investigation in phase I clinical trials. A phase I study of 57 relapsed/refractory CLL patients received up to 20 mg/kg IV of TRU-016 weekly for up to 12 doses. The agent was well tolerated with no dose-limiting toxicities (DLT) at the maximum dose level; therefore, the maximum tolerated dose was not achieved. In patients with 1 to 2 prior therapies, an ORR of 44% (7/16, all PR) was achieved with a 92% median reduction in peripheral lymphocytosis. In patients with at least 3 prior therapies (n = 41) no responses were achieved, but a 62% median reduction in lymphocyte count was observed.[106] In an expanded cohort of this study, 26 patients (7 treatment-naïve, 19 relapsed/refractory) received TRU-016 at doses of 10 mg/kg, 20 mg/kg, and 30 mg/kg IV weekly for 8 doses, followed by 4 monthly doses. The agent continued to show good tolerability, with infection (n = 4), neutropenia (n = 3), and febrile neutropenia (n = 2) as the most common grade 3/4 events. The ORR was 86% (6/7, all PR) and 17% (3/17) in the treatment-naïve and relapsed/refractory patients, respectively. However, 50% or greater reduction in peripheral lymphocytes was noted in 81% (17 of 21) of the patients newly enrolled on the expansion cohort.[107] Because of its success as a single agent, more phase I trials are under way or are planned for TRU-016 in combination with other agents, such as bendamustine and rituximab or rituximab in both relapsed/refractory and treatment-naïve CLL patients.

Other CD37 antibodies

Because of the tolerability and efficacy noted with TRU-016, other anti-CD37 mAbs are currently under investigation in vitro. 37.1 is a mouse/human chimeric IgG1 antibody similar to TRU-016 but with additional engineering of its Fc region. 37.2 is a humanized version of 37.1, which binds CD37 with low nanomolar affinity. In vitro studies with CLL cell lines show increased induction of direct cell death and improved CLL cell depletion from whole blood when compared with rituximab and alemtuzumab.[108] Both antibodies are currently entering phase I trials for CLL.

IMGN529 is an immunotoxin, which targets CD37 via conjugation of a CD37 antibody (K7153A) with a cytotoxic maytansinoid (DM1). K7153A is a novel CD37 antibody, which has demonstrated strong proapoptotic and direct cell-killing activity against NHL cell lines, and could mediate CDC and ADCC. In vitro experiments with purified peripheral blood mononuclear cells (PBMCs) and whole blood samples indicated that IMGN529 was more potent than rituximab or TRU-016, and was more specific than alemtuzumab at B-cell depletion. In vivo, IMGN529 demonstrated better antitumor activity than the K7153A antibody alone in NHL and CLL xenograft models in SCID mice.[109] As a consequence of these data, the antibody has entered phase I trials in NHL and will likely be explored in CLL.

CD40 ANTIBODIES

CD40 is a transmembrane protein of the tumor necrosis factor receptor family. CD40 is expressed on B cells from the pro-B to plasma cell stages, monocytes, macrophages, platelets, follicular dendritic cells, dendritic cells, eosinophils, and activated CD8+ T cells. In addition, CD40 is expressed in highly proliferative nonhematopoietic cells, such as epithelial and endothelial cells.[110] Of importance is that the protein is expressed on the vast majority of CLL cells.[111]

CD40 ligand (CD40L) is a soluble protein expressed on the surface of helper T cells, platelets, and NK cells. In normal B cells, the ligation of CD40 with CD40L activates the phosphoinositol-3 (PI3)-kinase pathway,[112,113] and nuclear factor κB (NF-κB)[114,115] which, in turn, disrupts apoptosis. A commonly seen pathologic feature of CLL cells is spontaneous apoptosis. In vitro, this PI3-kinase and NF-κB activation is demonstrated when CLL cells are treated with CD40L. Several groups have shown disruption of both spontaneous and drug-induced apoptosis in CLL cell lines.[114,115] Therefore, disrupting the CD40L-CD40 signaling axis is an attractive therapeutic target for the treatment of CLL.

Dacetuzumab (SGN-40)

Dacetuzumab is a humanized IgG1 mAb that targets CD40. Dacetuzumab induces ADCC and ADCP via interaction with Fc receptors on T cells, NK cells, monocytes, and macrophages.[110] In vitro, dacetuzumab mediates modest apoptosis when cross-linked and cytotoxicity through ADCC in CLL cell lines.[116] Initially, dacetuzumab was shown to be a weak agonist of normal B cells and there was some concern that the agent may also activate CLL cells, causing tumor flare or early disease progression.[110] However, in vitro data in CLL cells do not substantiate this concern.[116]

In a phase I trial dacetuzumab was given to 12 relapsed/refractory CLL patients at doses from 3 to 8 mg/kg. Although the agent was well tolerated with no DLTs or serious adverse events, no patients achieved response with monotherapy.[117] There is some interest in combining dacetuzumab with other chemoimmunotherapy agents to augment response in CLL. In vitro the immune modulating agent lenalidomide increases CD40 antigen expression on CLL cells and enhances CLL NK-cell activity toward antibody-laden tumor targets,[118] indicating that lenalidomide may be an attractive agent to use in combination of dacetuzumab. A recent phase IIb trial in relapsed/refractory diffuse large B-cell lymphoma patients comparing dacetuzumab with placebo when given in combination with rituximab, ifosfamide, carboplatin, and etoposide (R-ICE) therapy was terminated early, secondary to lack of added efficacy in the dacetuzumab arm. The clinical future of this antibody is unclear.

Lucatumumab (HCD-122, CHIR-12.12)

Lucatumumab is a human, recombinant IgG1 mAb, which targets CD40. Preclinical data indicate that lucatumumab is a potent antagonist that blocks signaling by CD40L. In vitro, the antibody mediates killing and elimination of tumor cells through ADCC and opsonization. In CLL cell lines, lucatumumab inhibits CD40L-induced cell protection from apoptosis, and is a more potent mediator of ADCC than is rituximab.[119]

In a recently published phase I trial, 26 relapsed/refractory CLL patients received lucatumumab at escalating doses weekly for 4 weeks. The maximum tolerated dose was found to be 3.0 mg/kg weekly after patients at higher dose levels experienced grade 3/4 asymptomatic, reversible elevations of amylase and lipase lasting for longer than 7 days. The agent was otherwise well tolerated. However, the clinical efficacy was limited, with only 1 patient achieving a nodular PR and the majority of patients (65.4%) demonstrating stable disease.[120] Future trials in CLL will likely involve lucatumumab in combination with other active agents.

CD19 ANTIBODIES

CD19 is a glycoprotein member of the Ig superfamily that is expressed on the cell membranes of follicular dendritic cells and B cells, from development until differentiation into plasma cells. CD19 regulates basal signal transduction thresholds in resting B cells via establishment of a novel Src-family kinase amplification loop. CD19 amplifies Src-family kinase activation following B-cell receptor ligation, which eventually leads to inhibition of B-cell signal transduction[121]

XmAb5574

XmAb5574 is a human, IgG1 mAb, with an engineered Fc portion with 2 amino acid substitutions that enhance its cytotoxic activity through higher affinity for the FcγIIIa portion of effector cells and decreased binding for FcγRIIb.[122] In vivo, XmAb5574 mediates potent ADCC, has moderate direct cytotoxicity and ADCP, and no CDC when used in CLL cell lines. The ADCC is mediated through NK cells by a granzyme B–dependent mechanism and is more potent than ADCC caused by rituximab in CLL cell lines. It was also noted that the addition of lenalidomide to XmAb5574 enhanced ADCC.[123] In nonhuman primates, infusion of XmAb5574 led to immediate and dose-related B-cell depletion along with sustained reduction of NK cells. The investigators of that study propose that effector-cell (possibly NK-cell) functions mediate the antibody's potency in monkeys, and enhancing these mechanisms will advance the progress of XmAb5574 in humans.[124] A phase I trial of XmAb5574 is currently under way in relapsed/refractory CLL patients (www.clinicaltrials.gov).

MDX-1342

MDX-1342 is a human mAb with an engineered Fc portion that is nonfucosylated (lacking fucose sugar units), with the goal of enhancing Fc-mediated effector function. In vitro, MDX-1342 demonstrated increased affinity for the FcγIIIa receptors and enhanced effector-cell function, which led to increased potency of ADCC and phagocytosis assays in CD-19 expressing cells when compared with its fucosylated counterpart. In vivo administration of MDX-1342 in nonhuman primates led to potent B-cell depletion.[125] Early data from a phase I trial of MDX-1342 in relapsed/refractory CLL has been reported. At the time of publication, 12 patients had received escalating doses of MDX-1342 (0.7–200 mg) IV weekly for 4 weeks. No serious adverse events were reported in the first 12 patients, with infusion reaction the most common event (n = 9, all grade 1/2). Nine patients were evaluable for response at the time of reporting and 1 patient achieved PR, 6 have stable disease, and 2 had to discontinue the study secondary to progressive disease.[126] This trial is currently suspended (www.clinicaltrials.gov).

HUMAN LEUKOCYTE ANTIGEN–DR ANTIBODIES

Human leukocyte antigen–DR (HLA-DR) is a subtype of a class II major histocompatibility complex (MHC) antigen that is expressed on B-cell malignancy tumor cells as well as normal B cells, monocytes/macrophages, dendritic cells, thymic epithelial cells, and activated T cells and endothelial cells[127] When stimulated by ligation of an antibody, these HLA molecules can affect growth differentiation and immunoglobulin synthesis of B lymphocytes, in addition to activation of caspase-dependent and caspase-independent cell death pathways.[128,129]

Apolizumab (Hu1D10, Remitogen)

Hu-1D10 is a humanized murine IgG1 mAb that targets HLA-DR. In vitro, apolizumab induced caspase-dependent apoptosis following cross-linking with concurrent activation of the AKT survival pathway in CLL cell lines.[128] In a phase I clinical trial, apolizumab was given to 23 patients (22 CLL, 1 acute lymphoblastic leukemia). DLTs at the highest dose level included aseptic meningitis and hemolytic uremia. Additional toxicities included infusion reactions, urticarial rash, and headache. Only 1 patient had a PR and 3 had stable disease. Owing to toxicity and limited efficacy, development of this antibody was discontinued.[130]

IMMU-114 (hL243γ4P)

IMMU-114 is a humanized pan-HLA-DR IgG4 antibody. In vitro, IMMU-114 demonstrated antigen-binding specificity, antiproliferative activity, and ability to induce apoptosis, with activation of the AKT survival pathway intact and CDC and ADCC activity abrogated[129] The same group found that IMMU-114 was consistently more cytotoxic in the lymphoma and MM cell lines (notably in the rituximab-resistant CLL line) than rituximab. In vivo, IMMU-114 induced long-term, disease-free survival in mice treated at early stages of disease in relatively rituximab-resistant models. Their data also indicated that IMMU-114–induced apoptosis occurs in activated, but not normal, resting B cells.[127] A phase I clinical trial of IMMU-114 in relapsed/refractory CLL is planned.

OTHER ANTIBODIES

Multiple other novel antibodies for the treatment of B-cell malignancies are currently in various stages of clinical development, including antibodies directed at CD74, PD1,

PDL1, CD200, CD38, BAFF-R, and CD22. To date these are either being developed in other diseases or are early in preclinical development.

SUMMARY

mAb therapies have changed the face of treatment for CLL patients. Many promising new mAbs are under development, which will likely show optimal efficacy in combination with other immunochemotherapy agents. In addition, there is great potential for combinations of these mAbs with other new ground-breaking therapies for CLL, such as agents targeting the B-cell receptor pathway (ibrutinib and GS-1101). Future development of these mAbs will likely continue to revolutionize therapy for CLL patients.

REFERENCES

1. Howlader N, Noone AM, Krapcho M. SEER Cancer Statistics Review, 1975-2009 (Vintage 2009 Populations), SEER stat fact sheet: chronic lymphocytic lymphoma. Based on November 2011 SEER data submission, posted to the SEER web site. 2012. Available at: http://seer.cancer.gov/statfacts/html/clyl.html. Accessed June 1, 2012.
2. Zenz T, Mertens D, Kuppers R, et al. From pathogenesis to treatment of chronic lymphocytic leukaemia. Nat Rev Cancer 2010;10(1):37–50.
3. Scott AM, Allison JP, Wolchok JD. Monoclonal antibodies in cancer therapy. Cancer Immun 2012;12:14.
4. Stashenko P, Nadler LM, Hardy R, et al. Characterization of a human B lymphocyte-specific antigen. J Immunol 1980;125(4):1678–85.
5. Press OW, Howell-Clark J, Anderson S, et al. Retention of B-cell-specific monoclonal antibodies by human lymphoma cells. Blood 1994;83(5):1390–7.
6. Li H, Ayer LM, Lytton J, et al. Store-operated cation entry mediated by CD20 in membrane rafts. J Biol Chem 2003;278(43):42427–34.
7. Uchida J, Lee Y, Hasegawa M, et al. Mouse CD20 expression and function. Int Immunol 2004;16(1):119–29.
8. Cragg MS, Morgan SM, Chan HT, et al. Complement-mediated lysis by anti-CD20 mAb correlates with segregation into lipid rafts. Blood 2003;101(3): 1045–52.
9. Simons K, Ehehalt R. Cholesterol, lipid rafts, and disease. J Clin Invest 2002; 110(5):597–603.
10. Ivanov A, Beers SA, Walshe CA, et al. Monoclonal antibodies directed to CD20 and HLA-DR can elicit homotypic adhesion followed by lysosome-mediated cell death in human lymphoma and leukemia cells. J Clin Invest 2009;119(8): 2143–59.
11. Byrd JC, Kitada S, Flinn IW, et al. The mechanism of tumor cell clearance by rituximab in vivo in patients with B-cell chronic lymphocytic leukemia: evidence of caspase activation and apoptosis induction. Blood 2002;99(3):1038–43.
12. Beum PV, Kennedy AD, Williams ME, et al. The shaving reaction: rituximab/CD20 complexes are removed from mantle cell lymphoma and chronic lymphocytic leukemia cells by THP-1 monocytes. J Immunol 2006;176(4):2600–9.
13. Clynes RA, Towers TL, Presta LG, et al. Inhibitory Fc receptors modulate in vivo cytotoxicity against tumor targets. Nat Med 2000;6(4):443–6.
14. Farag SS, Flinn IW, Modali R, et al. Fc gamma RIIIa and Fc gamma RIIa polymorphisms do not predict response to rituximab in B-cell chronic lymphocytic leukemia. Blood 2004;103(4):1472–4.

15. Anand M, Chodda SK, Parikh PM, et al. Dysregulated cytokine production by monocytes from chronic lymphocytic leukemia patients. Cancer Biother Radiopharm 1998;13(1):43–8.

16. McLaughlin P, Grillo-Lopez AJ, Link BK, et al. Rituximab chimeric anti-CD20 monoclonal antibody therapy for relapsed indolent lymphoma: half of patients respond to a four-dose treatment program. J Clin Oncol 1998;16(8):2825–33.

17. Jaglowski SM, Byrd JC. Rituximab in chronic lymphocytic leukemia. Semin Hematol 2010;47(2):156–69.

18. Ginaldi L, De Martinis M, Matutes E, et al. Levels of expression of CD19 and CD20 in chronic B cell leukaemias. J Clin Pathol 1998;51(5):364–9.

19. Ziegler HW, Kay NE, Zarling JM. Deficiency of natural killer cell activity in patients with chronic lymphocytic leukemia. Int J Cancer 1981;27(3):321–7.

20. Kay NE, Zarling JM. Impaired natural killer activity in patients with chronic lymphocytic leukemia is associated with a deficiency of azurophilic cytoplasmic granules in putative NK cells. Blood 1984;63(2):305–9.

21. Berinstein NL, Grillo-Lopez AJ, White CA, et al. Association of serum rituximab (IDEC-C2B8) concentration and anti-tumor response in the treatment of recurrent low-grade or follicular non-Hodgkin's lymphoma. Ann Oncol 1998;9(9): 995–1001.

22. Byrd JC, Murphy T, Howard RS, et al. Rituximab using a thrice weekly dosing schedule in B-cell chronic lymphocytic leukemia and small lymphocytic lymphoma demonstrates clinical activity and acceptable toxicity. J Clin Oncol 2001;19(8):2153–64.

23. O'Brien SM, Kantarjian H, Thomas DA, et al. Rituximab dose-escalation trial in chronic lymphocytic leukemia. J Clin Oncol 2001;19(8):2165–70.

24. Hainsworth JD, Litchy S, Barton JH, et al. Single-agent rituximab as first-line and maintenance treatment for patients with chronic lymphocytic leukemia or small lymphocytic lymphoma: a phase II trial of the Minnie Pearl Cancer Research Network. J Clin Oncol 2003;21(9):1746–51.

25. Schulz H, Klein SK, Rehwald U, et al. Phase 2 study of a combined immunochemotherapy using rituximab and fludarabine in patients with chronic lymphocytic leukemia. Blood 2002;100(9):3115–20.

26. Byrd JC, Peterson BL, Morrison VA, et al. Randomized phase 2 study of fludarabine with concurrent versus sequential treatment with rituximab in symptomatic, untreated patients with B-cell chronic lymphocytic leukemia: results from Cancer and Leukemia Group B 9712 (CALGB 9712). Blood 2003;101(1):6–14.

27. Byrd JC, Gribben JG, Peterson BL, et al. Select high-risk genetic features predict earlier progression following chemoimmunotherapy with fludarabine and rituximab in chronic lymphocytic leukemia: justification for risk-adapted therapy. J Clin Oncol 2006;24(3):437–43.

28. Byrd JC, Rai K, Peterson BL, et al. Addition of rituximab to fludarabine may prolong progression-free survival and overall survival in patients with previously untreated chronic lymphocytic leukemia: an updated retrospective comparative analysis of CALGB 9712 and CALGB 9011. Blood 2005;105(1):49–53.

29. Woyach JA, Ruppert AS, Heerema NA, et al. Chemoimmunotherapy with fludarabine and rituximab produces extended overall survival and progression-free survival in chronic lymphocytic leukemia: long-term follow-up of CALGB study 9712. J Clin Oncol 2011;29(10):1349–55.

30. Del Poeta G, Del Principe MI, Consalvo MA, et al. The addition of rituximab to fludarabine improves clinical outcome in untreated patients with ZAP-70-negative chronic lymphocytic leukemia. Cancer 2005;104(12):2743–52.

31. Tam CS, O'Brien S, Wierda W, et al. Long-term results of the fludarabine, cyclophosphamide, and rituximab regimen as initial therapy of chronic lymphocytic leukemia. Blood 2008;112(4):975–80.
32. Wierda W, O'Brien S, Wen S, et al. Chemoimmunotherapy with fludarabine, cyclophosphamide, and rituximab for relapsed and refractory chronic lymphocytic leukemia. J Clin Oncol 2005;23(18):4070–8.
33. Tsimberidou AM, Tam C, Abruzzo LV, et al. Chemoimmunotherapy may overcome the adverse prognostic significance of 11q deletion in previously untreated patients with chronic lymphocytic leukemia. Cancer 2009;115(2): 373–80.
34. Lin KI, Tam CS, Keating MJ, et al. Relevance of the immunoglobulin VH somatic mutation status in patients with chronic lymphocytic leukemia treated with fludarabine, cyclophosphamide, and rituximab (FCR) or related chemoimmunotherapy regimens. Blood 2009;113(14):3168–71.
35. Lamanna N, Kalaycio M, Maslak P, et al. Pentostatin, cyclophosphamide, and rituximab is an active, well-tolerated regimen for patients with previously treated chronic lymphocytic leukemia. J Clin Oncol 2006;24(10):1575–81.
36. Kay NE, Geyer SM, Call TG, et al. Combination chemoimmunotherapy with pentostatin, cyclophosphamide, and rituximab shows significant clinical activity with low accompanying toxicity in previously untreated B chronic lymphocytic leukemia. Blood 2007;109(2):405–11.
37. Fischer K, Cramer P, Busch R, et al. Bendamustine in combination with rituximab for previously untreated patients with chronic lymphocytic leukemia: a multicenter phase II trial of the German Chronic Lymphocytic Leukemia Study Group. J Clin Oncol 2012;30(26):3209–16.
38. Fischer K, Stilgenbauer S, Schweighofer CD, et al. Bendamustine in combination with rituximab (BR) for patients with relapsed chronic lymphocytic leukemia (CLL): a multicentre phase II trial of the German CLL Study Group (GCLLSG) [abstracts]. Blood (ASH Annual Meeting Abstracts) 2008; 112(11):330.
39. Hallek M, Fischer K, Fingerle-Rowson G, et al. Addition of rituximab to fludarabine and cyclophosphamide in patients with chronic lymphocytic leukaemia: a randomised, open-label, phase 3 trial. Lancet 2010;376(9747):1164–74.
40. Robak T, Dmoszynska A, Solal-Celigny P, et al. Rituximab plus fludarabine and cyclophosphamide prolongs progression-free survival compared with fludarabine and cyclophosphamide alone in previously treated chronic lymphocytic leukemia. J Clin Oncol 2010;28(10):1756–65.
41. Wu L, Adams M, Carter T, et al. lenalidomide enhances natural killer cell and monocyte-mediated antibody-dependent cellular cytotoxicity of rituximab-treated CD20+ tumor cells. Clin Cancer Res 2008;14(14):4650–7.
42. Badoux XC, Keating MJ, O'Brien S, et al. Final analysis of a phase 2 study of lenalidomide and rituximab in patients with relapsed or refractory chronic lymphocytic leukemia (CLL) [abstracts]. Blood (ASH Annual Meeting Abstracts) 2011;118(21):980.
43. James DF, Brown JR, Werner L, et al. Lenalidomide and rituximab for the initial treatment of patients with chronic lymphocytic leukemia (CLL) a multicenter study of the CLL research consortium [abstracts]. Blood (ASH Annual Meeting Abstracts) 2011;118(21):291.
44. Del Poeta G, Del Principe MI, Buccisano F, et al. Consolidation and maintenance immunotherapy with rituximab improve clinical outcome in patients with B-cell chronic lymphocytic leukemia. Cancer 2008;112(1):119–28.

45. Zecca M, De Stefano P, Nobili B, et al. Anti-CD20 monoclonal antibody for the treatment of severe, immune-mediated, pure red cell aplasia and hemolytic anemia. Blood 2001;97(12):3995–7.
46. Ghazal H. Successful treatment of pure red cell aplasia with rituximab in patients with chronic lymphocytic leukemia. Blood 2002;99(3):1092–4.
47. Gupta N, Kavuru S, Patel D, et al. Rituximab-based chemotherapy for steroid-refractory autoimmune hemolytic anemia of chronic lymphocytic leukemia. Leukemia 2002;16(10):2092–5.
48. D'Arena G, Laurenti L, Capalbo S, et al. Rituximab therapy for chronic lympho-cytic leukemia-associated autoimmune hemolytic anemia. Am J Hematol 2006; 81(8):598–602.
49. Hegde UP, Wilson WH, White T, et al. Rituximab treatment of refractory fludarabine-associated immune thrombocytopenia in chronic lymphocytic leukemia. Blood 2002;100(6):2260–2.
50. Maloney DG, Grillo-Lopez AJ, Bodkin DJ, et al. IDEC-C2B8: results of a phase I multiple-dose trial in patients with relapsed non-Hodgkin's lymphoma. J Clin Oncol 1997;15(10):3266–74.
51. Byrd JC, Waselenko JK, Maneatis TJ, et al. Rituximab therapy in hematologic malignancy patients with circulating blood tumor cells: association with increased infusion-related side effects and rapid blood tumor clearance. J Clin Oncol 1999;17(3):791–5.
52. Dervite I, Hober D, Morel P. Acute hepatitis B in a patient with antibodies to hepatitis B surface antigen who was receiving rituximab. N Engl J Med 2001; 344(1):68–9.
53. Carson KR, Focosi D, Major EO, et al. Monoclonal antibody-associated progres-sive multifocal leucoencephalopathy in patients treated with rituximab, natalizu-mab, and efalizumab: a review from the Research on Adverse Drug Events and Reports (RADAR) Project. Lancet Oncol 2009;10(8):816–24.
54. Teeling JL, Mackus WJ, Wiegman LJ, et al. The biological activity of human CD20 monoclonal antibodies is linked to unique epitopes on CD20. J Immunol 2006; 177(1):362–71.
55. Teeling JL, French RR, Cragg MS, et al. Characterization of new human CD20 monoclonal antibodies with potent cytolytic activity against non-Hodgkin lymphomas. Blood 2004;104(6):1793–800.
56. Pawluczkowycz AW, Beurskens FJ, Beum PV, et al. Binding of submaximal C1q promotes complement-dependent cytotoxicity (CDC) of B cells opsonized with anti-CD20 mAbs ofatumumab (OFA) or rituximab (RTX): considerably higher levels of CDC are induced by OFA than by RTX. J Immunol 2009;183(1): 749–58.
57. Coiffier B, Lepretre S, Pedersen LM, et al. Safety and efficacy of ofatumumab, a fully human monoclonal anti-CD20 antibody, in patients with relapsed or refractory B-cell chronic lymphocytic leukemia: a phase 1-2 study. Blood 2008;111(3):1094–100.
58. Wierda WG, Kipps TJ, Mayer J, et al. Ofatumumab as single-agent CD20 immu-notherapy in fludarabine-refractory chronic lymphocytic leukemia. J Clin Oncol 2010;28(10):1749–55.
59. Wierda WG, Padmanabhan S, Chan GW, et al. Ofatumumab is active in patients with fludarabine-refractory CLL irrespective of prior rituximab: results from the phase 2 international study. Blood 2011;118(19):5126–9.
60. Flinn IW, Harwin WN, Macias-Perez IM, et al. A phase II trial of ofatumumab for older patients and patients who refuse fludarabine-based regimens with

previously untreated chronic lymphocytic leukemia or small lymphocytic lymphoma [abstracts]. Blood (ASH Annual Meeting Abstracts) 2011;118(21): 3912.

61. Wierda WG, Kipps TJ, Durig J, et al. Chemoimmunotherapy with O-FC in previously untreated patients with chronic lymphocytic leukemia. Blood 2011; 117(24):6450–8.

62. Falchi L, Keating MJ, Badoux XC, et al. Phase II trial of the combination of ofatumumab and lenalidomide in patients with relapsed chronic lymphocytic leukemia (CLL) [abstracts]. J Clin Onc (ASCO Annual Meeting Abstracts) 2012;30(15 Suppl):6516.

63. Shanafelt TD, Lanasa MC, Zent CS, et al. Ofatumumab based chemoimmunotherapy (CIT) for patients with previously untreated CLL [abstracts]. Blood (ASH Annual Meeting Abstracts) 2011;118(21):3898.

64. Teichman ML, Ho VQ, Balducci L, et al. Efficacy of ofatumumab and high-dose methylprednisolone for the treatment of relapsed or refractory chronic lymphocytic leukemia (CLL) [abstracts]. Blood (ASH Annual Meeting Abstracts) 2011;118(21):4619.

65. Ujjani CS, Gehan EA, Ramzi P, et al. Ofatumumab and bendamustine in previously treated CLL and SLL [abstracts]. Blood (ASH Annual Meeting Abstracts) 2011;118(21):4615.

66. Jaglowski SM, Jones JA, Flynn JM, et al. A phase Ib/II study evaluating activity and tolerability of BTK inhibitor PCI-32765 and ofatumumab in patients with chronic lymphocytic leukemia/small lymphocytic lymphoma (CLL/SLL) and related diseases [abstracts]. J Clin Onc (ASCO Annual Meeting Abstracts) 2012;30(15 Suppl):6508.

67. Furman RR, Barrientos JC, Sharman JP, et al. A phase I/II study of the selective phosphatidylinositol 3-kinase-delta (PI3K{delta}) inhibitor, GS-1101 (CAL-101), with ofatumumab in patients with previously treated chronic lymphocytic leukemia (CLL) [abstracts]. J Clin Onc (ASCO Annual Meeting Abstracts) 2012;30(15 Suppl):6518.

68. Ferrara C, Stuart F, Sondermann P, et al. The carbohydrate at FcgammaRIIIa Asn-162. An element required for high affinity binding to non-fucosylated IgG glycoforms. J Biol Chem 2006;281(8):5032–6.

69. Alduaij W, Ivanov A, Honeychurch J, et al. Novel type II anti-CD20 monoclonal antibody (GA101) evokes homotypic adhesion and actin-dependent, lysosome-mediated cell death in B-cell malignancies. Blood 2011;117(17): 4519–29.

70. Laurenti L, De Padua L, D'Arena G, et al. New and old monoclonal antibodies for the treatment of chronic lymphocytic leukemia. Mini Rev Med Chem 2011;11(6): 508–18.

71. Niederfellner GJ, Lammens A, Schwaiger M, et al. Crystal structure analysis reveals that the novel type ii anti-CD20 antibody GA101 interacts with a similar epitope as rituximab and ocrelizumab but in a fundamentally different way [abstracts]. Blood (ASH Annual Meeting Abstracts) 2009;114(22):3726.

72. Zenz T, Volden M, Mast T, et al. In vitro activity of the Type II anti-CD20 antibody GA101 in refractory, genetic high-risk CLL [abstracts]. Blood (ASH Annual Meeting Abstracts) 2009;114(22):2379.

73. Patz M, Forcob N, Muller B, et al. Depletion of chronic lymphocytic leukemia cells from whole blood samples mediated by the anti-CD20 antibodies rituximab and GA101 [abstracts]. Blood (ASH Annual Meeting Abstracts) 2009; 114(22):2365.

74. Mossner E, Brunker P, Moser S, et al. Increasing the efficacy of CD20 antibody therapy through the engineering of a new type II anti-CD20 antibody with enhanced direct and immune effector cell-mediated B-cell cytotoxicity. Blood 2010;115(22):4393–402.

75. Dalle S, Reslan L, Besseyre de Horts T, et al. Preclinical studies on the mechanism of action and the anti-lymphoma activity of the novel anti-CD20 antibody GA101. Mol Cancer Ther 2011;10(1):178–85.

76. Salles G, Morschhauser F, Lamy T, et al. Phase 1 study results of the type II glycoengineered humanized anti-CD20 monoclonal antibody obinutuzumab (GA101) in B-cell lymphoma patients. Blood 2012;119(22):5126–32.

77. Morschhauser F, Cartron G, Lamy T, et al. Phase I study of RO5072759 (GA101) in relapsed/refractory chronic lymphocytic leukemia [abstracts]. Blood (ASH Annual Meeting Abstracts) 2009;114(22):884.

78. Cartron G, Morschhauser F, Thieblemont C, et al. Results from a phase II study of obinutuzumab (GA101) monotherapy in relapsed/refractory chronic lymphocytic leukemia [abstract 0101]. Haematologica (EHA Annual Meeting Abstracts) 2011;96(2 Suppl):39–40.

79. Sehn LH, Assouline SE, Stewart DA, et al. A phase 1 study of obinutuzumab induction followed by 2 years of maintenance in patients with relapsed CD20-positive B-cell malignancies. Blood 2012;119(22):5118–25.

80. Goldenberg DM, Rossi EA, Stein R, et al. Properties and structure-function relationships of veltuzumab (hA20), a humanized anti-CD20 monoclonal antibody. Blood 2009;113(5):1062–70.

81. Negrea OG, Allen SL, Rai KR, et al. Subcutaneous injections of low doses of humanized anti-cd20 veltuzumab for treatment of indolent B-cell malignancies [abstracts]. Blood (ASH Annual Meeting Abstracts) 2009;114(22):3757.

82. Jain N, Wierda W, Ferrajoli A, et al. A phase 2 study of yttrium-90 ibritumomab tiuxetan (Zevalin) in patients with chronic lymphocytic leukemia. Cancer 2009; 115(19):4533–9.

83. Jacene HA, Filice R, Kasecamp W, et al. Comparison of ^{90}Y-ibritumomab tiuxetan and ^{131}I-tositumomab in clinical practice. J Nucl Med 2007;48(11):1767–76.

84. Robak T, Robak E. New anti-CD20 monoclonal antibodies for the treatment of B-cell lymphoid malignancies. BioDrugs 2011;25(1):13–25.

85. Rossmann ED, Lundin J, Lenkei R, et al. Variability in B-cell antigen expression: implications for the treatment of B-cell lymphomas and leukemias with monoclonal antibodies. Hematol J 2001;2(5):300–6.

86. Ginaldi L, De Martinis M, Matutes E, et al. Levels of expression of CD52 in normal and leukemic B and T cells: correlation with in vivo therapeutic responses to Campath-1H. Leuk Res 1998;22(2):185–91.

87. Crowe JS, Hall VS, Smith MA, et al. Humanized monoclonal antibody CAMPATH-1H: myeloma cell expression of genomic constructs, nucleotide sequence of cDNA constructs and comparison of effector mechanisms of myeloma and Chinese hamster ovary cell-derived material. Clin Exp Immunol 1992;87(1): 105–10.

88. Hale G, Clark M, Waldmann H. Therapeutic potential of rat monoclonal antibodies: isotype specificity of antibody-dependent cell-mediated cytotoxicity with human lymphocytes. J Immunol 1985;134(5):3056–61.

89. Mone AP, Cheney C, Banks AL, et al. Alemtuzumab induces caspase-independent cell death in human chronic lymphocytic leukemia cells through a lipid raft-dependent mechanism. Leukemia 2006;20(2):272–9.

90. Lozanski G, Heerema NA, Flinn IW, et al. Alemtuzumab is an effective therapy for chronic lymphocytic leukemia with p53 mutations and deletions. Blood 2004;103(9):3278–81.
91. Stilgenbauer S, Dohner H. Campath-1H-induced complete remission of chronic lymphocytic leukemia despite p53 gene mutation and resistance to chemotherapy. N Engl J Med 2002;347(6):452–3.
92. Keating MJ, Flinn I, Jain V, et al. Therapeutic role of alemtuzumab (Campath-1H) in patients who have failed fludarabine: results of a large international study. Blood 2002;99(10):3554–61.
93. Stilgenbauer S, Zenz T, Winkler D, et al. Subcutaneous alemtuzumab in fludarabine-refractory chronic lymphocytic leukemia: clinical results and prognostic marker analyses from the CLL2H study of the German Chronic Lymphocytic Leukemia Study Group. J Clin Oncol 2009;27(24):3994–4001.
94. Hillmen P, Skotnicki AB, Robak T, et al. Alemtuzumab compared with chlorambucil as first-line therapy for chronic lymphocytic leukemia. J Clin Oncol 2007; 25(35):5616–23.
95. Wendtner CM, Ritgen M, Schweighofer CD, et al. Consolidation with alemtuzumab in patients with chronic lymphocytic leukemia (CLL) in first remission—experience on safety and efficacy within a randomized multicenter phase III trial of the German CLL Study Group (GCLLSG). Leukemia 2004;18(6): 1093–101.
96. O'Brien SM, Kantarjian HM, Thomas DA, et al. Alemtuzumab as treatment for residual disease after chemotherapy in patients with chronic lymphocytic leukemia. Cancer 2003;98(12):2657–63.
97. Byrd JC, Peterson BL, Rai KR, et al. Fludarabine followed by alemtuzumab consolidation for previously untreated chronic lymphocytic leukemia: final report of Cancer and Leukemia Group B study 19901. Leuk Lymphoma 2009;50(10): 1589–96.
98. Lin TS, Donohue KA, Byrd JC, et al. Consolidation therapy with subcutaneous alemtuzumab after fludarabine and rituximab induction therapy for previously untreated chronic lymphocytic leukemia: final analysis of CALGB 10101. J Clin Oncol 2010;28(29):4500–6.
99. Hainsworth JD, Vazquez ER, Spigel DR, et al. Combination therapy with fludarabine and rituximab followed by alemtuzumab in the first-line treatment of patients with chronic lymphocytic leukemia or small lymphocytic lymphoma: a phase 2 trial of the Minnie Pearl Cancer Research Network. Cancer 2008; 112(6):1288–95.
100. Horejsi V, Vlcek C. Novel structurally distinct family of leucocyte surface glycoproteins including CD9, CD37, CD53 and CD63. FEBS Lett 1991;288(1–2): 1–4.
101. Wright MD, Tomlinson MG. The ins and outs of the transmembrane 4 superfamily. Immunol Today 1994;15(12):588–94.
102. Schwartz-Albiez R, Dorken B, Hofmann W, et al. The B cell-associated CD37 antigen (gp40-52). Structure and subcellular expression of an extensively glycosylated glycoprotein. J Immunol 1988;140(3):905–14.
103. van Spriel AB, Puls KL, Sofi M, et al. A regulatory role for CD37 in T cell proliferation. J Immunol 2004;172(5):2953–61.
104. Zhao X, Lapalombella R, Joshi T, et al. Targeting CD37-positive lymphoid malignancies with a novel engineered small modular immunopharmaceutical. Blood 2007;110(7):2569–77.

105. Lapalombella R, Yeh YY, Wang L, et al. Tetraspanin CD37 directly mediates transduction of survival and apoptotic signals. Cancer Cell 2012;21(5): 694–708.

106. Furman RR, Andritsos L, Flinn IW, et al. Phase 1 dose escalation study of TRU-016, an anti-CD37 SMIPTM protein in relapsed and refractory CLL [abstracts]. Blood (ASH Annual Meeting Abstracts) 2010;116(21):56.

107. Awan FT, Pagel JM, Andritsos LA, et al. Phase 1 study of Tru-016, an anti-CD37 SMIP™ protein in naive and relapsed and/or refractory CLL patients [abstracts]. Blood (ASH Annual Meeting Abstracts) 2011;118(21):1792.

108. Krause G, Patz M, Isaeva P, et al. Action of novel CD37 antibodies on chronic lymphocytic leukemia cells. Leukemia 2012;26(3):546–9.

109. Deckert J, Chicklas S, Yi Y, et al. Potent B-cell depletion by IMGN529, a CD37-targeting antibody-maytansinoid conjugate for the treatment of B-Cell malignancies [abstracts]. Blood (ASH Annual Meeting Abstracts) 2011;118(21):3726.

110. Law CL, Gordon KA, Collier J, et al. Preclinical antilymphoma activity of a humanized anti-CD40 monoclonal antibody, SGN-40. Cancer Res 2005;65(18): 8331–8.

111. Damle RN, Ghiotto F, Valetto A, et al. B-cell chronic lymphocytic leukemia cells express a surface membrane phenotype of activated, antigen-experienced B lymphocytes. Blood 2002;99(11):4087–93.

112. Clayton E, Bardi G, Bell SE, et al. A crucial role for the p110delta subunit of phosphatidylinositol 3-kinase in B cell development and activation. J Exp Med 2002;196(6):753–63.

113. Cuni S, Perez-Aciego P, Perez-Chacon G, et al. A sustained activation of PI3K/NF-kappaB pathway is critical for the survival of chronic lymphocytic leukemia B cells. Leukemia 2004;18(8):1391–400.

114. Furman RR, Asgary Z, Mascarenhas JO, et al. Modulation of NF-kappa B activity and apoptosis in chronic lymphocytic leukemia B cells. J Immunol 2000;164(4): 2200–6.

115. Romano MF, Lamberti A, Tassone P, et al. Triggering of CD40 antigen inhibits fludarabine-induced apoptosis in B chronic lymphocytic leukemia cells. Blood 1998;92(3):990–5.

116. Lapalombella R, Gowda A, Joshi T, et al. The humanized CD40 antibody SGN-40 demonstrates pre-clinical activity that is enhanced by lenalidomide in chronic lymphocytic leukaemia. Br J Haematol 2009;144(6):848–55.

117. Furman RR, Forero-Torres A, Shustov A, et al. A phase I study of dacetuzumab (SGN-40, a humanized anti-CD40 monoclonal antibody) in patients with chronic lymphocytic leukemia. Leuk Lymphoma 2010;51(2):228–35.

118. Andritsos LA, Johnson AJ, Lozanski G, et al. Higher doses of lenalidomide are associated with unacceptable toxicity including life-threatening tumor flare in patients with chronic lymphocytic leukemia. J Clin Oncol 2008;26(15): 2519–25.

119. Luqman M, Klabunde S, Lin K, et al. The antileukemia activity of a human anti-CD40 antagonist antibody, HCD122, on human chronic lymphocytic leukemia cells. Blood 2008;112(3):711–20.

120. Byrd JC, Kipps TJ, Flinn IW, et al. Phase I study of the anti-CD40 humanized monoclonal antibody lucatumumab (HCD122) in relapsed chronic lymphocytic leukemia. Leuk Lymphoma 2012;53(11):2136–42.

121. Fujimoto M, Poe JC, Hasegawa M, et al. CD19 regulates intrinsic B lymphocyte signal transduction and activation through a novel mechanism of processive amplification. Immunol Res 2000;22(2–3):281–98.

122. Horton HM, Bernett MJ, Pong E, et al. Potent in vitro and in vivo activity of an Fc-engineered anti-CD19 monoclonal antibody against lymphoma and leukemia. Cancer Res 2008;68(19):8049–57.

123. Awan FT, Lapalombella R, Trotta R, et al. CD19 targeting of chronic lymphocytic leukemia with a novel Fc-domain-engineered monoclonal antibody. Blood 2010; 115(6):1204–13.

124. Zalevsky J, Leung IW, Karki S, et al. The impact of Fc engineering on an anti-CD19 antibody: increased Fcgamma receptor affinity enhances B-cell clearing in nonhuman primates. Blood 2009;113(16):3735–43.

125. Cardarelli PM, Rao-Naik C, Chen S, et al. A nonfucosylated human antibody to CD19 with potent B-cell depletive activity for therapy of B-cell malignancies. Cancer Immunol Immunother 2010;59(2):257–65.

126. Camacho LH, Joyce R, Brown JR, et al. A phase 1, open-label, multi-center, multiple-dose, dose-escalation study of MDX-1342 in patients with CD19-positive refractory/relapsed chronic lymphocytic leukemia [abstracts]. Blood (ASH Annual Meeting Abstracts) 2009;114(22):3425.

127. Stein R, Gupta P, Chen X, et al. Therapy of B-cell malignancies by anti-HLA-DR humanized monoclonal antibody, IMMU-114, is mediated through hyperactivation of ERK and JNK MAP kinase signaling pathways. Blood 2010;115(25): 5180–90.

128. Mone AP, Huang P, Pelicano H, et al. Hu1D10 induces apoptosis concurrent with activation of the AKT survival pathway in human chronic lymphocytic leukemia cells. Blood 2004;103(5):1846–54.

129. Stein R, Qu Z, Chen S, et al. Characterization of a humanized IgG4 anti-HLA-DR monoclonal antibody that lacks effector cell functions but retains direct antilymphoma activity and increases the potency of rituximab. Blood 2006;108(8): 2736–44.

130. Lin TS, Stock W, Xu H, et al. A phase I/II dose escalation study of apolizumab (Hu1D10) using a stepped-up dosing schedule in patients with chronic lymphocytic leukemia and acute leukemia. Leuk Lymphoma 2009;50(12):1958–63.

Phosphoinositide 3'-Kinase Inhibition in Chronic Lymphocytic Leukemia

Matthew S. Davids, MD, Jennifer R. Brown, MD, PhD*

KEYWORDS

- Lymphoid leukemia • Signaling therapies • Phosphoinositide 3'-kinase
- B-cell receptor

KEY POINTS

- Phosphoinositide 3'-kinase (PI3K) is a key node in B-cell receptor (BCR) signaling.
- The biology of PI3K signaling provides a strong rationale for targeting this kinase in CLL.
- Delta-isoform inhibitors such as GS1101 (formerly CAL-101), pan-PI3K inhibitors such as SAR245408 (S08), and dual pan-PI3K/mTOR inhibitors such as SAR245409 (S09) are all in development.
- Early-phase clinical trials have found these agents to be highly active and well tolerated.
- ZAP-70, *IGHV*, and CCL3 are all potential biomarkers for response to PI3K inhibitors.
- The place of PI3K inhibitors in the landscape of CLL therapy is evolving.

INTRODUCTION

Although chronic lymphocytic leukemia (CLL) usually responds well to initial chemotherapy, the disease inevitably relapses, and remains incurable by conventional therapy.[1] It has been hypothesized that after treatment, sanctuary sites such as the lymph nodes and bone marrow may harbor residual CLL cells that can later lead to relapse.[2] Indeed, the protective role of the CLL microenvironment may be a key to understanding why stroma-exposed CLL cells are protected from undergoing apoptosis in response to treatment. The B-cell receptor (BCR) pathway has been particularly identified as a key mediator of prosurvival signals in CLL cells.[3] Several novel kinase inhibitors are now in development to target various components of the BCR pathway.[4–7] A class effect of these BCR inhibitors is a "lymphocyte redistribution" phenomenon, whereby a majority of patients initially develop a transient

Department of Medical Oncology, Dana-Farber Cancer Institute, CLL Center, Harvard Medical School, 450 Brookline Avenue, Boston, MA 02215, USA
* Corresponding author. Dana-Farber Cancer Institute, CLL Center, Harvard Medical School, 450 Brookline Avenue, M232, Boston, MA 02215.
E-mail address: Jennifer_Brown@dfci.harvard.edu

Hematol Oncol Clin N Am 27 (2013) 329–339
http://dx.doi.org/10.1016/j.hoc.2012.12.002
0889-8588/13/$ – see front matter © 2013 Elsevier Inc. All rights reserved.

lymphocytosis while simultaneously achieving nodal reduction. This observation has led to the hypothesis that these agents may achieve their efficacy, at least in part, by mobilizing CLL cells out of sanctuary sites and into the peripheral blood, where they more readily die or can be killed by combination therapy.

Of the new agents targeting the BCR pathway, phosphoinositide 3′-kinase (PI3K) inhibitors are among the most promising. This article reviews the scientific rationale underlying PI3K inhibition in CLL, as well as data from recent and ongoing clinical trials of PI3K inhibitors in CLL. Also discussed are potential biological predictive markers for PI3K clinical response, as well as where PI3K inhibitors may fit into the evolving landscape of CLL therapy.

BIOLOGY OF PI3K IN CLL

Signaling cascades from several major pathways converge on PI3K, which serves as a key node regulating B-cell function and survival. Although there are 3 classes of PI3K isoforms, only class I isoforms are thought to be directly related to oncogenesis.[8] Within class I, PI3K isoforms can be further subdivided into class IA (PI3K-α, -β, and -δ) and class IB (PI3K-γ).[9] Although having shown that activating mutations in PI3K are very rare in CLL, we did identify amplification of *PIK3CA* in about 3.5% of CLL.[10,11] Furthermore, even in the absence of genetic activation, CLL cells generally express high levels of active PI3K (in particular the δ isoform[12]), and great interest has therefore focused on elucidating the role played by PI3K in the pathogenesis of the disease.

The 3 best characterized pathways that activate PI3K include the BCR, receptor tyrosine kinases (RTKs), and cytokine/chemokine receptors (**Fig. 1**). Of these, the BCR pathway is thought to play a dominant role in CLL. The BCR usually becomes activated in the presence of antigen (although tonic signaling has also been described[13]). Activated BCR recruits other kinases such as spleen tyrosine kinase (Syk) and Lyn kinase, which phosphorylate immunoreceptor tyrosine–based activation motifs (ITAMs) on the cytoplasmic immunoglobulin domains of the receptor.[14] Stimulated RTKs, cytokine, and chemokine receptors also cause autophosphorylation of the tyrosine residue on the ITAMs and subsequent PI3K activation in immune cells,[15] although the importance of these pathways in CLL is variable.

Stimulation of each of these 3 pathways sets off a chain of downstream molecular interactions, the net result of which is to create Src homology 2 (SH2)-binding domains capable of binding the p85 regulatory subunit of PI3K.[16] Once this binding occurs, p85 can no longer inhibit the p110 catalytic domain of PI3K, thereby leading to PI3K activation. One of the primary functions of activated PI3K in B cells is to convert phosphatidylinositol-3,4-biphosphate into phosphatidylinositol-3,4,5-triphosphate, leading to AKT phosphorylation, which then can go on to activate a wide variety of downstream kinases.[17] In addition to AKT, activated PI3K also promotes calcium mobilization and activation of other downstream kinases such as protein kinase C (PKC)-β, mammalian target of rapamycin (mTOR), and MAP kinase (ERK). These events promote increased proliferation of B cells, largely mediated by the upregulation of transcription factors such as nuclear factor κB (NF-κB) and nuclear factor of activated T cells (NFAT).[18]

Although substantial evidence indicates that PI3K activation inhibits both the extrinsic and intrinsic pathways of apoptosis, the precise mechanism of these interactions remains incompletely understood. Activated AKT likely interferes with FasL expression, thereby decreasing levels of this primary mediator of extrinsic apoptosis.[19] Activated AKT has also been hypothesized to affect the intrinsic mitochondrial

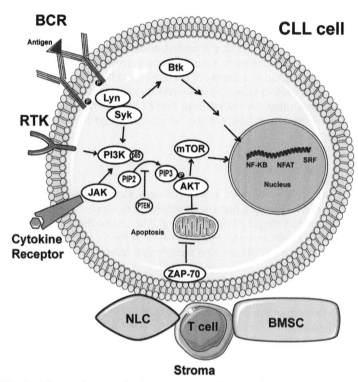

Fig. 1. PI3K signaling and molecular interactions in the CLL cell. Three important pathways converge on PI3K signaling, including the B-cell receptor (BCR), thought to be the dominant pathway in CLL, as well as receptor tyrosine kinases (RTKs) and cytokine/chemokine receptors. The BCR usually becomes activated in the presence of antigen (although tonic signaling has also been described). Activated BCR recruits other kinases such as spleen tyrosine kinase (Syk) and Lyn kinase, which phosphorylate immunoreceptor tyrosine–based activation motifs (ITAMs) on the cytoplasmic immunoglobulin domains of the receptor. RTKs can be stimulated by a variety of ligands, and also lead to autophosphorylation of the tyrosine residue on the ITAM. Stimulated cytokine and chemokine receptors can activate Janus-activated kinase (JAK) tyrosine kinases, which phosphorylate tyrosine residues in proteins such as gp130 and inflammatory response system (IRS) family members. These tyrosine-phosphorylated proteins interact with SH2 domains of the p85 subunit of PI3K, thereby activating the p110 kinase activity, which is normally inhibited in the p85-p110 complex. This activation results in the conversion of phosphatidylinositol-4,5-biphosphate (PIP2) to phosphatidylinositol-3,4,5-triphosphate (PIP3), which has several downstream effects, many of which are mediated by AKT. The net result of PI3K activation is to promote CLL cell survival and proliferation, largely through activation of nuclear transcription factors such as nuclear factor κB, nuclear factor of activated T cells (NFAT), and serum response factor (SRF). These effects can be modulated by nearby stromal cells including T cells, nurse-like cells (NLC), and bone marrow stromal cells (BMSC). mTOR, mammalian target of rapamycin; PTEN, phosphatase and tensin homolog.

pathway of apoptosis by increasing the amount of the proapoptotic protein BAD that is sequestered by 14-3-3, a regulatory protein that by binding BAD limits its ability to promote apoptosis, thereby pushing the cell farther from the threshold of apoptosis (ie, decreasing "priming" for apoptosis).[20] Other interactions between AKT and the mitochondrial pathway of apoptosis are likely, and this remains an active area of investigation.

Beyond its direct effects on promoting B-cell proliferation and inhibiting apoptosis, activated PI3K also has a profound influence on B-cell trafficking by promoting CLL cell chemotaxis toward CXCL12/13, migration beneath stromal cells, and upregulation of CLL cell chemokine secretion.[21] Once CLL cells enter the stromal microenvironment, they become bathed in a variety of protective mediators such as CD40L, fibronectin, and B-cell activating factor, all of which likely send prosurvival signals through PI3K. We have shown that the net effect of these stromal interactions is to decrease CLL cell mitochondrial apoptotic priming, which may lead to resistance to a wide variety of therapies.[22]

INHIBITION OF PI3K IN CLL

Given the key role that PI3K plays in CLL pathophysiology, the potential efficacy of small-molecule PI3K inhibitors has been widely recognized. Several different PI3K inhibitors are in various stages of development, and can be divided into 2 main categories: δ-isoform specific and pan-PI3K inhibitors. A third category of dual inhibitors targeting both PI3K and mTOR are also being investigated.

PI3K-δ Inhibition

Preclinical

Because the δ isoform of the p110 catalytic subunit of PI3K is the predominant form expressed in leukocytes,[23] a δ-isoform–specific PI3K inhibitor was the first logical target to pursue and is currently the furthest along in clinical development. GS1101 (formerly CAL-101) is a small molecule that specifically and potently inhibits the δ isoform of PI3K.[6] The drug has been shown to induce apoptosis in primary CLL cells ex vivo in a time-dependent and dose-dependent manner.[12] In vitro, GS1101 partially reverses the chemoresistance observed in stroma-exposed CLL cells and also reduces CLL cell chemotaxis into stroma.[22,24] Of importance, GS1101 alone can induce a modest degree of apoptosis even in the presence of stroma.[21,22]

Given its ability to release CLL cells from protective stroma niches, in vitro studies have been performed to determine which drugs might best complement the activity of GS1101 by blocking other pathways that contribute to CLL cell survival. The drug does appear to have at least additive effects in killing when combined with commonly used CLL chemotherapies such as fludarabine and bendamustine.[21]

Recent preclinical work has focused on developing rational combinations of GS1101 by utilizing agents with complementary but targeted mechanisms of action. One such approach combined pharmacologic inhibition of PI3K-δ with lenalidomide, an immunomodulatory agent known to induce tumor flare at low doses and to have modest clinical activity in patients with relapsed refractory CLL.[25] Pharmacologic inhibition (or siRNA knockdown) of PI3K-δ was found to abrogate CLL cell activation and to reduce costimulatory molecule expression, as well as gene expression of vascular endothelial growth factor and basic fibroblast growth factor, which are thought to contribute to CLL survival in stroma.[26,27] These findings suggest that combining GS1101 with lenalidomide might limit tumor flare and potentially augment the clinical activity of lenalidomide in patients with CLL.

We studied another approach of combining GS1101 with the BH3-mimetic drug ABT-737 to increase apoptotic killing of stroma-exposed CLL cells.[22] In vitro, stroma-exposed CLL cells were highly resistant to ABT-737 and only underwent modest levels of apoptotic killing with GS1101 alone. The combination of GS1101 and ABT-737 led to rapid and significant CLL cell killing. GS1101 was also shown to lead to release of CLL cells from stroma, thereby increasing the level of CLL cell apoptotic priming, which may have accounted for their increased susceptibility to killing by BH3 mimetics. Ongoing investigation is needed to confirm whether these observations hold true in the clinic.

Clinical

GS1101 (formerly CAL-101) GS1101 was first evaluated in a large phase I study of approximately 190 patients with relapsed refractory hematologic malignancies.[28] The CLL subjects in this study (n = 55) were heavily pretreated (median 5 prior therapies) and the majority (82%) had bulky lymphadenopathy. The most common symptomatic adverse event was grade 3 or higher pneumonia in 24% of patients. Grade 3 or higher hematological laboratory abnormalities included neutropenia (24%), thrombocytopenia (11%), and anemia (8%), which in most cases were not considered GS1101 related. Nodal partial response was seen in greater than 80% of patients, but the overall response rate was a modest 24% owing to the fact that more than half of the patients had an early, transient elevation in lymphocyte count thought to be related to mobilization of lymphocytes out of stroma. This redistribution lymphocytosis was associated with nodal response and did not represent disease progression, but it did preclude many patients from meeting the International Workshop on CLL (iwCLL) response criteria.[29] Patients did not appear to have any ill effects from persistent lymphocytosis. High-risk patients such as those with del(17p), at least initially, had clinical benefit similar to those with standard-risk disease. The median progression-free survival reported thus far is 16 months, and 21 patients remain under study after 1 year with continued benefit, suggesting that responses to GS1101 can be durable. Given the important role that chemokines such as CCL3, CCL4, and CXCL13 play in the CLL microenvironment, it was notable that patients on GS1101 in this study experienced a rapid decline in plasma concentrations of these chemokines.[21] In addition, constitutive phosphorylation at AKT T308 was observed at baseline and was completely abrogated by GS1101. Both of these observations suggest pharmacodynamic inhibition of activated PI3K signaling.

GS1101 has substantial single agent-activity, but the effect of the drug in mobilizing CLL cells from stroma also makes it a natural partner for combination studies, several of which are now under way. Initial data from a phase I study of GS1101 in combination with rituximab or bendamustine in patients with relapsed refractory CLL were recently presented.[30] These combinations have been well tolerated and have shown an impressive overall response rate of greater than 75% (by iwCLL criteria) in the initial 27 patients under study. Lymphocyte redistribution has been less apparent, particularly with bendamustine, likely because mobilized CLL cells are killed rapidly. Registration studies for GS1101 are now under way, and other novel combinations with chemotherapy, antibodies, or other small-molecule inhibitors will also be explored in both the front-line and relapsed settings.

Pan-PI3K Inhibition

Like PI3Kδ, the other class IA PI3K isoforms p110-α and p110-β as well as the class IB isoform p110-γ, are also expressed in leukocytes, including CLL cells; however, because of their widespread expression in other cell types, pan-PI3K inhibitors were expected to have too much toxicity to move forward into the clinic. Early animal data did suggest important potential toxicities including hyperglycemia caused by inhibition of PI3K-α in the β-islet cells of the pancreas.[31] However, the introduction of pan-PI3K inhibitors into clinical trials in solid tumors demonstrated that these compounds were relatively well tolerated,[32] and raised the possibility of exploring their use in CLL.

We recently showed through an integrative genomic analysis that not only is PI3K-α expressed in CLL cells, but some CLL patients may also have amplification of the *PI3KCA* gene that leads to enrichment of the α subunit in their CLL cells.[11] α-Subunit enrichment in this subset of CLL patients could theoretically render their disease resistant to a δ-isoform–specific inhibitor. Furthermore, upregulation of alternative PI3K isoforms while on treatment with a PI3Kδ-specific inhibitor would be one possible way for patients to acquire drug resistance over time. These considerations raise the possibility that a pan-PI3K inhibitor may even have activity superior to that of a δ-isoform inhibitor.

Moreover, p110-γ is known to be the predominant PI3K isoform expressed in T cells. For example, p110-γ isoform knockout mice have an isolated T-cell defect that, while not embryonically lethal, does confer significant immune dysfunction.[33] Given the critical role played by T cells in providing prosurvival signals to CLL cells in the microenvironment, p110-γ isoform inhibition may significantly disrupt the CLL microenvironment, thereby facilitating CLL cell death.

Clinical

SAR245408 (S08) SAR245408 (S08) is a class I pan-PI3K inhibitor that was previously found to be well tolerated in patients with solid tumors.[32] This initial study of 68 patients with solid tumors found a dose-limiting toxicity (DLT) of grade 3 rash (4%) when dosing was scheduled on days 1 to 21 in 28-day cycles. When the schedule was switched to continuous daily dosing, no further DLTs were observed. SAR245408 (S08) was found to inhibit both the PI3K and ERK signaling pathways, suggesting that the drug was pharmacodynamically active. An arm focused on relapsed CLL and lymphoma was added to this study, and 25 patients in total were enrolled. At the first report, of 7 CLL/SLL patients, 5 were evaluable. In these 5 patients with refractory CLL, SAR245408 (S08) was well tolerated.[34] Although none of the 5 patients met formal iwCLL criteria for response, 3 patients (60%) benefited from a nodal partial response with transient lymphocytosis and remained on treatment at 12 to 18 months' follow-up. Although these early results in CLL have been promising, the availability of SAR245408 (S08) for clinical trials is currently limited because of a change in the drug formulation.

Dual PI3K/mTOR Inhibition

Preclinical

CLL cells may also develop resistance to a δ-isoform–specific PI3K inhibitor through activation of the RAS/MEK/ERK pathway, which eventually leads to mTOR activation.[35] The disappointing activity of mTOR inhibitors as monotherapy in CLL[5] has raised the question of whether PI3K preferentially activates alternative downstream messengers such as NF-κB or PKC-β, thereby leading to resistance to mTOR inhibition. A drug able to inhibit both PI3K and mTOR would have the potential to overcome this type of resistance mechanism. Furthermore, because PI3K inhibitors directly induce apoptosis in CLL cells, and mTOR inhibitors primarily cause induction of growth arrest, these complementary mechanisms of action further justify the potential utility of such a combined blockade approach. Therefore, a dual pan-PI3K/mTOR inhibitor has the potential to be highly active in CLL.

Clinical

SAR245409 (S09) SAR245509 (S09) is a small-molecule dual PI3K/mTOR inhibitor currently being evaluated in clinical trials, which although primarily a pan-PI3K inhibitor, does have some activity against mTOR. In a PTEN-deficient mantle-cell lymphoma cell line, the drug inhibited PI3K and ERK, and led to a marked decrease in proliferation markers such as Ki-67.[36] SAR245509 (S09) was relatively well tolerated in a phase I dose-escalation study of patients with advanced solid tumors.[37] A phase I dose-expansion cohort of 16 patients with non-Hodgkin lymphoma found the most common related adverse events to be nausea (25%), elevated liver enzymes (18.8%), and diarrhea (12.5%). Two patients with mantle-cell lymphoma remained on study with clinical benefit for over 1 year.[36] The drug is therefore now being explored at the recommended phase II dose of 50 mg twice daily in a large, multicenter phase II study in patients with CLL, follicular, and mantle-cell lymphomas. A phase I study of SAR245509 (S09) in combination with bendamustine and/or rituximab in the same patient population is also under way.

PREDICTING RESPONSE TO PI3K INHIBITION

Nodal response rates have been high in the early trials of GS1101, yet a substantial minority of patients either does not respond or progresses relatively shortly after starting on therapy. Therefore, in parallel with ongoing clinical trials of PI3K inhibitors are efforts to develop predictive biomarkers for response to these drugs. Both conventional CLL prognostic markers (such as ZAP-70 and immunoglobulin heavy chain [*IGHV*] status) and novel biomarkers are currently being evaluated.

ZAP-70 is a cytoplasmic tyrosine kinase, normally associated with the T-cell receptor, which is aberrantly upregulated in the malignant B cells of a subset of patients with CLL.[38] ZAP-70 positivity (defined as >20% expression) is associated with activation of the BCR pathway, unmutated *IGHV* status, and clinically more aggressive CLL. ZAP-70 may also increase CLL cell responsiveness to the chemokines CCL19, CCL21, and CXCL12, thereby leading to increased CLL cell motility.[39] Given these observations that increased ZAP-70 expression is associated with signaling through the BCR pathway, it will be interesting to see whether PI3K inhibitors will be more effective in patients with ZAP-70 positive CLL.

Unmutated *IGHV* status predicts a shorter time to first treatment and overall worse prognosis compared with mutated *IGHV* status.[40] Preclinical data have suggested that mutation status may serve as a biomarker of response to PI3K inhibition. In response to immunoglobulin M–mediated BCR stimulation in vitro, functional gene groups including signal transduction, transcription, cell-cycle regulation, and cytoskeletal organization were all upregulated in unmutated but not mutated CLL cases.[41] Furthermore, *IGHV* unmutated CLL cells cultured ex vivo are more prone to spontaneous apoptosis and are more dependent on stromal prosurvival signals from cell-to-cell contact and soluble factors in comparison with mutated CLL cells.[42] We have also shown that *IGHV* unmutated CLL cells have increased levels of mitochondrial apoptotic priming when compared with their mutated counterparts.[22] All of these observations suggest that patients with unmutated *IGHV* would benefit preferentially from PI3K inhibitors in comparison with mutated patients, and detailed reports from the clinical trials of PI3K inhibitors should demonstrate whether this is true.

Novel biomarkers of response to PI3K inhibition are also in development. Of these the leading candidate is CCL3, a chemokine produced by both normal and malignant lymphocytes that acts through the chemokine receptors CCR1 and CCR5 as a chemoattractant for other lymphocytes and adaptive immune cells.[43] When the BCR pathway is activated, CCL3 is secreted in high levels by CLL cells,[44] particularly in lymph node–derived CLL,[45] suggesting that stroma enhances CCL3 expression. Based on these observations, agents that target the BCR pathway and disrupt stromal support signals should theoretically lead to decreased CCL3 levels. Indeed,

PI3K-δ inhibition[21] has been shown to decrease CLL cell secretion of CCL3 in a nurse-like cell model in vitro. Moreover, patients treated with GS1101 were found to normalize their CCL3 levels in the peripheral blood after 28 days.[21] These preclinical and clinical findings make CCL3 a promising predictive biomarker for PI3K inhibitors; however, it should be noted that because nearly all patients normalized CCL3 levels, it is not clear that CCL3 level alone will be predictive of clinical response. In addition to measurement of CCL3, future trials will also incorporate evaluations of genetic biomarkers, such as the novel mutations SF3B1, NOTCH1, MYD88, and others recently described in CLL.[10,46,47]

It is hoped that utility of both conventional and novel biomarkers will help to optimize the use of PI3K inhibitors by targeting the use of these agents to those patients who will benefit most. Using these agents in high-risk CLL patients who typically have short-lived responses to chemotherapy, especially those who are ZAP-70 positive and IGHV unmutated, may potentially represent an important therapeutic advance in CLL.

SUMMARY

An improved understanding of the key molecular pathways fueling the survival and growth of CLL cells is an important advance that heralds the development of selective, well-tolerated, and effective therapies. PI3K, within the BCR pathway, is a key node being targeted. The unique pattern of nodal response with redistribution lymphocytosis observed with BCR pathway inhibitors, including PI3K inhibitors, may serve as a pharmacodynamic marker and also facilitate potent combination therapies. Given that the iwCLL 2008 response criteria were devised before the lymphocyte redistribution effect of BCR pathway antagonists became known, the currently reported formal response rates for these agents underestimate their clinical benefit. For this reason, leading investigators have proposed modifying the traditional response criteria to recognize the benefits patients derive from nodal response in the presence of persistent lymphocytosis.[48] Given the significant toxicities associated with modern chemoimmunotherapy regimens, the approval of BCR pathway–targeted agents such as PI3K inhibitors would represent a new therapeutic paradigm. If PI3K inhibitors could be used either as monotherapy or in combination with other novel agents to achieve long-term disease remission without the toxicity and inconvenience of chemotherapy, this would provide significant benefit for CLL patients, particularly for those unable to tolerate chemoimmunotherapy, such as older patients or those with comorbidities.

Despite the excitement surrounding these new agents, several important questions need to be addressed in future studies. For example, which approach to PI3K inhibition will strike the best balance between efficacy and toxicity: δ-isoform selective or pan-PI3K inhibitors? Why are certain patients resistant to PI3K inhibitors at baseline, and which resistance mechanisms will evolve in patients who initially respond to treatment? How durable will the responses observed in early-phase trials turn out to be? Will PI3K inhibitors be effective enough as monotherapy or in combination with antibodies to obviate chemotherapy in CLL, or will they need to be combined with chemotherapy to achieve a durable effect? Is there a role for PI3K inhibitors as maintenance in the post-chemoimmunotherapy or post–allogeneic stem cell transplantation setting?

These challenging but important questions will need to be answered with carefully constructed clinical trials. Equally essential to the successful future development of PI3K inhibitors will be the correlative studies embedded within these trials, which will help us learn how best to combine novel agents, and what mechanisms of resistance may arise. PI3K inhibitors are one of several exciting new approaches to the treatment of CLL. Moving forward, the expected approval of such targeted therapies will be a major advance for patients with CLL.

REFERENCES

1. Chiorazzi N, Rai KR, Ferrarini M. Chronic lymphocytic leukemia. N Engl J Med 2005;352(8):804–15.
2. Burger JA, Ghia P, Rosenwald A, et al. The microenvironment in mature B-cell malignancies: a target for new treatment strategies. Blood 2009;114(16): 3367–75.
3. Stevenson FK, Caligaris-Cappio F. Chronic lymphocytic leukemia: revelations from the B-cell receptor. Blood 2004;103(12):4389–95.
4. Friedberg JW, Sharman J, Sweetenham J, et al. Inhibition of Syk with fostamatinib disodium has significant clinical activity in non-Hodgkin lymphoma and chronic lymphocytic leukemia. Blood 2010;115(13):2578–85.
5. Zent CS, LaPlant BR, Johnston PB, et al. The treatment of recurrent/refractory chronic lymphocytic leukemia/small lymphocytic lymphoma (CLL) with everolimus results in clinical responses and mobilization of CLL cells into the circulation. Cancer 2010;116(9):2201–7.
6. Lannutti BJ, Meadows SA, Herman SE, et al. CAL-101, a p110delta selective phosphatidylinositol-3-kinase inhibitor for the treatment of B-cell malignancies, inhibits PI3K signaling and cellular viability. Blood 2011;117(2):591–4.
7. Honigberg LA, Smith AM, Sirisawad M, et al. The Bruton tyrosine kinase inhibitor PCI-32765 blocks B-cell activation and is efficacious in models of autoimmune disease and B-cell malignancy. Proc Natl Acad Sci U S A 2010;107(29): 13075–80.
8. Hawkins PT, Anderson KE, Davidson K, et al. Signalling through Class I PI3Ks in mammalian cells. Biochem Soc Trans 2006;34(Pt 5):647–62.
9. Vanhaesebroeck B, Ali K, Bilancio A, et al. Signalling by PI3K isoforms: insights from gene-targeted mice. Trends Biochem Sci 2005;30(4):194–204.
10. Wang L, Lawrence MS, Wan Y, et al. SF3B1 and other novel cancer genes in chronic lymphocytic leukemia. N Engl J Med 2011;365(26):2497–506.
11. Brown JR, Hanna M, Tesar B, et al. Integrative genomic analysis implicates gain of PIK3CA at 3q26 and MYC at 8q24 in chronic lymphocytic leukemia. Clin Cancer Res 2012;18(14):3791–802.
12. Herman SE, Gordon AL, Wagner AJ, et al. Phosphatidylinositol 3-kinase-delta inhibitor CAL-101 shows promising preclinical activity in chronic lymphocytic leukemia by antagonizing intrinsic and extrinsic cellular survival signals. Blood 2010;116(12):2078–88.
13. Monroe JG. ITAM-mediated tonic signalling through pre-BCR and BCR complexes. Nat Rev Immunol 2006;6(4):283–94.
14. Reth M. Antigen receptors on B lymphocytes. Annu Rev Immunol 1992;10: 97–121.
15. Koyasu S. The role of PI3K in immune cells. Nat Immunol 2003;4(4):313–9.
16. Chantry D, Vojtek A, Kashishian A, et al. p110δ, a novel phosphatidylinositol 3-kinase catalytic subunit that associates with p85 and is expressed predominantly in leukocytes. J Biol Chem 1997;272(31):19236–41.
17. So L, Fruman DA. PI3K signalling in B- and T-lymphocytes: new developments and therapeutic advances. Biochem J 2012;442(3):465–81.

18. Shinohara H, Kurosaki T. Comprehending the complex connection between PKCbeta, TAK1, and IKK in BCR signaling. Immunol Rev 2009;232(1): 300–18.

19. Uriarte SM, Joshi-Barve S, Song Z, et al. Akt inhibition upregulates FasL, down-regulates c-FLIPs and induces caspase-8-dependent cell death in Jurkat T lymphocytes. Cell Death Differ 2005;12(3):233–42.

20. She QB, Solit DB, Ye Q, et al. The BAD protein integrates survival signaling by EGFR/MAPK and PI3K/Akt kinase pathways in PTEN-deficient tumor cells. Cancer Cell 2005;8(4):287–97.

21. Hoellenriegel J, Meadows SA, Sivina M, et al. The phosphoinositide 3′-kinase delta inhibitor, CAL-101, inhibits B-cell receptor signaling and chemokine networks in chronic lymphocytic leukemia. Blood 2011;118(13):3603–12.

22. Davids MS, Deng J, Wiestner A, et al. Decreased mitochondrial apoptotic priming underlies stroma-mediated treatment resistance in chronic lymphocytic leukemia. Blood 2012;120:3501–9.

23. Vanhaesebroeck B, Welham MJ, Kotani K, et al. P110delta, a novel phosphoinositide 3-kinase in leukocytes. Proc Natl Acad Sci U S A 1997;94(9):4330–5.

24. Niedermeier M, Hennessy BT, Knight ZA, et al. Isoform-selective phosphoinositide 3′-kinase inhibitors inhibit CXCR4 signaling and overcome stromal cell-mediated drug resistance in chronic lymphocytic leukemia: a novel therapeutic approach. Blood 2009;113(22):5549–57.

25. Herman SE, Lapalombella R, Gordon AL, et al. The role of phosphatidylinositol 3-kinase-delta in the immunomodulatory effects of lenalidomide in chronic lymphocytic leukemia. Blood 2011;117(16):4323–7.

26. Lee YK, Shanafelt TD, Bone ND, et al. VEGF receptors on chronic lymphocytic leukemia (CLL) B cells interact with STAT 1 and 3: implication for apoptosis resistance. Leukemia 2005;19(4):513–23.

27. Konig A, Menzel T, Lynen S, et al. Basic fibroblast growth factor (bFGF) upregulates the expression of bcl-2 in B cell chronic lymphocytic leukemia cell lines resulting in delaying apoptosis. Leukemia 1997;11(2):258–65.

28. Furman RR, Byrd JC, Brown JR, et al. CAL-101, an isoform-selective inhibitor of phosphatidylinositol 3-kinase P110d demonstrates clinical activity and pharmacodynamic effects in patients with relapsed or refractory chronic lymphocytic leukemia. Blood (ASH Annual Meeting Abstracts), November 2010;116:55.

29. Hallek M, Cheson BD, Catovsky D, et al. Guidelines for the diagnosis and treatment of chronic lymphocytic leukemia: a report from the International Workshop on Chronic Lymphocytic Leukemia updating the National Cancer Institute-Working Group 1996 guidelines. Blood 2008;111(12):5446–56.

30. Sharman J, de Vos S, Leonard J, et al. A phase 1 study of the selective PI3K inhibitor CAL-101 (GS-1101) in combination with rituximab and/or bendamustine in patients with relapsed or refractory CLL. Blood (ASH Annual Meeting Abstracts), November 2011;118:1787.

31. Luo J, Manning BD, Cantley LC. Targeting the PI3K-Akt pathway in human cancer: rationale and promise. Cancer Cell 2003;4(4):257–62.

32. Edelman G, Bedell G, Shapiro SS, et al. A phase I dose-escalation study of XL147 (SAR245408), a PI3K inhibitor administered orally to patients with advanced malignancies. J Clin Oncol (ASCO Annual Meeting Abstracts), 2010;28:15s:3004.

33. Martin AL, Schwartz MD, Jameson SC, et al. Selective regulation of CD8 effector T cell migration by the p110 gamma isoform of phosphatidylinositol 3-kinase. J Immunol 2008;180(4):2081–8.

34. Brown JR, Davids MS, Rodon J, et al. Phase I trial of SAR245408 (S08), a pan-PI3K inhibitor, in patients with CLL and lymphoma. Blood (ASH Annual Meeting Abstracts), November 2011;118:2683.

35. Drakos E, Rassidakis GZ, Medeiros LJ. Mammalian target of rapamycin (mTOR) pathway signalling in lymphomas. Expert Rev Mol Med 2008;10:e4.

36. Papadopoulos K, Abrisqueta P, Chambers G, et al. A phase I dose escalation expansion cohort study of the safety, pharmacokinetics and pharmacodynamics of SAR245409 (S09), an orally administered PI3K/mTOR inhibitor, in patients with lymphoma. Blood (ASH Annual Meeting Abstracts), November 2011;118:1608.

37. Lorusso P, Markman J, Tabernero R, et al. A phase I dose-escalation study of the safety, pharmacokinetics (PK), and pharmacodynamics of XL765, a PI3K/TORC1/TORC2 inhibitor administered orally to patients (pts) with advanced solid tumors. J Clin Oncol (ASCO Annual Meeting Abstracts), 2009;27:15s:3502.

38. Wiestner A, Rosenwald A, Barry TS, et al. ZAP-70 expression identifies a chronic lymphocytic leukemia subtype with unmutated immunoglobulin genes, inferior clinical outcome, and distinct gene expression profile. Blood 2003;101(12):4944–51.

39. Richardson SJ, Matthews C, Catherwood MA, et al. ZAP-70 expression is associated with enhanced ability to respond to migratory and survival signals in B-cell chronic lymphocytic leukemia (B-CLL). Blood 2006;107(9):3584–92.

40. Hamblin TJ, Davis Z, Gardiner A, et al. Unmutated Ig V(H) genes are associated with a more aggressive form of chronic lymphocytic leukemia. Blood 1999;94(6):1848–54.

41. Guarini A, Chiaretti S, Tavolaro S, et al. BCR ligation induced by IgM stimulation results in gene expression and functional changes only in IgV H unmutated chronic lymphocytic leukemia (CLL) cells. Blood 2008;112(3):782–92.

42. Coscia M, Pantaleoni F, Riganti C, et al. IGHV unmutated CLL B cells are more prone to spontaneous apoptosis and subject to environmental prosurvival signals than mutated CLL B cells. Leukemia 2011;25(5):828–37.

43. Schall TJ, Bacon K, Camp RD, et al. Human macrophage inflammatory protein alpha (MIP-1 alpha) and MIP-1 beta chemokines attract distinct populations of lymphocytes. J Exp Med 1993;177(6):1821–6.

44. Burger JA, Quiroga MP, Hartmann E, et al. High-level expression of the T-cell chemokines CCL3 and CCL4 by chronic lymphocytic leukemia B cells in nurse-like cell cocultures and after BCR stimulation. Blood 2009;113(13):3050–8.

45. Herishanu Y, Perez-Galan P, Liu D, et al. The lymph node microenvironment promotes B-cell receptor signaling, NF-kappaB activation, and tumor proliferation in chronic lymphocytic leukemia. Blood 2011;117(2):563–74.

46. Puente XS, Pinyol M, Quesada V, et al. Whole-genome sequencing identifies recurrent mutations in chronic lymphocytic leukaemia. Nature 2011;475(7354):101–5.

47. Borchmann P, Eichhorst B, Hellmann M, et al. Hematology 2008. Dtsch Med Wochenschr 2008;133(25–26):1400–4 [in German].

48. Cheson BD, Byrd JC, Rai KR, et al. Novel targeted agents and the need to refine clinical end points in chronic lymphocytic leukemia. J Clin Oncol 2012;30(23):2820–2.

Chimeric Antigen Receptor Therapy for Chronic Lymphocytic Leukemia: What are the Challenges?

Marco L. Davila, MD, PhD, Renier Brentjens, MD, PhD*

KEYWORDS

- Chimeric antigen receptor • Chronic lymphocytic leukemia • CD19
- Adoptive cell therapy • Cell engineering

KEY POINTS

- Numerous targeted therapies are being developed for patients with chronic lymphocytic leukemia (CLL).
- CAR-modified T cells targeting CD19 expressed by normal and malignant B cells is a unique therapy, and recent results from 4 different trials highlight the dramatic potential of this therapy for patients with relapsed CLL.
- Because adoptive transfer of chimeric antigen receptor–modified T cells is a novel approach to cancer therapy, there are issues for the medical oncologist to consider when evaluating current and future clinical trials for patients with CLL.

INTRODUCTION

Chronic lymphocytic leukemia (CLL) is the target for numerous new investigational drugs and immunotherapies. Unique among these is the genetic modification of T cells to B-cell antigens through the gene transfer of a chimeric antigen receptor (CAR), which is composed of an antigen-binding component fused to T-cell signaling domains. A patient's own T cells are genetically modified and then adoptively transferred back to the patient to mediate killing of malignant, and normal, B cells. Over the past 10 years, work initiated at the authors' center[1] has transitioned this technology from preclinical models to clinical trials, with evidence of promising results.[2–7] However, there are important details that should be considered when evaluating and comparing the various CAR-modified T cells under study, because this therapy is unlike any traditionally used by the medical oncologist. The goal of this article is to

Disclosures: None.
Funded by: NIH K08CA148821 (MLD) and R01CA138738 (RB).
Leukemia Service, Department of Medicine, Memorial Sloan-Kettering Cancer Center, 1275 York Avenue, New York, NY, USA
* Corresponding author.
E-mail address: brentjer@mskcc.org

Hematol Oncol Clin N Am 27 (2013) 341–353
http://dx.doi.org/10.1016/j.hoc.2012.12.004
0889-8588/13/$ – see front matter © 2013 Elsevier Inc. All rights reserved.

describe and evaluate these details, including CAR design, T-cell production and dose, prior conditioning chemotherapy regimens, and tumor burden, and to discuss how they may affect the treatment response in patients with CLL.

RESULTS OF CLINICAL TRIALS

Clinical outcomes of 16 patients with CLL treated with CAR-modified T cells targeted to the B-cell–specific CD19 antigen have recently been reported from 4 trials conducted at various academic medical centers.[2–7] The National Cancer Institute (NCI) reported their results concerning 4 patients with relapsed CLL treated with flu-darabine and cyclophosphamide followed by CD19-targeted CAR-modified T cells. These patients, previously treated with an average of 4 chemotherapy regimens, had variable anti-CD19 responses including a complete remission (CR) of greater than 15 months' duration. In addition, several patients developed anticipated B-cell aplasia as a consequence of their treatment and exhibited systemic serum cytokine elevations consistent with robust CAR-modified T-cell activation. Investigators at the University of Pennsylvania (UPenn)[3,4] reported the results of 3 CLL patients treated with CD19-targeted CAR-modified T cells, of whom 2 patients had relapsed disease and 1 patient was chemotherapy-naïve, treated with bendamustine or pentostatin plus cyclophosphamide as conditioning therapy before T-cell infusion. Two of the patients had ongoing CR while the third achieved a partial remission (PR). Similar to the clinical outcomes at the NCI, 1 of these patients experienced a prolonged (>6 months) B-cell aplasia. The authors recently reported the largest cohort of CLL patients treated with CD19-targeted T cells (**Fig. 1**).[2] Outcomes in these patients included objective responses with lymph node reductions and B-cell aplasia.[2] Further-more, this trial included a unique secondary end point evaluating the requirement for conditioning therapy before gene-modified T-cell infusion. Lastly, investigators at the Baylor College of Medicine reported the results of 6 patients with B-cell malignancies, 1 of whom had CLL.[7] Although no objective response was detected, the patient did have stable disease (SD) for 10 months after T-cell infusion. Of note, this trial did not include prior conditioning chemotherapy.

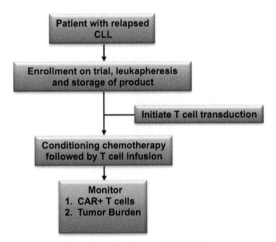

Fig. 1. Memorial Sloan-Kettering Cancer Center (MSKCC) treatment schema using CAR-modified T cells for patients with relapsed CLL. Patients with relapsed CLL are eligible for enrollment, leukapheresis, and infusion with CAR-modified T cells after treatment with conditioning chemotherapy.

Overall, the toxicities reported among the different trials were quite similar and included fevers, rigors, hypotension, and B-cell aplasia.[2-6] These toxicities began approximately 1 to 21 days after initial T-cell infusion. Furthermore, the toxicities appeared to be coincident with peaks in cytokine production.[2-6] Collectively, in 2 of these patients their symptoms resolved and cytokine levels decreased after initiation of steroid therapy.[3]

All of the reported trials present clinical evidence to support in vivo CD19-targeted T-cell efficacy. However, closer inspection of results and comparison of the trials focusing on elements of CAR design, T-cell production, and patient selection allows for a better understanding regarding disparities in results from the individual trials, providing insight for more rational designs of future CARs and therapeutic clinical trials. Furthermore, this discussion will allow the medical oncologist to critically evaluate the multiple clinical trials involving gene-modified T-cell therapy available for their patients with CLL (**Table 1**).

CAR DESIGN

CARs are generally classified as being of first-generation, second-generation, or third-generation design. This classification relates to the signal transduction domains incorporated within the CAR (**Fig. 2**). First-generation CARs most commonly consist of a CD3ζ signaling element, which when combined with an anti-CD19 single chain variable fragment (scFv) successfully redirects T cells to mediate killing of B cells in vitro and in vivo in immunodeficient preclinical animal models.[1,8] However, these first-generation CARs ultimately have been found to have limited in vivo efficacy, with little evidence of T-cell persistence in these models.[9-11] The reason for this limited efficacy is related to T-cell biology: T cells are optimally activated when they encounter antigen for the first time if they receive two signals, one mediated by CD3ζ (signal 1) and the other mediated by a costimulatory receptor, most commonly CD28 (signal 2).[1] This 2-signal paradigm for efficient T-cell activation could be recapitulated through second-generation CARs that included costimulatory T-cell cytoplasmic signal domains proximal to CD3ζ cytoplasmic signal domains (see **Fig. 2**).[9,10] T cells modified to express second-generation CARs demonstrated enhanced in vivo tumor killing and persistence. While CD28 is the most commonly used costimulatory signaling domain, others have modified second-generation CARs to include the costimulatory signal domains of 41BB, OX40, DAP10, and CD27.[10,12,13] Studies have demonstrated that additional signal domains enhance gene-modified T-cell function by increasing cytokine secretion and enhancing T-cell proliferation and persistence.[12-14] Third-generation anti-CD19 CARs, which have 2 costimulatory domains combined with CD3ζ, demonstrate impressive results in preclinical animal models, but have not been evaluated in CLL patients to date.[15,16]

Comparison of anti-CD19 CARs using different monoclonal antibody (mAb) derived scFvs have not been performed, although one could speculate that if the binding affinities of the scFvs were significantly different it could affect CAR-mediated T-cell activation and consequent B-cell killing. To this end, studies at the Memorial Sloan-Kettering Cancer Center (MSKCC) used a different scFv, derived from the SJ25C1 hybridoma, in comparison with studies at the NCI and UPenn wherein the anti-CD19 CAR used a scFv derived from the FMC63 hybridoma.

The 4 clinical trials involving CLL patients have all used second-generation CARs, but the clinical trial results reported by Savoldo and colleagues[7] are unique for directly infusing a mixture of T cells genetically modified with a first-generation CD3ζ CAR and a second-generation CAR including the CD28 costimulatory domain. In a cohort of

Table 1
Active clinical trials for adults with CLL

Clinical Trial Identifier	CAR	Gene Transfer	Disease Status	T-Cell Escalation	Conditioning Therapy	Trial Site
NCT00586391	19z[a] vs 1928z	γ-Retrovirus	Relapsed	Yes	CY	Dallas, TX
NCT00709033	192[b] vs 1928z	γ-Retrovirus	Relapsed	Yes	CY	Dallas, TX
NCT00924326	1928z	γ-Retrovirus	Relapsed	No	CY + FLU Interleukin-2[c]	Washington, DC
NCT00968760[d]	1928z	Electroporation with SB transposase	Relapsed	Yes	BEAM + R ± Interleukin-2	Houston, TX
NCT01653717	1928z	Electroporation with SB transposase	8 weeks from last chemo	Yes	CY + FLU	Houston, TX
NCT01416974	1928z	γ-Retrovirus	MRD[e]	Yes	CY	New York, NY
NCT00466531	1928z	γ-Retrovirus	Relapsed	Yes	CY	New York, NY
NCT01029366	19BBz	Lentivirus	Relapsed	No	Investigators' choice	Philadelphia, PA

Listed are currently accruing clinical trials using autologous CAR-modified T cells targeted to the CD19 antigen for patients with CLL.
Abbreviations: CY, cyclophosphamide; FLU, fludarabine; MRD, minimal residual disease; SB, Sleeping Beauty.
[a] Patients are infused with a mixture of T cells modified with either the 19z or 1928z CAR.
[b] Patients are infused with a mixture of T cells modified with either the 19z or 1928z CAR. The 19z CARs are transduced into EBV+ T cells, whereas the 1928z CARs are transduced into normal peripheral, polyclonal T cells.
[c] Interleukin-2 is not given as a lymphodepleting agent but as a T-cell growth factor.
[d] This is the only trial listed in which the T cells are administered as part of an autologous stem cell transplant.
[e] This trial is evaluating CAR-modified T cells as a consolidation regimen. Patients treated with an initial chemotherapy regimen and who have residual disease after completing this regimen are infused with 1928z+ T cells.

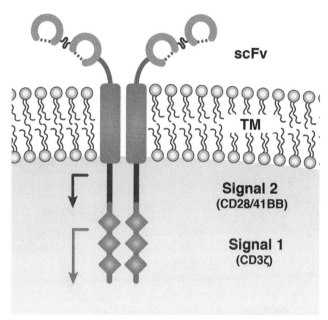

Fig. 2. The chimeric antigen receptor. Most CARs are composed of the antigen-binding domains of an scFv, fused to the transmembrane (TM) region of a protein such as CD8, which is fused to signal transduction domains normally associated with a T-cell receptor. The scFv binds an antigen and T-cell activation is mediated in part by the 2 signal-transduction domains. The 3 diamonds represent the 3 immunoreceptor tyrosine-based activation motifs present within CD3ζ.

46 patients (1 with CLL), investigators clearly demonstrated that T cells with second-generation CARs enhanced persistence and/or expansion when compared with T cells modified with a first-generation CAR.

Investigators at UPenn have the only trial for CLL patients using a CAR that has a costimulatory domain other than CD28, namely 41BB.[3,4] At present the only direct comparison of anti-CD19 second-generation CARs with a CD28 or 41BB costimulatory domain (19-28z vs 19-bbz) is in preclinical models, and the results documenting protection against B-cell malignancies have been contradictory, possibly because the anti-CD19 scFvs were derived from different mAbs.[10,12]

T-CELL PRODUCTION

In most trials, CAR-modified T cells are generated ex vivo and include an initial activation step followed by a gene-transfer step (**Fig. 3**). All trials activate T cells with agonistic mAb-mediated CD3 stimulation with or without additional CD28 costimulation.[2–7] In 3 of the reported clinical trials gammaretroviral vectors were used for gene transfer, whereas studies from UPenn used lentiviral vectors. However, given the small number of patients treated to date on these trials, it is not yet possible to assess the superiority of one viral transfer system over the other. Although in theory lentiviral gene transfer may increase safety given prior reports of leukemogenic integration sites associated with gammaretroviruses, in these cases the cells transduced were hematopoietic stem cells, not mature T cells.[17,18] To date, there have been no reports of insertional oncogenesis with gammaretroviral vectors in the context of genetically

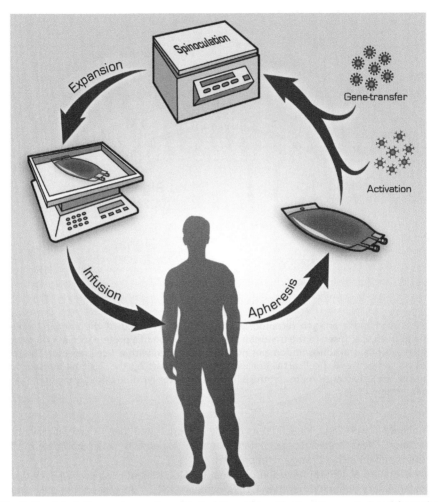

Fig. 3. T-cell isolation and gene-transfer. Peripheral blood leukocytes are isolated from the patient and T cells are enriched and activated from this leukapheresis product with anti-CD3 and/or anti-CD28 ligation. Gene transfer can be accomplished by retroviral transduction (depicted here with spinoculation), electroporation, RNA transfection, or via transposase activity. Afterward, CAR-modified T cells are expanded, in this example with a Wave Bioreactor, and ultimately adoptively transferred back into the patient.

modified mature lymphocytes. In fact, a recent report identified no long-term sequelae in 43 subjects infused with gammaretroviral transduced T cells in several clinical trials evaluating patients after an 11-year follow-up period.[19]

Another important consideration with respect to CAR-modified T-cell technologies is how efficiently and rapidly gene-targeted T cells can be produced. This point is highlighted by 2 trials for lymphoma patients that involved the genetic modification of T cells targeted to the CD20 antigen; an anti-CD20 CAR gene was introduced through electroporation and the cells were subsequently expanded after drug selection.[20,21] No objective responses were noted, and a valid concern regarding these modest clinical outcomes was related to the long culture period required to produce the T cells, potentially resulting in "exhausted" T cells with limited proliferative potential following infusion.[22] By contrast, all CLL trials using retroviral vectors generated the requisite T-cell dose within 1 to 3 weeks, and consisted of T cells that seem to have retained proliferative capacity.

An optimal anti-CD19 T-cell product would be expected to provide immediate tumor control, by way of direct cytotoxicity, but also to have the ability to generate long-term memory cells to mediate subsequent tumor immunosurveillance. Studies at MSKCC and the NCI characterized the immunophenotype of the final T-cell product and confirmed the expression of memory markers (CD62L 4%–78%, CCR7 1%–37%), suggesting that these T cells had retained proliferative potential and the capacity to become long-term memory cells.[2,5,6]

T-CELL DOSE, TUMOR BURDEN, AND CONDITIONING TREATMENT AS PREDICTORS FOR OPTIMAL CAR-MODIFIED T-CELL FUNCTION

Unlike standard therapeutic drugs, T cells have a completely different dynamic regulating their half-life and efficacy. For example, T cells ideally have the potential to proliferate and persist long after adoptive transfer, making the half-life of these T cells incalculable and their effects indefinite. Scholler and colleagues[19] estimated the half-life of retrovirally gene-modified T cells infused into patients to be longer than 16 years at the least. When CAR-modified T-cell trials were being developed as a therapy for CLL and other indolent B-cell malignancies, preclinical and clinical studies identified major determinants for T-cell function to be T-cell dose, tumor (or antigen) burden, and/or prior conditioning with chemotherapy or radiation therapy.[10,23,24] Reflecting on currently published clinical results, the authors are now able to comment on how each of these variables appear to affect CAR-modified T-cell function in patients with CLL.

T-cell dose is an intriguing variable because it is possible that T cells will expand after transfer into optimally conditioned patients by homeostatic proliferation or in response to a pro-proliferative cytokine profile.[22] Therefore, as the T-cell dose increases, T-cell expansion may plateau or decrease if limited by available cytokines or space in lymphoid tissues for expansion.[25] To this end, results from these trials do not identify any correlation between T-cell dose and clinical outcome.[2–7] Specifically, an optimal antitumor response achieved at UPenn was in a patient treated with a T-cell dose 40 to 80 times lower than that infused into the other 2 patients reported in this cohort.[3,4] Similarly, in the authors' studies at MSKCC, better objective responses in a lower dose cohort were noted when compared with patients treated at a 3-fold higher CAR-modified T-cell dose.[2] Therefore, based on currently published reports there does not appear to be a correlation between T-cell dose and clinical outcome within a large range of clinically meaningful treatment doses (2×10^5 to 3.1×10^7 CAR+ T cells/kg).

The authors speculate that the T-cell dose required for a positive clinical outcome may be affected by tumor burden. In fact, they have previously reported an inverse correlation between tumor burden and persistence of CAR-modified T cells in CLL patients treated on their protocol.[2] A similar inverse rank order is noted among the 3 CLL patients treated at UPenn. The best response in these studies, a CR with long-term B-cell aplasia, was observed in the patient with the lowest estimated tumor burden, whereas a more modest PR response was noted in the patient with the greatest estimated tumor burden.[3,4] These comparisons were assisted by the measurement of CLL tumor burden, calculated as the sum of the nodal tumor mass, blood tumor mass, and bone marrow tumor mass.[3] A similar calculation for CLL tumor burden performed retrospectively on the authors' treated patients was consistent with an inverse correlation between tumor burden and clinical outcome (data not shown). How the function of CAR-modified T cells is regulated by antigen and/or tumor burden is unknown, but it is reasonable to speculate that infused T cells may be rendered nonfunctional through tolerance or exhaustion in the context of excessive tumor bulk and/or CD19 antigen expressed on normal B cells.

If tumor burden is an important regulator of clinical outcome it follows that conditioning with chemotherapy or radiation therapy may enhance CAR-modified T-cell function, in part through debulking tumor mass before CAR-modified T-cell infusion. Preclinical studies of CAR-modified T cells targeting B-cell malignancies in immunocompetent mice suggest that optimal anti-CD19 T-cell cytotoxic function and subsequent persistence is enhanced by lymphodepleting conditioning therapy before adoptive T-cell transfer.[24,26–28] Conditioning regimens used in these studies are variable and include γ-irradiation, cyclophosphamide chemotherapy, and anti-CD20 mAb immunotherapy. Though diverse, all these conditioning regimens have the ability to readily lymphodeplete mice. One recent preclinical study found that in the presence of overwhelming antigen, CAR+ T cells were sequestered in the lung and subsequently eliminated before encounter with tumor.[24] This mechanism is likely most relevant when CAR-modified T cells target an abundant self-antigen such as CD19, which is expressed on normal B cells, but does not exclude other mechanisms attributed to conditioning regimens enhancing the function of adoptively transferred T cells such as homeostatic proliferation, cytokine sinks, and regulatory T-cell depletion.[22]

Given the preclinical findings with respect to conditioning regimens, all reported clinical trials using CD19-targeted T cells into CLL patients with the exception of the trial conducted by Savoldo and colleagues[7] have been designed to include conditioning chemotherapy before CAR-modified T-cell infusion. The MSKCC clinical trial is the only one to date to compare cohorts of patients treated with and without prior conditioning chemotherapy.[2] The results of 8 CLL patients included 3 patients treated with CAR-modified T cells alone and 5 patients treated with cyclophosphamide and then CAR-modified T cells. Inclusion of cyclophosphamide conditioning chemotherapy before T-cell infusion was associated with increased T-cell persistence and improved clinical outcomes despite this cohort being infused with a lower dose of CAR-modified T cells than the nonconditioned cohort. It must be noted that patients treated with cyclophosphamide conditioning in the MSKCC studies had previously been treated with this agent as part of prior multi-chemotherapeutic regimens for their CLL. Therefore, the relapsed CLL tumor cells were likely resistant to cyclophosphamide. This assumption is further supported by an absence of tumor lysis, no decrease in absolute lymphocyte count, and no decrease in lymphadenopathy after infusion of the cyclophosphamide before infusion of the CAR-modified T cells. Therefore, the potential benefit of this conditioning therapy would be related to lymphodepletion of nonmalignant chemosensitive normal B cells to reduce the CD19 antigen burden. By contrast, 2 of the patients reported by UPenn were treated with chemotherapeutic regimens not previously used in these patients, and the other was treated with a regimen they were currently responding to; all the regimens used are known to be highly active in CLL.[3,4] Long-term effects, such as B-cell aplasia 10 months after treatment, are likely to be related to CAR-modified T cells; however, in these patients it is difficult to differentiate the observed tumor reduction mediated by highly active chemotherapy regimens from those mediated by the subsequently infused CAR-modified T cells. For example, one of the patients treated at UPenn was induced into a CR after treatment with bendamustine and CAR-modified T cells, but this patient had recovery of normal B cells and immunoglobulin G serum levels.[3,4] So it would be difficult to determine the role played by bendamustine in inducing a CR in this particular patient. The NCI conditioned its 4 CLL patients with a combination of fludarabine and high-dose cyclophosphamide before infusion with CAR-modified T cells.[5,6] Both drugs are highly active against CLL, so the relative contributions of the chemotherapy and T cells in the overall tumor reduction remain difficult to assess.

The results from the clinical trials complement those from preclinical animal models demonstrating that prior conditioning therapy is critical to the subsequent anti-CD19 efficacy of CAR-modified T cells. Nevertheless, the trials reported to date have created new questions, which need to be addressed in future clinical studies. What is the optimal conditioning regimen? Should the goal of the conditioning treatment be merely lymphodepletion or should it also mediate substantial antitumor activity? Which of these variables enhance the efficacy of one conditioning regimen relative to another?

Based on the available published clinical data of anti-CD19 CAR T-cell therapy, the most active antitumor conditioning chemotherapy regimens are those that mediate tumor lysis, because these regimens are associated with the best clinical outcomes. Therefore, the authors believe that most trials should include a tumor-responsive conditioning chemotherapy regimen, which in turn reduces tumor bulk, enhances tumor antigen presentation to foster endogenous antitumor immune responses, and enhances the persistence and function of adoptively transferred CAR-modified T cells. Although the use of highly active chemotherapy regimens may blur the role of the CAR-modified T cells in the antitumor response, the latter may be assessed, in part, by predicted CAR T-cell–mediated long-term B-cell aplasia, persistence of CAR-modified T cells, and loss of detectable clonal CLL tumor cell immunoglobulin heavy-chain rearrangement.

FUTURE DIRECTIONS

Promising clinical trial results have established the potential of anti-CD19 CAR-modified T-cell therapy for patients with CLL and have spurred the clinical investigation of this technology at multiple academic medical centers, with currently 8 clinical trials using this technology enrolling patients with CLL (see **Table 1**). The optimal costimulatory domain for targeting CLL may ultimately be addressed by a planned clinical trial at UPenn, Children's Hospital of Pennsylvania, and MSKCC funded by an NIH Special Translational Research Acceleration Project (STRAP) award (**Fig. 4**). In these studies, patients will be evaluated after infusion with two populations of T cells: one modified with a 19-28z CAR, derived from MSKCC, and the other modified with the UPenn 19-BBz CAR. Detection of both CAR-modified T-cell populations by quantitative polymerase chain reaction may assess whether either T-cell population expands better and/or persists longer in vivo. In addition, lentiviral and gammaretroviral production systems will be compared head to head in these studies, with respect to gene-transfer efficacy and CAR-modified T-cell persistence.

Six of the currently open trials are performing T-cell dose escalations to determine the maximum tolerated T-cell dose. Although clinical evidence suggests that T-cell dose may not be a critical variable for optimal T-cell function, these trials will allow the comparison of toxicities and benefits among multiple cohorts of patients treated under similar conditions. The results may finally suggest an acceptable dose of CAR-modified T cells, balancing toxicities and clinical outcomes.

This review highlights the importance of tumor burden and effective tumor debulking conditioning regimens. At present, ongoing trials do not optimally evaluate tumor burden before and after treatment. However, use of the tumor-burden calculation for CLL described by Kalos and colleagues[3] will allow for the reporting of tumor burden at

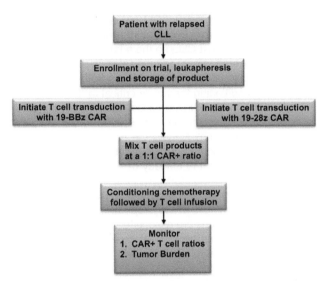

Fig. 4. MSKCC and University of Pennsylvania (UPenn) treatment schema comparing 19-28z and 19-BBz CAR-modified T cells in patients with relapsed CLL. Patients with relapsed CLL at MSKCC or UPenn are eligible for enrollment, leukapheresis, and infusion with CAR-modified T cells after treatment with conditioning chemotherapy. The patients are infused with a mixture of CAR-modified T cells composed of an equal ratio of 19-28z+ T cells to 19-BBz+ T cells. Transduction of the 19-28z CAR occurs by gammaretroviral transduction, whereas transduction of the 19-BBz CAR occurs by lentiviral transduction. Production of both T-cell groups occurs at the Good Manufacturing Practice facility located within the medical center treating the patient. Enhanced T-cell persistence and/or proliferation will be determined by measuring the ratio of both CAR-modified T-cell groups in treated patients.

the time of treatment and retrospective analyses of antitumor responses. Universal use of the CLL tumor-burden calculation may allow prospectively a more rigorous evaluation of the suggested inverse correlation between tumor burden and CAR-modified T-cell antitumor efficacy.

The clear preclinical and clinical evidence arguing for effective conditioning chemotherapy before CAR-modified T-cell infusion is reflected by the fact that all currently open clinical trials include some form of conditioning therapy before T-cell infusion (see **Table 1**). Variability of these conditioning regimens is quite broad, spanning single-agent cyclophosphamide to a 5-drug regimen used in the context of an autologous stem cell transplant. Although current comparison of clinical trial outcomes are unlikely to identify an optimal conditioning regimen, it may help to further validate the role of prior conditioning to enhance or optimize subsequently transferred CAR-modified T cells. Ultimately, future clinical trials designed to compare conditioning regimens may need to be conducted to prospectively identify an ideal regimen.

Initial first-in-man clinical trials using CAR-modified T cells treated only CLL patients with relapsed and/or chemorefractory disease. Despite this poor-prognosis patient population, there were clear instances of impressive clinical outcomes. Given the previously inferred inverse correlation between tumor burden and anti-CD19 CAR-modified T-cell antitumor efficacy, the authors have recently opened a trial at MSKCC that uses anti-CD19 CAR-modified T cells as a consolidation regimen for CLL following completion of initial upfront chemotherapy. This trial is exclusively for CLL patients with detectable or minimal residual disease (PR or MRD) after completing standard front-line chemotherapy (**Fig. 5**). The goal of this trial is to generate complete molecular remissions in patients with PR or MRD following upfront chemotherapy. The results from this trial could support the application of CAR-modified T cells at an earlier stage of disease progression if periods of remission are increased. Results from this upfront trial could have a major impact on the treatment of patients with CLL by increasing the number of patients with complete molecular remissions, long-term disease control, and/or delaying the start of subsequent salvage therapies.

In conclusion, the early reports from these trials in patients with relapsed and/or refractory CLL clearly demonstrate the potential of CAR-modified T-cell therapy. Significant work lies ahead, and a cooperative effort between academic medical centers will be required to determine the optimal CAR design, prior conditioning regimen, and gene-transfer methodology to rationally design second-generation clinical trials to treat CLL patients with optimized CAR-modified T cells. With a sustained collaborative effort by academic medical centers to this end, the medical oncologist may soon have an established novel and potentially curative approach for the treatment of CLL.

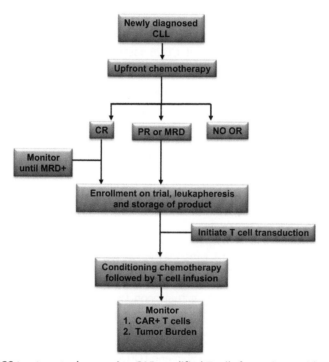

Fig. 5. MSKCC treatment schema using CAR-modified T cells for patients with residual CLL. This trial is open at MSKCC for patients with newly diagnosed CLL. Patients receive a complete course of standard combination chemotherapy after developing an indication for treatment. Afterward, patients are stratified based on response to treatment. Patients with no response or stable disease (NO OR) are not eligible for the trial. Patients with a partial remission or minimal residual disease (PR or MRD) are eligible for enrollment, CAR-modified T-cell production, and conditioning followed by infusion with T cells. Patients with a CR are monitored for relapse by flow cytometry or by a quantitative polymerase chain reaction for the immunoglobulin heavy-chain rearrangement associated with the CLL tumor cells. Detection of MRD makes the patient eligible for enrollment and treatment with CAR-modified T cells as above.

REFERENCES

1. Brentjens RJ, Latouche JB, Santos E, et al. Eradication of systemic B-cell tumors by genetically targeted human T lymphocytes co-stimulated by CD80 and interleukin-15. Nat Med 2003;9:279.
2. Brentjens RJ, Riviere I, Park JH, et al. Safety and persistence of adoptively transferred autologous CD19-targeted T cells in patients with relapsed or chemotherapy refractory B-cell leukemias. Blood 2011;118:4817.
3. Kalos M, Levine BL, Porter DL, et al. T cells with chimeric antigen receptors have potent antitumor effects and can establish memory in patients with advanced leukemia. Sci Transl Med 2011;3:95ra73.
4. Porter DL, Levine BL, Kalos M, et al. Chimeric antigen receptor-modified T cells in chronic lymphoid leukemia. N Engl J Med 2011;365:725.
5. Kochenderfer JN, Dudley ME, Feldman SA, et al. B-cell depletion and remissions of malignancy along with cytokine-associated toxicity in a clinical trial of anti-CD19 chimeric-antigen-receptor-transduced T cells. Blood 2011;119(12): 2709–20.
6. Kochenderfer JN, Wilson WH, Janik JE, et al. Eradication of B-lineage cells and regression of lymphoma in a patient treated with autologous T cells genetically engineered to recognize CD19. Blood 2010;116:4099.
7. Savoldo B, Ramos CA, Liu E, et al. CD28 costimulation improves expansion and persistence of chimeric antigen receptor-modified T cells in lymphoma patients. J Clin Invest 2011;121:1822.
8. Cooper LJ, Topp MS, Serrano LM, et al. T-cell clones can be rendered specific for CD19: toward the selective augmentation of the graft-versus-B-lineage leukemia effect. Blood 2003;101:1637.
9. Kowolik CM, Topp MS, Gonzalez S, et al. CD28 costimulation provided through a CD19-specific chimeric antigen receptor enhances in vivo persistence and antitumor efficacy of adoptively transferred T cells. Cancer Res 2006; 66:10995.
10. Brentjens RJ, Santos E, Nikhamin Y, et al. Genetically targeted T cells eradicate systemic acute lymphoblastic leukemia xenografts. Clin Cancer Res 2007;13: 5426.
11. Brocker T, Karjalainen K. Signals through T cell receptor-zeta chain alone are insufficient to prime resting T lymphocytes. J Exp Med 1995;181:1653.
12. Milone MC, Fish JD, Carpenito C, et al. Chimeric receptors containing CD137 signal transduction domains mediate enhanced survival of T cells and increased antileukemic efficacy in vivo. Mol Ther 2009;17:1453.
13. Song DG, Ye Q, Poussin M, et al. CD27 costimulation augments the survival and antitumor activity of redirected human T cells in vivo. Blood 2012;119:696.
14. Maher J, Brentjens RJ, Gunset G, et al. Human T-lymphocyte cytotoxicity and proliferation directed by a single chimeric TCRzeta/CD28 receptor. Nat Biotechnol 2002;20:70.
15. Carpenito C, Milone MC, Hassan R, et al. Control of large, established tumor xenografts with genetically retargeted human T cells containing CD28 and CD137 domains. Proc Natl Acad Sci U S A 2009;106:3360.
16. Zhong XS, Matsushita M, Plotkin J, et al. Chimeric antigen receptors combining 4-1BB and CD28 signaling domains augment PI3kinase/AKT/Bcl-XL activation and CD8+ T cell-mediated tumor eradication. Mol Ther 2010;18:413.
17. Fischer A, Abina SH, Thrasher A, et al. LMO2 and gene therapy for severe combined immunodeficiency. N Engl J Med 2004;350:2526.

18. Hacein-Bey-Abina S, Von Kalle C, Schmidt M, et al. LMO2-associated clonal T cell proliferation in two patients after gene therapy for SCID-X1. Science 2003;302:415.
19. Scholler J, Brady TL, Binder-Scholl G, et al. Decade-long safety and function of retroviral-modified chimeric antigen receptor T cells. Sci Transl Med 2012;4:132ra53.
20. Jensen MC, Popplewell L, Cooper LJ, et al. Antitransgene rejection responses contribute to attenuated persistence of adoptively transferred CD20/CD19-specific chimeric antigen receptor redirected T cells in humans. Biol Blood Marrow Transplant 2010;16:1245.
21. Till BG, Jensen MC, Wang J, et al. CD20-specific adoptive immunotherapy for lymphoma using a chimeric antigen receptor with both CD28 and 4-1BB domains: pilot clinical trial results. Blood 2012;119:3940.
22. Restifo NP, Dudley ME, Rosenberg SA. Adoptive immunotherapy for cancer: harnessing the T cell response. Nat Rev Immunol 2012;12:269.
23. Dudley ME, Yang JC, Sherry R, et al. Adoptive cell therapy for patients with metastatic melanoma: evaluation of intensive myeloablative chemoradiation preparative regimens. J Clin Oncol 2008;26:5233.
24. James SE, Orgun NN, Tedder TF, et al. Antibody-mediated B-cell depletion before adoptive immunotherapy with T cells expressing CD20-specific chimeric T-cell receptors facilitates eradication of leukemia in immunocompetent mice. Blood 2009;114:5454.
25. Ho WY, Blattman JN, Dossett ML, et al. Adoptive immunotherapy: engineering T cell responses as biologic weapons for tumor mass destruction. Cancer Cell 2003;3:431.
26. Pegram HJ, Lee JC, Hayman EG, et al. Tumor-targeted T cells modified to secrete IL-12 eradicate systemic tumors without need for prior conditioning. Blood 2012;119(18):4133–41.
27. Kochenderfer JN, Yu Z, Frasheri D, et al. Adoptive transfer of syngeneic T cells transduced with a chimeric antigen receptor that recognizes murine CD19 can eradicate lymphoma and normal B cells. Blood 2010;116:3875.
28. Cheadle EJ, Hawkins RE, Batha H, et al. Natural expression of the CD19 antigen impacts the long-term engraftment but not antitumor activity of CD19-specific engineered T cells. J Immunol 2010;184:1885.

The Evolving Role of Stem Cell Transplantation in Chronic Lymphocytic Leukemia

Peter Dreger, MD, On behalf of the European Group for Blood and Marrow Transplantation (EBMT)

KEYWORDS

- Allogeneic stem cell transplantation • Chronic lymphocytic leukemia
- Minimal residual disease • Nonrelapse mortality

KEY POINTS

- Novel forms of (reduced intensity) conditioning have resulted in dramatic reduction of early morbidity and mortality of allogeneic stem cell transplantation (alloSCT), making this procedure now suitable for comorbid and elderly patients.
- This "new" alloSCT is working particularly well in chronic lymphocytic leukemia (CLL) based on strong graft-versus-leukemia efficacy.
- New alloSCT is effective also in poor-risk CLL and can provide long-term disease-free survival.
- Preliminary evidence suggests that alloSCT indeed can change the natural history of poor-risk CLL, and novel CLL-targeting drugs may have the potential to further improve transplant outcome.

To improve the prognosis of patients with poor-risk chronic lymphocytic leukemia (CLL), efforts to develop effective treatment strategies have focused on autologous and allogeneic stem cell transplantation (SCT) more than 20 years ago.[1,2] The rationale for this was the assumption that intensive myeloablative treatment might be able to eradicate the leukemic clones, thereby curing the disease. However, myeloablative treatment is associated with profound nonhematopoietic toxicity, making this procedure often intolerable for elderly and comorbid individuals who represent most patients with CLL. Moreover, recent mature results from studies on autologous stem cell transplantation (autoSCT) and T-cell depleted allogeneic stem cell transplantation (alloSCT) have suggested that myeloablative therapy alone is generally not sufficient to cure CLL.[3–5]

After it had been recognized that in CLL the antileukemic effect of alloSCT is largely, if not entirely, due to the graft-versus-leukemia (GVL) activity conferred with the

Department of Medicine V, University of Heidelberg, Im Neuenheimer Feld 410, 69120 Heidelberg, Germany
E-mail address: peter.dreger@med.uni-heidelberg.de

Hematol Oncol Clin N Am 27 (2013) 355–369
http://dx.doi.org/10.1016/j.hoc.2013.01.007
0889-8588/13/$ – see front matter © 2013 Elsevier Inc. All rights reserved.

hematopoietic stem cell graft[6–9] and that engraftment and GVL activity can be achieved without preceding myeloablative treatment,[10–12] the avenues for a completely new form of allogeneic transplant were opened.[13] This "new" alloSCT is fundamentally different from the traditional myeloablative transplant, is applicable to a large proportion of the CLL target population, and represents the most effective and only curative treatment of CLL available today. Its clinical effectiveness relies on the initiation of cellular immune therapy permanently active in the patient, thereby providing a treatment modality that is in a biologic sense completely different from any other cytotoxic or immunologic therapy. Accordingly, the numbers of (nonmyeloablative) allotransplants for CLL are steadily increasing, making CLL now the most frequent indication for alloSCT among all lymphomas in the European Group for Blood and Marrow Transplantation (EBMT) registry. In contrast, autoSCT is rapidly declining (**Fig. 1**).

This overview summarizes the knowledge characterizing the efficacy and tolerability of modern alloSCT strategies in CLL and describes the resulting role of alloSCT in the current therapeutic arsenal for CLL.

EVIDENCE FOR EFFICACY OF NEW ALLOSCT IN CLL

The basis of new (nonmyeloablative or reduced-intensity conditioning [RIC]) alloSCT in CLL is that GVL effects are active. Evidence for GVL efficacy in CLL derives from the observation that, in contrast to autoSCT or other intensive therapies, the relapse incidence seems to decrease over time after RIC alloSCT. Accordingly, all larger studies on RIC alloSCT in CLL show a plateau at 40% to 50% in the disease-free survival curve (**Table 1**). Furthermore, GVL activity in CLL is indicated by a reduced relapse risk in the presence of chronic graft-versus-host disease (GVHD),[14–16] and an increased relapse risk associated with the use of T-cell depletion.[3,17]

The most convincing proof of the GVL principle in CLL comes from studies analyzing the kinetics of minimal residual disease (MRD) after RIC alloSCT. MRD denotes a disease burden remaining after specific therapy, which is detectable only at a subclinical level. For CLL, this is defined as a contamination of 5 CLL cells or less per nanoliter of peripheral blood in the absence of clinical signs or symptoms of the disease. Patients showing less than 1 CLL cell in 10,000 benign leukocytes in peripheral blood or bone marrow are considered as being MRD negative.[18]

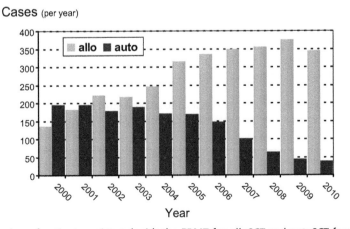

Fig. 1. Number of patients registered with the EBMT for alloSCT and autoSCT for CLL.

Table 1
Efficacy of prospective clinical trials on RIC alloSCT in CLL

	Dreger et al,[25] 2010	Sorror et al,[24] 2008	Brown et al,[22] 2012	Khouri et al,[49] 2011	Michallet et al,[50] 2011
N	90	82	76	86	40
Conditioning regimen	Nonmyeloablative (fludarabine-cyclophosphamide ± antithymocyte globulin)	Nonmyeloablative (fludarabine—low-dose total body irradiation)	Reduced intensity (fludarabine-busulfan)	Nonmyeloablative (fludarabine-cyclophosphamide-rituximab)	Nonmyeloablative (fludarabine-cyclophosphamide-rituximab)
Alternative donors[a] (%)	59	37	63	50	0
Relapse incidence (%)	40 (4 y)	38 (5 y)	40 (5 y)	nr	22 (3 y)
Progression-free survival (%)	42 (4 y)	39 (5 y)	43 (5 y)	36 (5 y)	46 (3 y)
Overall survival (%)	70 (4 y)	50 (5 y)	63 (5 y)	51 (5 y)	55 (3 y)
Follow-up (y)	3.8 (0.6–8.5)	5 (0.9–7.3)	5.1	3.1 (0.9–10.9)	2.3 (0.3–5.9)

Abbreviation: nr, not reported.
[a] Donors other than siblings with identical HLA antigen.

In CLL, MRD can be quantified even at low levels by sensitive (>10E4) polymerase chain reaction– or flow cytometry–based assays. We analyzed MRD kinetics in 43 patients who had undergone RIC alloSCT within the prospective CLL3X trial of the German CLL Study Group (GCLLSG) or a pilot study and remained event-free 1 year after alloSCT. Of these, 32 patients had become MRD negative at 1 year after transplant, while in 11 patients the MRD level did not decrease below the threshold of detection until this landmark. Achievement of MRD negativity was clearly linked to immune intervention, such as tapering of immunosuppression or donor lymphocyte infusions (**Fig. 2**). Absence of detectable MRD 1 year after alloSCT was strongly associated with a reduced risk of clinical relapse (hazard ratio [HR], 0.037; 95% confidence interval [CI], 0.008–0.18; $P<.0001$).[16] Similar observations were reported by other investigators.[15,19]

Altogether, MRD kinetics studies consistently indicate that permanent MRD negativity after alloSCT for CLL can be reached in the context of immunomodulating intervention. Both the durability of MRD remission and its sensitivity to immunomodulation strongly suggest that GVL activity is effective in CLL. GVL activity in CLL seems to be closely correlated to chronic GVHD, implying that it essentially depends on allogeneic effects with broader specificity rather than on a CLL-specific reactivity of donor GVL effector cells.

> In summary, clinical trials and MRD studies provide clear evidence that GVL is working in CLL and can provide long-term MRD-free survival in up to 50% of patients undergoing RIC alloSCT.

RISKS AND TOLERABILITY OF NEW ALLOSCT IN CLL

The core feature of modern alloSCT strategies is that their tolerability has dramatically increased in comparison with traditional conditioning based on standard-dose total body irradiation or myeloablative doses of oral busulfan. Together with a tremendous improvement of supportive treatment (eg, antiemetics, antibiotics, and cytomegalovirus monitoring) during the past decade, this makes a huge difference for the patients especially during the early transplant phase (ie, conditioning, transplant, and aplasia): higher-grade nausea and mucositis affects only a small minority of patients undergoing RIC, and although grade 3 to 4 infections still occur in up to 60% of the patients, only few result in life-threatening complications (**Table 2**). Accordingly, the early death

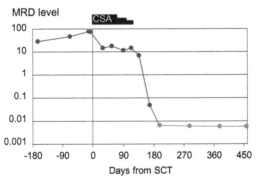

Fig. 2. MRD kinetics in a patient with poor-risk CLL during RIC (real-time polymerase chain reaction). Red dots indicate MRD positivity, green dots MRD negativity.

Table 2
Toxicity of prospective clinical trials on RIC alloSCT in CLL

	Dreger et al,[25] 2010	Sorror et al,[24] 2008	Brown et al,[22] 2012	Khouri et al,[49] 2011	Michallet et al,[50] 2011
N	90	82	76	86	40
Conditioning regimen	Nonmyeloablative (fludarabine–cyclophosphamide ± antithymocyte globulin)	Nonmyeloablative (fludarabine—low-dose total body irradiation)	Reduced intensity (fludarabine–busulfan)	Nonmyeloablative (fludarabine–cyclophosphamide–rituximab)	Nonmyeloablative (fludarabine–cyclophosphamide–rituximab)
Mucositis grade 3–4 (%)	6	12	nr	nr	<5
Infection grade 3–4 (%)	55	60	nr	nr	48
Early death (within 100 d from alloSCT) (%)	2	<10	<3	3	0
Nonrelapse mortality (%)	23 (4 y)	23 (5 y)	16 (5 y)	17 (1 y)	27 (3 y)
Acute GVHD 2–4 (3–4) (%)	45 (14)	nr (16–23)	30 (17)	37 (7)	44 (23)
Extensive chronic GVHD (%)	55	49–53	48	56	29
Follow-up (y)	3.8 (0.6–8.5)	5 (0.9–7.3)	5.1	3.1 (0.9–10.9)	2.3 (0.3–5.9)

Abbreviation: nr, not reported.

rate (ie, death within the first 100 days after alloSCT) has dramatically decreased from up to 40% in the old days of traditional conditioning down to less than 3% with RIC (see **Table 2**). This rate has to be taken into account when considering the risk of dying with and without transplant. Thus, undergoing conditioning for alloSCT for CLL is no longer a "hell ride" with a 30% risk of not leaving the ward alive. It is clear that the prospective studies on RIC alloSCT represent selected patients and not intent-to-treat analyses from the time of relapse or transplant indication, implying that they should be biased in favor of a more favorable patient population in comparison to studies on nontransplant salvage trials in poor-risk CLL. However, even with this in mind it might be justified to state that with modern conditioning and appropriate supportive care, the hospitalization phase for alloSCT could be not less safe than other aggressive salvage therapies in patients with poor-risk CLL.

Despite the remarkable improvements in terms of early fatalities, nonrelapse mortality (NRM) after RIC alloSCT for CLL still mounts up to 15% to 25% during the first 2 posttransplant years. This scenario seems to be largely due to complications of acute and chronic GVHD. Although some studies suggest that patients exposed to RIC might be less prone to acute GVHD than those who underwent traditional myeloablative conditioning,[20–22] higher-grade acute GVHD still affects up to 20% of patients after RIC alloSCT for CLL (see **Table 2**). Moreover, about half the surviving patients suffer from extensive chronic GVHD, which can contribute to late NRM.

Apart from its impact on NRM, chronic GVHD is the major determinant of long-term morbidity affecting quality of life (QOL) after alloSCT. At least 25% of survivors experience impaired life satisfaction during the first posttransplant years, with chronic GVHD being a robust predictor of reduced QOL.[23] However, in many affected patients, clinical symptoms of chronic GVHD decrease over time. In their series of 82 patients, Sorror and colleagues[24] observed a 5-year cumulative incidence of extensive chronic GVHD of 49% for related and 53% for unrelated recipients. Overall, in an increasing proportion of patients chronic GVHD resolved during follow-up, allowing discontinuation of therapeutic immunosuppression after a median of 25 months. Similar observations were made in the GCLLSG trial, in which one-third of the patients originally experiencing chronic GVHD were off systemic immunosuppression 1 year after transplant.[25] Planned QOL analyses at baseline and 12 months postalloSCT were available for 24 of the patients who were event-free at 1 year after transplant. In spite of the high chronic GVHD risk, 58% of the patients reported the maximum QOL (Spitzer) score 12 months posttransplant (vs 48% at baseline), 32% of the patients reported an increase of their QOL score at 12 months compared with baseline, and only 14% reported a decreased score (GCLLSG, data on file).

In conclusion, transplant-related long-term morbidity after alloSCT for CLL can be significant but is mainly restricted to those patients who have ongoing active chronic GVHD. The morbidity caused by alloSCT for patients with poor-risk CLL must be weighed against the morbidity due to uncontrolled disease and palliative treatment associated with nontransplant salvage strategies.

It has to be emphasized that the good tolerability of RIC alloSCT allows offering the procedure to older (up to 70 years of age) and comorbid patients who represent the CLL target population. From 1991 to 2010, in the EBMT registry the proportion of patients who underwent RIC increased from 0 to more than 60% of all patients registered for alloSCT for lymphoma. During the same time interval, the fraction of patients older than 50 years who underwent allograft increased from 5% to 38%. Most recently, the 1-year NRM of the age group 61 to 70 years was still less than 25% (**Fig. 3**).

In summary, RIC has resulted in a dramatic reduction of early morbidity and mortality of alloSCT in CLL, making this procedure now suitable for comorbid and elderly patients. Because up to 20% of patients who undergo allograft experience severe acute GVHD, long-term NRM in all prospective trials on RIC alloSCT still ranges from 15% to 25%. Long-term morbidity and QOL is largely determined by chronic GVHD (which is also the most important prerequisite for CLL eradication).

INDICATIONS OF ALLOSCT IN CLL IN 2013

In 2006, the EBMT worked out a consensus on indications for alloSCT in CLL, stating that alloSCT is a reasonable treatment option for eligible patients with previously treated, poor-risk CLL.[26] Criteria for poor-risk CLL according to this "EBMT transplant consensus" are purine-analog refractoriness, relapse within 2 years after purine-analog combination therapy, and CLL with TP53 lesion requiring treatment (**Box 1**).

Since then, a huge body of novel treatment modalities has been studied in the indications covered by the EBMT transplant consensus. These comprise rituximab–purine analog or bendamustine combination regimens, alemtuzumab-containing regimens, and new drugs, such as flavopiridol, lenalidomide, and ibrutinib. Second, published experience with RIC alloSCT has largely increased during the past 7 years, allowing much better conclusions about allotransplant efficacy and safety in defined situations. Therefore, evaluation of alloSCT indication in 2013 requires addressing 3 key questions: first, do the new treatment options have the potential to change the natural course of poor-risk CLL, thereby making alloSCT unnecessary; second, is there valid evidence that alloSCT indeed can improve the otherwise fatal course of poor-risk CLL; third, which other factors apart from the principle disease-related risk determine the outcome of alloSCT in CLL?

Is Poor-risk CLL Still Poor Risk?

del 17p and TP53 mutations
Fludarabine-cyclophosphamide (FC)-rituximab (FCR) has been shown to improve overall survival in CLL when administered as first-line therapy, but even this highly effective combination does not seem to be capable of improving the dismal natural

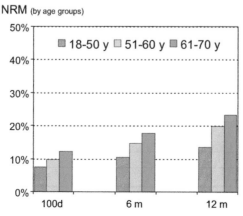

Fig. 3. NRM of patients undergoing alloSCT for lymphoma registered with the EBMT between 2006 and 2010 by age groups.

Box 1
Criteria for poor-risk disease according to the EBMT CLL transplant consensus

- Nonresponse or early relapse (within 12 months) after purine analog–containing therapy
- Relapse (within 24 months) after purine-analog combination therapy or treatment of similar efficacy (ie, autoSCT)
- p53 deletion/mutation (del 17p13) requiring treatment

Data from Dreger P, Corradini P, Kimby E, et al. Indications for allogeneic stem cell transplantation in chronic lymphocytic leukemia: the EBMT Transplant Consensus. Leukemia 2007;21:12–7.

---

course of patients with del 17p-deleted CLL.[27,28] Similarly, FC-ofatumumab,[29] bendamustine-rituximab,[30] alemtuzumab (even in combination with fludarabine or high-dose steroids),[31] flavopiridol,[32] and lenalidomide[33] do not provide sustained disease control in patients with 17p- (**Table 3**). Promising results were reported for the Bruton tyrosine kinase inhibitor ibrutinib, alone or in combination with bendamustine and rituximab. The ibrutinib-bendamustine-rituximab regimen yielded a 71% response rate in 7 patients with relapsed or refractory 17p- CLL. However, the observation time was too short to conclude on long-term efficacy.[34]

It was unclear at the time when the EBMT transplant consensus was released if patients with TP53 mutations in the absence of 17p- indeed have a poor prognosis. In the meantime, post hoc analyses from prospective trials have provided sound evidence that patients with TP53 mutation have a natural course as bad as those with 17p-.[35,36]

Purine-analog refractoriness

Similarly, these new agents and drug combinations do not provide significant disease control when administered to patients with fludarabine-refractory disease (see **Table 3**).

Table 3
Results of novel regimens in 17p- and fludarabine-refractory CLL

Regimen	17p- (First-line Only)				Fludarabine-refractory			
	n	ORR	PFS	Reference	n	ORR	PFS	Reference
FCR	22	68%	18% (3 y)	28	54	56%	8 mo	51
Bendamustin + rituximab	8	38%	8 mo	52	22	46%	15 mo[a]	30
Alemtuzumab	11	64%	11 mo	53	103	34%	8 mo	31
Alemtuzumab + steroids	31	100%		54	31	47%		54
Alemtuzumab + FCR (CFAR)					80	65%	11 mo	55
Ofatumumab					138	47%–58%	6 mo	56
Ofatumumab + FC	8	63%	3 mo	29				
Flavopiridol[b]	16	25%	nr	32	40	31%	12 mo[b]	32

Abbreviations: FCR, fludarabine-cyclophosphamide-rituximab; nr, not reported; ORR, overall response rate; PFS, progression-free survival.

[a] Median duration of response of responding patients.
[b] Salvage treatment only.

Early relapse after intensive pretreatment

There are no detailed studies showing the effect of individual salvage regimens in this risk group. However, the overall outlook of patients early after administration of FCR or FC is poor. In a post hoc analysis of patients relapsing within the CLL8 trial, the overall survival after start of salvage treatment of those patients whose disease recurred within the second year after end-of-study treatment was about 2 years and thereby comparable to that of truly refractory patients.[37] Similarly, time to FCR failure was a significantly adverse factor for survival after first salvage treatment in 114 patients relapsing after FCR in a study from the MD Anderson Cancer Center, with a median survival of less than 2 years in those 34 patients who had treatment failure within the first 3 years.[38]

In addition, novel potential clinical and biologic risk factors indicating a poor outcome with conventional immunochemotherapy have emerged recently, such as MRD response[39,40] and mutations of the driver genes SF3B1, NOTCH1, and BIRC3.[41–44] However, further prospective validation of these markers is needed before definite conclusions on their prognostic value can be drawn.

Can alloSCT Improve the Outcome of Poor-risk CLL?

del 17p and TP53 mutations

Data from randomized trials or prospective trials focusing on patients with TP53 lesions are not available. However, subset data from prospective phase 2 studies as well as a larger registry analysis[17] strongly suggest that long-term disease control can be achieved in 30% to 45% of patients with 17p- referred to alloSCT (**Table 4**). A post hoc analysis of the GCLLSG CLL3X trial indicates that this is also true for patients with TP53 mutation in the absence of 17p-.[45]

Purine-analog refractoriness

The published phase 2 evidence indicates that alloSCT can overcome the poor prognostic impact of purine-analog refractoriness if the patient can be put into a state of sensitive disease by other measures before transplant (see **Table 4**).

Table 4
Prognostic factors for progression-free survival in prospective clinical trials on RIC alloSCT in CLL

	Dreger et al,[25] 2010	Sorror et al,[24] 2008	Brown et al,[22] 2012	Khouri et al,[49] 2011	Michallet et al,[50] 2011
N	90	82	76	86	40
Higher age	++ (>55)	−[a]	++ (>65)	−[a]	−
Comorbidity score	nr	++[a]	++ (>0)	−[a]	nr
Alternative donors[b]	−	−[a]	−	−[a]	nr
High number of pretreatment lines	nr	−	−	−[a]	nr
Purine-analog refractoriness	−	−	−	nr	nr
Unresponsive disease at SCT	++	++[c]	++	−	−
17p-	−	−[a]	−	nr	nr

Abbreviations: −, not significant; ++, significantly predicting adverse outcome; nr, not reported.
[a] Tested by univariate analysis only.
[b] Donors other than siblings with identical HLA antigen.
[c] Defined as lymphadenopathy >5 cm at SCT.

Early relapse after intensive pretreatment

There is no structured data available on the specific effect of alloSCT in this subset. However, because the prognosis of these patients with conventional salvage treatment is not worse than that of fludarabine-refractory patients and there is no fundamental biologic difference between patients with early relapse and those who are truly fludarabine-refractory, it can be anticipated that alloSCT is at least as effective as in true purine-analog refractoriness. A preliminary single-center analysis confirms this assumption.[46]

Which Other Factors Determine the Outcome of alloSCT in CLL?

A significantly unfavorable effect of matched unrelated donors (MUDs) could not be found in any of the prospective RIC studies listed in **Table 4**, indicating that this factor has only limited clinical implications, if any, in CLL. Accordingly, a matched sibling donor should be preferred for alloSCT in CLL whenever possible, but a MUD is a reasonable alternative if a sibling with identical HLA antigen is not available.[47] In contrast, active or unresponsive disease at the time of alloSCT, advanced age, and a high comorbidity index reproducibly predicted an unfavorable outcome of alloSCT for CLL. Although not perfectly matching the differential impact reported for these factors in the prospective trials, the EBMT transplant risk score aggregating age, disease status, time from diagnosis, donor source, and donor-recipient sex combination was found to be an important survival predictor in a retrospective study.[47]

> In summary, it seems that poor-risk CLL remains poor-risk CLL despite the advent of numerous new treatment options and that alloSCT is the only treatment with the potential of providing long-term disease control in this condition, thereby confirming the indications for alloSCT in CLL as defined in the EBMT CLL transplant consensus. In addition to the principal disease risk, patient-related risk factors, such as age, comorbidity, and actual disease activity, have to be considered when the decision about alloSCT is made.

WHEN SHOULD ALLOSCT IN CLL BE PERFORMED?

Because the eligibility for allotransplant in CLL is largely defined by the quality of response to therapy, alloSCT is never indicated as part of the first-line treatment of CLL except for those few patients who have del 17p- with treatment indication (third EBMT criterion); this implies that transplant should not be considered too early. On the other hand, the larger RIC prospective trials suggest that in CLL the results of alloSCT are considerably impaired if the disease is not in remission at the time of transplant due to nodal bulk and/or chemotherapy resistance (see **Table 4**). Thus, alloSCT should be performed before CLL has advanced to a status of complete refractoriness or large resistant tumor burden in order not to miss the "window of opportunity" for a successful outcome.

> In summary, in eligible patients alloSCT should be considered as soon as one of the EBMT criteria is met.

CAN ALLOSCT CHANGE THE NATURAL COURSE OF POOR-RISK CLL?

Although there is no doubt from the published CLL transplant studies that alloSCT can largely improve the prognosis of individual poor-risk patients, it is unclear to what extent alloSCT can affect the natural history of the patient population with aggressive CLL and what its overall clinical value for the treatment armory of CLL might be. This question can be properly addressed only by prospective trials comparing alloSCT with nontransplant strategies in defined clinical risk situations by intention to treat. It is crucial for such comparisons that patients are followed up from the time of reaching transplant indication as triggered by need for treatment rather than from the time of alloSCT. A trial planned by the GCLLSG to address this question could not be launched because of the extremely complex regulatory requirements for clinical trials involving unrelated donors, which are currently effective in Germany.

A retrospective study from Heidelberg comparing patients with poor-risk CLL with transplant indication according to the EBMT criteria in a donor-versus-no-donor landmark analysis suggested a survival advantage for those patients for whom a donor could be found.[46] However, this single retrospective analysis from a single center has to be regarded as preliminary. A survival advantage of alloSCT over nontransplant strategy in patients with relapsed CLL was also concluded from a systematic metaanalysis using a Markov decision model.[48] Due to its artificial design, however, this study also has serious limitations.

Nevertheless, these results are encouraging, confirm the current important role of alloSCT in the treatment of poor-risk CLL, and warrant further studies in this field. It is hoped that the new drugs that are about to enter the therapeutic arena in CLL will help improve the results of alloSCT by reducing the tumor load before transplant and/or eradicating MRD posttransplant.

REFERENCES

1. Rabinowe SN, Soiffer RJ, Gribben JG, et al. Autologous and allogeneic bone marrow transplantation for poor prognosis patients with B-cell chronic lymphocytic leukemia. Blood 1993;82:1366–76.
2. Khouri IF, Keating MJ, Vriesendorp HM, et al. Autologous and allogeneic bone marrow transplantation for chronic lymphocytic leukemia: preliminary results. J Clin Oncol 1994;12:748–58.
3. Gribben JG, Zahrieh D, Stephans K, et al. Autologous and allogeneic stem cell transplantation for poor risk chronic lymphocytic leukemia. Blood 2005;106: 4389–96.
4. Michallet M, Dreger P, Sutton L, et al. Autologous hematopoietic stem cell transplantation in chronic lymphocytic leukemia: results of European intergroup randomized trial comparing autografting versus observation. Blood 2011;117:1516–21.
5. Dreger P, Dohner H, McClanahan F, et al. Early autologous stem cell transplantation for chronic lymphocytic leukemia: long-term follow-up of the GCLLSG CLL3 trial. Blood 2012;119:4851–9.
6. Mehta J, Powles R, Singhal S, et al. Clinical and hematologic response of chronic lymphocytic and prolymphocytic leukemia persisting after allogeneic bone marrow transplantation with the onset of acute graft-versus-host disease: possible role of graft-versus-leukemia. Bone Marrow Transplant 1996;17:371–5.
7. Mattsson J, Uzunel M, Remberger M, et al. Minimal residual disease is common after allogeneic stem cell transplantation in patients with B cell chronic lymphocytic leukemia and may be controlled by graft-versus-host disease. Leukemia 2000;14:247–54.
8. Pavletic ZS, Arrowsmith ER, Bierman PJ, et al. Outcome of allogeneic stem cell transplantation for B cell chronic lymphocytic leukemia. Bone Marrow Transplant 2000;25:717–22.

9. Ben Bassat I, Raanani P, Gale RP. Graft-versus-leukemia in chronic lymphocytic leukemia. Bone Marrow Transplant 2007;39:441–6.

10. Slavin S, Nagler A, Naparstek E, et al. Nonmyeloablative stem cell transplantation and cell therapy as an alternative to conventional bone marrow transplantation with lethal cytoreduction for the treatment of malignant and nonmalignant hematologic diseases. Blood 1998;91:756–63.

11. Khouri IF, Keating M, Korbling M, et al. Transplant-lite: induction of graft-versus-malignancy using fludarabine-based nonablative chemotherapy and allogeneic blood progenitor-cell transplantation as treatment for lymphoid malignancies. J Clin Oncol 1998;16:2817–24.

12. McSweeney PA, Niederwieser D, Shizuru JA, et al. Hematopoietic cell transplantation in older patients with hematologic malignancies: replacing high-dose cytotoxic therapy with graft-versus-tumor effects. Blood 2001;97:3390–400.

13. Champlin R, Khouri I, Kornblau S, et al. Reinventing bone marrow transplantation: reducing toxicity using nonmyeloablative, preparative regimens and induction of graft-versus-malignancy. Curr Opin Oncol 1999;11:87–95.

14. Toze CL, Galal A, Barnett MJ, et al. Myeloablative allografting for chronic lymphocytic leukemia: evidence for a potent graft-versus leukemia effect associated with graft-versus-host disease. Bone Marrow Transplant 2005;36:825–30.

15. Farina L, Carniti C, Dodero A, et al. Qualitative and quantitative polymerase chain reaction monitoring of minimal residual disease in relapsed chronic lymphocytic leukemia: early assessment can predict long-term outcome after reduced intensity allogeneic transplantation. Haematologica 2009;94:654–62.

16. Böttcher S, Ritgen M, Dreger P. Allogeneic stem cell transplantation for chronic lymphocytic leukemia: lessons to be learned from minimal residual disease studies. Blood Rev 2011;25:91–6.

17. Schetelig J, van Biezen A, Brand R, et al. Allogeneic hematopoietic cell transplantation for chronic lymphocytic leukemia with 17p deletion: a retrospective EBMT analysis. J Clin Oncol 2008;26:5094–100.

18. Hallek M, Cheson BD, Catovsky D, et al. Guidelines for the diagnosis and treatment of chronic lymphocytic leukemia: a report from the International Workshop on Chronic Lymphocytic Leukemia (IWCLL) updating the National Cancer Institute Working Group (NCI-WG) 1996 guidelines. Blood 2008;111: 5446–56.

19. Moreno C, Villamor N, Esteve J, et al. Clinical significance of minimal residual disease, as assessed by different techniques, after stem cell transplantation for chronic lymphocytic leukemia. Blood 2006;107:4563–9.

20. Mielcarek M, Martin PJ, Leisenring W, et al. Graft-versus-host disease after nonmyeloablative versus conventional hematopoietic stem cell transplantation. Blood 2003;102:756–62.

21. Jagasia M, Arora M, Flowers ME, et al. Risk factors for acute GVHD and survival after hematopoietic cell transplantation. Blood 2012;119:296–307.

22. Brown JR, Kim HT, Armand P, et al. Long-term follow-up of reduced-intensity allogeneic stem cell transplantation for chronic lymphocytic leukemia: prognostic model to predict outcome. Leukemia 2012. [Epub ahead of print].

23. Pidala J, Anasetti C, Jim H. Quality of life after allogeneic hematopoietic cell transplantation. Blood 2009;114:7–19.

24. Sorror ML, Storer BE, Sandmaier BM, et al. Five-year follow-up of patients with advanced chronic lymphocytic leukemia treated with allogeneic hematopoietic cell transplantation after nonmyeloablative conditioning. J Clin Oncol 2008;26: 4912–20.

25. Dreger P, Döhner H, Ritgen M, et al. Allogeneic stem cell transplantation provides durable disease control in poor-risk chronic lymphocytic leukemia: long-term clinical and MRD results of the GCLLSG CLL3X trial. Blood 2010;116: 2438–47.

26. Dreger P, Corradini P, Kimby E, et al. Indications for allogeneic stem cell transplantation in chronic lymphocytic leukemia: the EBMT transplant consensus. Leukemia 2007;21:12–7.

27. Tam CS, O'Brien S, Wierda W, et al. Long-term results of the fludarabine, cyclophosphamide, and rituximab regimen as initial therapy of chronic lymphocytic leukemia. Blood 2008;112:975–80.

28. Hallek M, Fischer K, Fingerle-Rowson G, et al. Addition of rituximab to fludarabine and cyclophosphamide in patients with chronic lymphocytic leukaemia: a randomised, open-label, phase 3 trial. Lancet 2010;376:1164–74.

29. Wierda WG, Kipps TJ, Durig J, et al. Chemoimmunotherapy with O-FC in previously untreated patients with chronic lymphocytic leukemia. Blood 2011;117: 6450–8.

30. Fischer K, Cramer P, Busch R, et al. Bendamustine combined with rituximab in patients with relapsed and/or refractory chronic lymphocytic leukemia: a multicenter phase II trial of the German Chronic Lymphocytic Leukemia Study Group. J Clin Oncol 2011;29:3559–66.

31. Stilgenbauer S, Zenz T, Winkler D, et al. Subcutaneous alemtuzumab in fludarabine-refractory chronic lymphocytic leukemia: clinical results and prognostic marker analyses from the CLL2H trial of the GCLLSG. J Clin Oncol 2009;27:3994–4001.

32. Lanasa MC, Andritsos L, Brown JR, et al. Interim analysis of EFC6663, a multicenter phase 2 study of Alvocidib (flavopiridol), demonstrates clinical responses among patients with fludarabine refractory CLL. ASH Annual Meeting Abstracts. Blood 2010;116:58.

33. Badoux XC, Keating MJ, Wen S, et al. Lenalidomide as initial therapy of elderly patients with chronic lymphocytic leukemia. Blood 2011;118:3489–98.

34. O'Brien S, Barrientos J, Flinn I, et al. Combination of the Bruton's tyrosine kinase (BTK) inhibitor ibrutinib (PCI-32765) with bendamustine/rituximab is active and tolerable in patients with relapsed or refractory (R/R) chronic lymphocytic leukemia/small lymphocytic lymphoma (CLL/SLL): interim results of a phase Ib/II study [abstract]. Proceedings of ASCO 2012.

35. Zenz T, Eichhorst B, Busch R, et al. TP53 mutation and survival in chronic lymphocytic leukemia. J Clin Oncol 2010;28:4473–9.

36. Gonzalez D, Martinez P, Wade R, et al. Mutational status of the TP53 gene as a predictor of response and survival in patients with chronic lymphocytic leukemia: results from the LRF CLL4 trial. J Clin Oncol 2011;29:2223–9.

37. Zenz T, Busch R, Fink AM, et al. Genetics of patients with F-refractory CLL or early relapse after FC or FCR: results from the CLL8 trial of the GCLLSG. Blood (ASH Annual Meeting Abstracts) 2010;116:2427.

38. Keating MJ, Wierda W, Tam CS. Long term outcome following treatment failure of FCR chemoimmunotherapy as initial therapy for chronic lymphocytic leukemia [abstract]. Blood (ASH Annual Meeting Abstracts) 2009;114:940–1.

39. Moreton P, Kennedy B, Lucas G, et al. Eradication of minimal residual disease in B-cell chronic lymphocytic leukemia after alemtuzumab therapy is associated with prolonged survival. J Clin Oncol 2005;23:2971–9.

40. Bottcher S, Ritgen M, Fischer K, et al. Minimal residual disease quantification is an independent predictor of progression-free and overall survival in chronic

lymphocytic leukemia: a multivariate analysis from the randomized GCLLSG CLL8 trial. J Clin Oncol 2012;30:980–8.

41. Wang L, Lawrence MS, Wan Y, et al. SF3B1 and other novel cancer genes in chronic lymphocytic leukemia. N Engl J Med 2011;365:2497–506.

42. Balatti V, Bottoni A, Palamarchuk A, et al. NOTCH1 mutations in CLL associated with trisomy 12. Blood 2012;119:329–31.

43. Rossi D, Rasi S, Fabbri G, et al. Mutations of NOTCH1 are an independent predictor of survival in chronic lymphocytic leukemia. Blood 2012;119: 521–9.

44. Rossi D, Fangazio M, Rasi S, et al. Disruption of BIRC3 associates with fludara-bine chemorefractoriness in TP53 wild-type chronic lymphocytic leukemia. Blood 2012;119:2854–62.

45. Zenz T, Dreger P, Dietrich S, et al. Allogeneic stem cell transplantation can over-come the adverse prognostic impact of TP53 mutation in chronic lymphocytic leukemia (CLL): results from the GCLLSG CLL3x trial. Blood (ASH Annual Meeting Abstracts) 2010;116:2357.

46. Herth I, Hegenbart U, Dietrich S, et al. First evidence that alloSCT can improve the natural course of poor-risk chronic lymphocytic leukemia (CLL) as defined by the EBMT consensus criteria: a retrospective donor vs no donor comparison [abstract]. Bone Marrow Transplant 2012;47(Suppl 1):S43–4.

47. Michallet M, Sobh M, Milligan D, et al. The impact of HLA matching on long-term transplant outcome after allogeneic hematopoietic stem cell transplantation for CLL: a retrospective study from the EBMT registry. Leukemia 2010;24: 1725–31.

48. Kharfan-Dabaja MA, Pidala J, Kumar A, et al. Comparing efficacy of reduced-toxicity allogeneic hematopoietic cell transplantation with conventional chemo-(immuno) therapy in patients with relapsed or refractory CLL: a Markov decision analysis. Bone Marrow Transplant 2012;47:1164–70.

49. Khouri IF, Bassett R, Poindexter N, et al. Nonmyeloablative allogeneic stem cell transplantation in relapsed/refractory chronic lymphocytic leukemia: long-term follow-up, prognostic factors, and effect of human leukocyte histocompatibility antigen subtype on outcome. Cancer 2011;117:4679–88.

50. Michallet M, Sobh M, Morisset S, et al. Rituximab in allogeneic HSCT for advanced chronic lymphocytic leukemia with fludarabine + total body irradiation conditioning: results of a phase II prospective multicenter study (ITAC 02-02) [abstract]. Bone Marrow Transplant 2011;46(Suppl 1):S43–4.

51. Badoux XC, Keating MJ, Wang X, et al. Fludarabine, cyclophosphamide and rituximab chemoimmunotherapy is highly effective treatment for relapsed patients with CLL. Blood 2011;117:3016–24.

52. Fischer K, Cramer P, Busch R, et al. Bendamustine in combination with rituximab for previously untreated patients with chronic lymphocytic leukemia: a multicenter phase II trial of the German Chronic Lymphocytic Leukemia Study Group. J Clin Oncol 2012;30:3209–16.

53. Hillmen P, Skotnicki AB, Robak T, et al. Alemtuzumab compared with chlorambu-cil as first-line therapy for chronic lymphocytic leukemia. J Clin Oncol 2007;25: 5616–23.

54. Stilgenbauer S, Cymbalista F, Leblond V, et al. Subcutaneous alemtuzumab combined with oral dexamethasone, followed by alemtuzumab maintenance or allo-SCT in CLL with 17p- or refractory to fludarabine - interim analysis of the CLL2O trial of the GCLLSG and FCGCLL/MW. Blood (ASH Annual Meeting Abstracts) 2010;116:920.

55. Badoux XC, Keating MJ, Wang X, et al. Cyclophosphamide, fludarabine, rituximab and alemtuzumab (CFAR) as salvage therapy for heavily pre-treated patients with chronic lymphocytic leukemia. Blood 2011;118:2085–93.
56. Wierda WG, Kipps TJ, Mayer J, et al. Ofatumumab as single-agent CD20 immunotherapy in fludarabine-refractory chronic lymphocytic leukemia. J Clin Oncol 2010;28:1749–55.

Index

Note: Page numbers of article titles are in **boldface** type.